MOTOR NEUROBIOLOGY OF THE SPINAL CORD

METHODS & NEW FRONTIERS IN NEUROSCIENCE

Series Editors
Sidney A. Simon, Ph.D.
Miguel A.L. Nicolelis, M.D., Ph.D.

Published Titles

Apoptosis in Neurobiology
Yusuf A. Hannun, M.D., Professor/Biomedical Research and Department Chairman/
Biochemistry and Molecular Biology, Medical University of South Carolina
Rose-Mary Boustany, M.D., tenured Associate Professor/Pediatrics and Neurobiology,
Duke University Medical Center

Methods for Neural Ensemble Recordings
Miguel A.L. Nicolelis, M.D., Ph.D., Associate Professor/Department of Neurobiology,
Duke University Medical Center

Methods of Behavioral Analysis in Neuroscience
Jerry J. Buccafusco, Ph.D., Professor/Pharmacology and Toxicology,
Professor/Psychiatry and Health Behavior, Medical College of Georgia

Neural Prostheses for Restoration of Sensory and Motor Function
John K. Chapin, Ph.D., MCP and Hahnemann School of Medicine
Karen A. Moxon, Ph.D., Department of Electrical and Computer Engineering,
Drexel University

Computational Neuroscience: Realistic Modeling for Experimentalists
Eric DeSchutter, M.D., Ph.D., Department of Medicine, University of Antwerp

Methods in Pain Research
Lawrence Kruger, Ph.D., Professor Emeritus/Neurobiology, UCLA School of Medicine

MOTOR NEUROBIOLOGY OF THE SPINAL CORD

Edited by Timothy C. Cope

CRC Press

Boca Raton   London   New York   Washington, D.C.

The top image is an alpha motor neuron in the lumbrosacral spinal cord of an adult cat stained with Rhodamine - dextran. The image is courtesy of R.E.W. Fyffe and F.J. Alvarez, Department of Anatomy, Wright State University. The lower image is a muscle spindle from a normal rat medial gastrocnemius muscle.The spindle has been stained with PGP 9.5 (green) and with SMI 311 (red). The image is courtesy of T. Cope, M. Pinter, and A. Shirley, Department of Physiology, Emory University School of Medicine, with special thanks to H. Rees and A. Levey, Department of Neurology, Emory University School of Medicine, for the use of the confocal microscope.

Library of Congress Cataloging-in-Publication Data

Motor neurobiology of the spinal cord / edited by Timothy C. Cope.
    p. cm. -- (Methods & new frontiers in neuroscience)
    Includes bibliographical references and index.
    ISBN 0-8493-0006-1 (alk. paper)
        1. Spinal cord--Research--Methodology. 2. Motor neurons--Research--Methodology.
    I. Cope, Timothy C., 1953- II. Methods & new frontiers in neuroscience series

QP371 .M68 2001
612.8'3--dc21   2001025610

Visit the CRC Press Web site at www.crcpress.com

© 2001 by CRC Press LLC

No claim to original U.S. Government works
International Standard Book Number 0-8493-0006-1
Library of Congress Card Number 2001025610
Printed in the United States of America 1 2 3 4 5 6 7 8 9 0
Printed on acid-free paper

Methods & New Frontiers in Neuroscience

Series Editors
Sidney A. Simon, Ph.D.
Miguel A.L. Nicolelis, M.D., Ph.D.

Our goal in creating the Methods & New Frontiers in Neuroscience Series is to present the insights of experts on emerging experimental techniques and theoretical concepts that are, or will be, at the vanguard of neuroscience. Books in the series cover topics ranging from methods to investigate apoptosis to modern techniques for neural ensemble recordings in behaving animals. The series also covers new and exciting multidisciplinary areas of brain research, such as computational neuroscience and neuroengineering, and describes breakthroughs in classical fields such as behavioral neuroscience. We want these to be the books every neuroscientist will use in order to get acquainted with new methodologies in brain research. These books can be given to graduate students and postdoctoral fellows when they are looking for guidance to start a new line of research.

Each book is edited by an expert and consists of chapters written by the leaders in a particular field. Books are richly illustrated and contain comprehensive bibliographies. Chapters provide substantial background material relevant to the particular subject. Hence, they are not just "methods books." They contain detailed "tricks of the trade" and information as to where these methods can be safely applied. In addition, they include information about where to buy equipment and websites that are helpful in solving both practical and theoretical problems.

We hope that as the volumes become available the effort put in by us, the publisher, the book editors, and individual authors will contribute to the further development of brain research. The extent that we achieve this goal will be determined by the utility of these books.

Preface

There is no more direct connection between cell biology and animal behavior than that found between motoneurons and movement. Alpha motoneurons are the final common pathway from the central nervous system to the skeletomuscular system, and the synaptic input that converges on motoneurons and causes them to fire necessarily results in the generation of muscle force. Thus, all properties of motoneurons and their synaptic inputs can be interpreted in direct relation to the tasks of producing movement and posture. For many of us, it is this linkage between cells and behavior that motivates study of spinal motoneurons and their synaptic inputs. Others of us are allured by the unique experimental accessibility of the spinal sensorimotor system that favors study of neural processes, which we presume to represent processes in other, less accessible parts of the CNS. Still others are attracted to motor behavior itself and to the underlying neural mechanisms that account for movement function and dysfunction.

All chapters in this book present new methods and/or concepts in motor neurobiology of the spinal cord. The focus on innovative approaches is certainly fitting to our book's parent series, entitled *Methods & New Frontiers in Neuroscience*. Nonetheless, readers will note that several of the topics addressed here have been the subject of considerable experimental and scholarly attention for many years. Should this realization generate questions about the suitability of these topics in a series on frontiers in neuroscience, we recommend the assertions made by Ragnar Granit in his 1972 essay entitled "Discovery and Understanding." Dr. Granit argues "... that 'discovery' and 'understanding' really are different concepts and are not arbitrarily differentiated. There is in discovery a quality of uniqueness tied to a particular moment in time, while understanding goes on and on from level to level of penetration and insight and thus is a process that lasts for years ...".* Several of the chapters in this book present ongoing efforts to achieve understanding of some long-studied, yet incompletely understood issues.

In addition to those directly interested and/or participating in studies of the motor neurobiology of the spinal cord, neurobiologists with different interests and in other fields may find this book useful. As enticement we refer the reader to arguments made by Dr. Patricia Churchland in her book, *Neurophilosophy*. There she argues persuasively against the notion of a dualistic brain, in which mind and brain structure are two different things. In parallel, she argues against the notion that "... brain processes that make for cognition are one sort of thing and that the brain processes that contribute to motor control belong to an entirely different category." She goes on to say that, "If we want to understand the fundamental principles of cognition, ... we may need to understand their origins in sensorimotor control."**

---

* Granit R., Discovery and understanding, *Ann. Rev. Physiol.*, 34, 1, 1972.
** Churchland, P.S., *Neurophilosophy: Toward a Unified Science of the Mind-Brain*, Rumelhart, D.E., Feldman, J.A., and Hayes, P. J., Eds., MIT Press, Boston, 1989.

About the Editor

Timothy C. Cope is a professor of physiology and a member of the Neuroscience Program at Emory University in Atlanta, Georgia, where he lives with his wife, Meredith and children Russ, Audrey, and Cassie. He earned B.S. and M.S. degrees from the University of California at Los Angeles and a Ph.D. in physiology from Duke University in 1980. Following postdoctoral studies at the University of Washington and the University of California at Los Angeles from 1980–1983, he held faculty positions at the University of Texas, Southwestern Medical School and at Hahnemann University.

Dr. Cope's research focuses on sensorimotor integration in the spinal cord. His published work includes studies of motor-unit function, motoneuron recruitment order and rate modulation, and central synaptic transmission between spinal motoneurons and primary sensory afferents. He has been particularly interested in the adaptations following injuries to the central and peripheral nervous systems.

Contributors

Jacob B. Andersen
Center for Sensory-Motor Interaction
Aalborg University
Aalborg, Denmark

Anne Bekoff
Department of EPO Biology
  and Center for Neuroscience
University of Colorado
Boulder, Colorado

Charles R. Buck
Center for Molecular Medicine
  and Molecular Core,
Alzheimer's Disease Center
Emory University School of Medicine
Atlanta, Georgia

Timothy C. Cope
Department of Physiology
Emory University School of Medicine
Atlanta, Georgia

Linda C. Cork
Department of Comparative Medicine
Stanford University School of Medicine
Stanford, California

Joseph R. Fetcho
Department of Neurobiology
  and Behavior
SUNY at Stony Brook
Stony Brook, New York

Robert E. W. Fyffe
Center for Brain Research and
  Department of Anatomy
Wright State University School
  of Medicine
Dayton, Ohio

Sandra M. Garraway
Department of Physiology
Emory University
Atlanta, Georgia

Sherril L. Green
Department of Comparative Medicine
Stanford University School of Medicine
Stanford, California

Michael Grey
Center for Sensory-Motor Interaction
Aalborg University
Aalborg, Denmark

Thomas M. Hamm
Division of Neurobiology
Barrow Neurological Institute
St. Joseph's Hospital and
  Medical Center
Phoenix, Arizona

C. J. Heckman
Department of Physiology and
  Department of Physical Medicine and
  Rehabilitation
Northwestern University Medical
  School
Chicago, Illinois

Shawn Hochman
Department of Physiology
Emory University
Atlanta, Georgia

Michel Ladouceur
Center for Sensory-Motor Interaction
Aalborg University
Aalborg, Denmark

Robert H. Lee
Department of Physiology and
  Department of Physical Medicine and
  Rehabilitation
Northwestern University Medical
  School
Chicago, Illinois

Victoria MacDermid
CIHR Group in Sensory-Motor Systems
Department of Physiology
Queen's University
Kingston, Ontario, Canada

David W. Machacek
Department of Physiology
Emory University
Atlanta, Georgia

Martha L. McCurdy
Department of Kinesiology
University of Wisconsin
Madison, Wisconsin

Monica Neuber-Hess
CIHR Group in Sensory-Motor Systems
Department of Physiology
Queen's University
Kingston, Ontario, Canada

T. Richard Nichols
Department of Physiology
Spinal Cord Research Center
Emory University
Atlanta, Georgia

Jens B. Nielsen
Department of Medical Physiology
University of Copenhagen
Copenhagen, Denmark

Steve I. Perlmutter
Department of Physiology and
  Biophysics and Regional Primate
  Research Center
University of Washington
Seattle, Washington

Martin. J. Pinter
Department of Physiology
Emory University School of Medicine
Atlanta, Georgia

Randall K. Powers
Department of Physiology and
  Biophysics
School of Medicine
University of Washington
Seattle, Washington

Yifat Prut
Department of Physiology and
  Biophysics and Regional Primate
  Research Center
University of Washington
Seattle, Washington

Mark M. Rich
Department of Neurology
Emory University School of Medicine
Atlanta, Georgia

P. Kenneth Rose
CIHR Group in Sensory-Motor Systems
Department of Physiology
Queen's University
Kingston, Ontario, Canada

Kevin Seburn
The Jackson Laboratory
Bar Harbor, Maine

Andrew A. Sharp
Department of Environmental,
  Population and Organismic Biology
University of Colorado
Boulder, Colorado
and
Department of Cellular and Stuctural
  Biology
University of Colorado Health Sciences
  Center
Denver, Colorado

Barbara L. Shay
Department of Physiology
University of Manitoba
Winnipeg, Manitoba, Canada

Thomas Sinkjær
Center for Sensory-Motor Interaction
Aalborg University
Aalborg, Denmark

Tamara V. Trank
Naval Health Research Center
San Diego, California

Kemal S. Türker
Department of Physiology
University of Adelaide
Adelaide, Australia

Vladimir V. Turkin
Division of Neurobiology
Barrow Neurological Institute
St. Joseph's Hospital and Medical
  Center
Phoenix, Arizona

Michael Voigt
Center for Sensory-Motor Interaction
Aalborg University
Aalborg, Denmark

Table of Contents

Introduction

The field of spinal motor neurobiology has grown dramatically over the last decade. One can argue that our understanding of spinal motoneurons and functionally related interneurons at both the cellular and systems levels advanced during the past 10 years as much as at any time since neurobiologists, including Sir Charles Sherrington, David Lloyd, and John Eccles established the foundations of the field. It was a relatively simple task, therefore, to identify topics to fill this book. By contrast, it was not easy to restrict the number of topics and contributors. The chief guiding principle used to select contributions to the book was one of providing a broad description of recent conceptual and technical advances in the field. This principle is met by chapters which collectively cover topics ranging from genetics to kinematics, examining cells, tissues, or whole animals, in species ranging from fish to humans that are normal, injured, or diseased, using techniques including immunocytochemisty, optical imaging, and electrical and mechanical analyses. Despite the breadth of coverage, our book is not comprehensive. Fortunately, the reader can compensate for some of our omissions by looking at recent books, including, *Neuronal Mechanisms for Generating Locomotor Activity,* O. Kiehn, R.M. Harris-Warrick, L.M. Jordan, H. Hultborn, and N. Kudo, Eds., 1998, and *Presynaptic Inhibition and Neural Control,* P. Rudomin, R. Romo, and L. Mendell, Eds., 1998.

The reader will find that each chapter is a rich source of information relevant to a variety of issues. Indeed, these features made it difficult to sequence the chapters, which might have been arranged in several ways other than the one chosen. The versatility expressed by each chapter also defies adequate description. Nonetheless, the following few comments describing each chapter are offered to give the reader a rough notion of content.

The book begins with a chapter from Joe Fetcho that focuses on the neural circuits involved in swimming movements in fish. Discussion of the information using conventional electrophysiological and anatomical techniques is followed by introduction to new optical and genetic methods. The next group of three chapters focuses attention on the integrative properties of motoneuron dendrites and/or the synaptic inputs they receive. Specific details about the distribution and density of various synapses, receptors, and ion channels are examined morphologically by Robert Fyffe, pharmacologically by Shawn Hochman and co-authors, and electrophysiogically by Bob Lee and C.J. Heckman. The two chapters that follow address analyses of motoneuron firing: Randy Powers and Kemal Türker describe advances in measuring and interpreting synaptic effects on human motoneuron discharge, while Tom Hamm and co-authors evaluate correlation in the frequency domain and its value in discovering the organization of neural circuits involved in rhythmic motor patterns in the cat spinal cord. Subsequently, Steve Perlmutter and Yifat Prut describe their studies of spinal interneuron responses recorded in association with hand movements made by awake, behaving monkeys. Two other chapters examine the role of sensory feedback in modulating motor output: Andrew Sharp and Anne Beckoff describe how specific sensory modalities contribute to the development of motility in chick embryos, while Thomas Sinkjær and co-workers report on the effects of proprioception on human gait. The book ends with four chapters examining the responses of motoneurons and segmental motor circuits to injury and disease. Marty Pinter and co-authors promote the notion that dysfunction at the neuromuscular junction results in muscular weakness far in advance of neural degeneration in a mutant dog. In the next chapter, Ken Rose and co-authors present evidence that cutting the axons of motoneurons supplying neck muscles in cats causes the motoneuron's dendrites to acquire axon-like characteristics, thereby raising questions about the molecular polarity of motoneurons and the pleural potentiality of their neuritic projections. Tim Cope and co-authors explore the potential role of afferent activity, neurotrophins, and glutamate receptors in enhancing central synaptic strength following peripheral nerve injury. Finally, Richard Nichols and Tim Cope present findings that challenge traditional notions about specific spinal reflexes that are released by spinal cord injury.

I am sincerely grateful to all contributing authors for their efforts, responsiveness, and success in generating high quality chapters. Thanks also to Miguel Nicolelis for his invitation to produce a book in this series, and to Barbara Norwitz, Tiffany Lane, and Pat Roberson at CRC Press for their assistance. High praise and gratitude go to Anne Shirley and her assistants, Katie Bannister and Amy Gandhi, for their conscientious efforts in communicating with authors and organizing incoming materials.

1 Optical and Genetic Approaches toward Understanding Spinal Circuits

Joseph R. Fetcho

CONTENTS

1.1 OVERVIEW

This chapter deals with our understanding of the circuits for movement in spinal cord. The emphasis is on what is missing in our knowledge of spinal circuits. There are significant gaps in our understanding and it is helpful to consider why it is that these gaps exist and what the prospects are for using new technologies and model systems to fill them. The conclusion is that most of the limitations in our understanding are a consequence of those of technique and model systems. The available techniques and accepted models have provided wonderful accounts of some aspects of spinal circuits, but at the same time they have limited the questions we are equipped to ask and in doing so have shaped the boundaries of our understanding of motor circuits. This is about to change. New models and, more importantly, new optical and genetic methods are opening our work to entire classes of questions that were previously inaccessible. These approaches will impact not only studies of spinal cord, but systems neurobiology more generally. The result will be a more complete picture of the link between circuits and behavior in vertebrates than ever before.

The following account deals first with some of what we do know and why we know it, which forms a basis for understanding why there are important gaps in our knowledge. The chapter moves on to define some of those gaps and to lay out the new technological developments that offer ways to attack these problems. As the work in my laboratory has dealt largely with the circuits for escape and swimming movements in fishes, most of the examples are drawn from studies of these systems. The issues raised are broad ones though, extending not just to other spinal motor circuits, but to neuronal circuits in general, whether in spinal cord or in the brain.

1.2 WHAT WE KNOW AND WHY WE KNOW IT

The approach to motor circuit analysis is a fairly standard one, pioneered in the invertebrate systems and applied to vertebrates with much success in the extensive studies of the spinal rhythm generators for swimming in frog tadpoles and lampreys.[1-6] Usually it centers around a fictive preparation in which the motor behavior of interest can be elicited in a paralyzed animal and monitored by extracellular recordings from motor nerves. The goal is to arrive at a neural circuit which accounts for the activation pattern of the motoneurons and, by extension, the motor behavior of interest.

Some features of circuit organization are especially accessible by the application of current technology to these fictive preparations. Neurons can be filled by backfilling with any number of markers, including horseradish peroxidase and a suite of fluorescent labels, to identify the cell types present in spinal cord. Similar labels injected intracellularly allow for a detailed examination of the morphology of individual cells. Single cell recording by intracellular (sharp electrode) or patch recording makes accessible the cellular properties of individual neurons to explore both their ion channels and, via pairwise recording, the synaptic connections of cells in the spinal cord. By combining these physiological tools with pharmacological and immunocytochemical ones, it is possible to understand the transmitter phenotypes of the neurons and explore the receptors involved in circuits.

Studies of the spinal circuits for swimming and escape in fishes and amphibians have applied these established techniques to great advantage.[7-10] The strategy is to first attempt to identify neurons that participate in the behavior by eliciting the fictive form of the movement while recording intracellularly from spinal neurons.

The cells then can be filled with a dye to identify them and establish the set of active neurons and their patterns of activity. Since it is important that the critical cells be identified, there are significant advantages to using this approach in relatively simple systems with few cell types, where it is likely that any potential participants in spinal cord can be identified. It is no wonder, therefore, that the most successful models here have been *Xenopus* tadpoles, which have been studied at a developmental stage at which there are few types of spinal neurons, and lampreys, which have a comparatively simple spinal cord with large neurons. In both of these preparations, spinal interneurons rhythmically active in swimming were identified by intracellular recording and then filled for morphological study. Using a similar approach in goldfish, the neurons active in escape circuits have been identified by activation of the large reticulospinal Mauthner cell to mimic initiation of an escape in a fictive preparation while simultaneously recording from spinal neurons to identify and fill those activated.[11–13]

In addition to identification of the cells, single cell recordings under voltage clamp allow a dissection of the ion channel composition of the neurons.[14] The ion channels, of course, determine the firing properties of the neurons. Differences in the firing properties of cells can profoundly influence the role of those cells in a circuit and in turn the resulting motor output, so the exploration of channels is a key part of understanding the circuit function.

Identification of the interneurons active in the behavior and their membrane and ion channel properties is not enough, of course. Information about their connectivity is critical as it defines the circuit. This is typically obtained by pair-wise recordings.[7,8,12,13,15] In the best case, these recordings are from unambiguously identified pre- and postsynaptic cells. Through a combination of pair-wise physiology and pharmacology, particular interneurons can be identified as excitatory or inhibitory, their postsynaptic targets can be determined, the receptors on the postsynaptic cells identified, and the kinetics of the postsynaptic responses defined.

The application of these morphological and physiological tools provides an account of the potential cell types and circuitry that might produce the motor pattern being studied. The information these techniques provide is absolutely essential for an understanding of the circuits. But, while essential, it is not enough. The cells and the circuitry must be linked in a compelling way to the motor pattern and ultimately to the behavior. This is where our current approaches begin to falter.

1.3 THE JUST-SO STORY PROBLEM

The problem of linking circuits to motor output and behavior is illustrated by an example from our studies of escape networks in goldfish. The escape behavior in fish is one in which the fish turns very rapidly away from a threatening stimulus. This behavior is thought to be initiated by the firing of a hindbrain neuron, the Mauthner cell, whose cell body is located in the brain and whose axon crosses in the hindbrain and then extends the length of the spinal cord.[16,17] Over 10 years ago, we set out to identify the spinal outputs of the Mauthner cell that might underlie the behavior.

A couple of key features of the behavior were of interest. First, there is a massive, rapid motor output on the side of the active Mauthner axon. Second, activating both Mauthner cells leads to no motor output, suggesting some sort of reciprocal inhibition in the pathways.[18] In studies for which we searched for and filled neurons postsynaptic to the Mauthner cell, we found that the Mauthner neuron directly excites very large, so-called primary motoneurons, which innervate fast muscle fibers. It also monosynaptically excites two classes of interneurons.[11] An interneuron with a descending axon on the same side as the Mauthner axon is excited via a chemical synapse. An interneuron with a commissural axon is excited by the Mauthner axon via an electrical synapse. In further studies using pairwise recording, we showed that the descending interneuron is excitatory and excites primary motoneurons via electrical synapses.[13] Similar work showed that the commissural interneuron is inhibitory and inhibits contralateral motoneurons and interneurons.[12]

These identified cells could potentially account for key features of the behavior. The massive motoneuron activity might be a consequence of the direct and indirect excitatory connections of the Mauthner cell with motoneurons, while the contralateral inhibition could block motor activity on the opposite side. Thus, we could, in a way, account for the behavior with a simple just-so story in which a big bend to one side is produced by the direct and indirect excitation of motoneurons to get massive motor output, while opposing contralateral activity was blocked by commissural cells. This sounds great, but we must recognize that it is simply a just-so story until we have some more causal links between the neurons and behavior. These are not easy to come by, but are essential to really understand the production of the behavior.

For example, even though the direct excitation of motoneurons by the Mauthner cell likely contributes to the initial bend, it is impossible to know with standard approaches what the difference is between the contribution to the behavior of the direct excitation of motoneurons vs. the contribution of the indirect excitation of the motoneurons through the identified excitatory interneurons. This is difficult to establish for many reasons. In part, key pieces of information are missing and are hard to get with standard approaches. First, we have little idea of exactly how many of the interneurons there are. We do not know how strong they are (except for the very few studied with pair-wise recording) or how they are distributed along cord. We do not know how much of the population is activated in the behavior and how that activity might vary in association with known variability in the escape bend. Other reticulospinal neurons participate in the behavior along with the Mauthner cell and how those other pathways interact with those of the Mauthner cell at the level of motoneurons and interneurons is unknown.[19–22] Finally, there is no way of selectively and specifically removing the class of excitatory interneurons from the circuit to test its behavioral contribution. All of these problems compound the difficulty of pinning down the behavioral significance of the cell type in the circuit.

1.4 MODELING AS A TOOL

A common approach to evaluating the role of the neurons in generating the motor pattern (beyond telling a just-so story) has been to use modeling. The strategy is to use the information provided by the cellular studies to build a network containing cells and connectivity that mimic as closely as possible those in the real animal.[23,24] If the resulting network can reproduce the motor output of the animal, then there is more confidence that the relevant circuitry has been identified. The modeling certainly provides evidence that the cells and circuits could potentially generate the right pattern. In principle, if all of the details of the cells and connectivity put into the model come from the animal, then if the model can reproduce the natural motor output, the case for the contribution of the neurons is fairly strong. Of course, rarely is all the information available and often there must be substantial simplifications and/or guesses about some components in the model. To the extent that parameters in the model are not based on the animal, the usefulness of the model as a "test" of the function of neurons in the circuit is reduced. This is simply because there might be many combinations of neurons and parameters that can produce a particular motor output; the questions are which ones really do it in the animal and what is the role of each cell in producing the motor pattern and behavior? It is not that the modeling is not useful as a guide to thinking about the circuit and potential experiments, but it is not a true test of the behavioral role of the components of the circuit. Some sort of perturbations of neurons in the animal, perhaps inspired by a model, have to be done to properly test the behavioral contribution of the cells.

1.5　THE GENERALITY OF THE PROBLEM OF MONITORING AND PERTURBING ACTIVITY IN NEURONAL POPULATIONS

Many of the same issues arise in studies of all motor circuits that contain a number of any particular cell type (which includes almost every vertebrate circuit). We have the model systems and experimental tools to obtain detailed information about the morphology and physiological properties of individual cells and their connectivity, but moving from that to what the cells contribute behaviorally is a formidable and largely failed or ignored task. The situation with regard to Renshaw cells in mammalian spinal cord captures the essence of the problem in another system. We know much about the physiology and morphology of Renshaw cells, which provide a feedback inhibition of motoneurons, but there is, remarkably enough, still not a clear understanding of their role in behavior.[25] How can this be so long after their identification?

These gaps remain because it is difficult to monitor the activity in populations of neurons of identified type during behavior and even more difficult to perturb that activity. This is true almost everywhere in the nervous system, but is especially so in spinal cord where the interneurons of different types are intermingled and so are not accessible even to tools such as electrode arrays that are useful for monitoring population activity when a cell type is grouped together. Still, we need to understand the correlations between the activity in the populations and the behavior, as individual cells contribute very little. These correlations can then, along with cellular and connectivity information, form a basis for hypotheses about the behavioral contributions of the neurons that must somehow be tested by perturbation of activity in a cell-specific way.

1.6 WHY IS IT SO HARD TO TEST THE CONTRIBUTION OF NEURONS TO MOTOR PATTERNS AND BEHAVIOR IN VERTEBRATES?

The contribution of particular neurons to motor patterns has been examined successfully in invertebrate models.[26-28] What then precludes such tests among vertebrates? The problem centers largely around the number of neurons involved in the different systems and the accessibility of the neurons. In those invertebrate systems where the most compelling tests of neuronal function have been accomplished, such as in the stomatogastric system of crustaceans or the nervous system of nematodes, the number of neurons in the motor circuits of interest is small. Individual cells can be removed from the circuit by laser killing them either in isolated ganglia from crustaceans or in intact nematodes. It is even possible to artificially alter the connectivity of neurons in very simple invertebrate circuits by using the dynamic clamp.[29] The consequences of the ablation or alterations in connectivity then can be assessed to determine the contribution of the neurons or their synaptic connections to a motor pattern or to a behavior.

The ability to use single cell ablations depends both on having neurons that are accessible enough to be targeted specifically with a laser and on having few cells, so that enough of a cell type can be removed to impact on the motor behavior. Both of these pose severe problems for applying this method in vertebrates. Most vertebrates are not transparent like nematodes, so it is not possible to simply focus a laser into the animal onto cells in the nervous system to kill them. Even isolating the nervous system, as is done in some invertebrate systems, does not help very much because the myelination in vertebrates produces much light scattering which makes laser targeting more difficult. If the neurons could be individually targeted, there are usually so many cells of any type that removing them one at a time is unrealistic. Neurons clustered in a nucleus could, in principle, be removed with a more gross aspiration, chemical, or electrolytic lesion, but such nuclei rarely consist of a single cell type. It is critical that the contribution of one and only one cell type be affected to test its functional role.

1.7 OPTICAL AND GENETIC METHODS OFFER A POTENTIAL SOLUTION

The major gaps in our understanding, therefore, center around knowing what the activity is in populations of identified neurons and linking that activity in a compelling way to behavior. One strategy for attacking these problems is to use a combination of optical and genetic approaches. Recent technical developments offer the possibility of using optical and genetic tools to monitor and perturb activity in particular populations of neurons in intact vertebrates. The potential of these approaches to complement and extend the results from studies of cellular and synaptic studies is only beginning to be realized as new preparations and techniques are introduced. Our work has focused on the development of a larval zebrafish preparation which is especially suitable for combining optical and genetic approaches. The following sections first introduce this preparation and its advantages through examples from our work. The last section deals with the work of others showing how optical and genetic approaches are proving powerful for exploring neuronal function in mammals as well.

1.8 THE LARVAL ZEBRAFISH MODEL

Our frustrations with the "just so" stories of neuronal function in our own work and most other studies of spinal circuits contributed to our move toward a new preparation in which the activity and behavioral contribution of neuronal populations could potentially be tested. We chose to study larval zebrafish for several reasons. Zebrafish were already well established as a model for developmental studies, thanks largely to a group in Oregon started by George Streisinger.[30,31] One of the great advantages for developmental work was the transparency of the fish early in life, which allowed the growth of neurons to be imaged *in vivo*. This same transparency allows neurons to be visualized throughout the nervous system of the intact fish for more than 2 weeks after the animals hatch, making zebrafish particularly amenable to optical studies of neuronal function. The genetics of zebrafish were also blossoming with the production of many mutant lines and the first evidence for the feasibility of making transgenic fish.[32-36] Finally, zebrafish were closely related to the goldfish we had studied with electrophysiological methods in the past, so the results from zebrafish would complement the previous goldfish work. Our first studies, described in the next two sections, took advantage of the transparency of the fish to image neuronal activity in the intact animal and to ablate neurons with a laser to test their contributions to behavior.

1.9 IMAGING NEURONAL ACTIVITY IN ZEBRAFISH

In order to monitor activity with optical methods, it is important to have an indicator that will signal when the neurons are active. The most commonly used ones are voltage and calcium indicators. The current voltage dyes are very phototoxic when imaging single cells, making them less useful in experiments where a number of experimental trials are required. As better voltage indicators become available, they will likely be a tool of choice since they provide a direct measure of membrane potential. In the meantime, we have used fluorescent calcium indicators to monitor neuronal activity because calcium rises in active neurons, calcium indicators have large signals, neurons can be backfilled with the indicators, and the calcium indicators are less phototoxic than voltage dyes.

Our approach was based upon the initial work of Michael O'Donovan which showed that neurons could be backfilled with calcium indicators.[37] Injections of one of these indicators (calcium green coupled to a 10,000 mol wt dextran) into the muscle or spinal cord of 5-day-old larval zebrafish produce brightly labeled neurons that can easily be visualized in the spinal cord or brain of the living animal with confocal microscopy.[21,38] An example of some spinal interneurons is shown in Fig. 1.1. Fish with labeled cells are partially embedded in agar to restrain them.

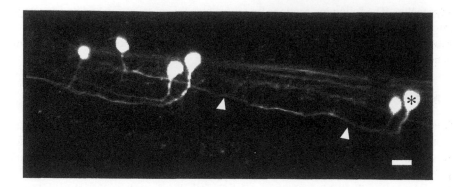

FIGURE 1.1 Morphology of spinal interneurons filled with calcium green and observed in the live fish. Circumferential descending interneurons (CiD cells) in a lateral view of spinal cord (dorsal is up). Asterisk marks the soma, and arrowheads mark the axon of one of a longitudinal array of CiD cells. The axons extend ventrally from the soma, then run caudally and dorsally to join a dorsolateral axonal bundle that contains the axons of the array of CiD cells. Rostral is to the right. Scale bar = 10 μm.

Then, the neurons of interest are imaged while a behavior is elicited. Confocal images of the fluorescence of the cells are collected while the movements of the fish are also monitored with a high speed (1000 frame/s) digital camera. The active cells show increases in calcium and therefore fluorescence during the behavior, as illustrated in Color Figure 1.* The neurons involved in the behavior thus light up when they are active.

The advantages of the approach are that one can monitor different neurons simply by focusing on different filled cells, and a group of cells in the same optical section can be imaged simultaneously to assess population activity. Finally, one obtains data not only about the activity of the cells, but also about their morphology because confocal optical sections through the neurons allow for a 3-D reconstruction of the live cells studied physiologically. We have used this approach to study the activation of spinal motoneurons, spinal interneurons, and hindbrain neurons during movements.[21,38,39] Our efforts have dealt mostly with the activation of neurons in escape behaviors, although we have also examined neurons during swimming movements.

Much of our work has focused on hindbrain neurons involved in escapes.[21,22] The hindbrain is segmentally organized, with similar reticulospinal neurons in successive hindbrain segments.[40] One of the segmental sets of reticulospinal cells includes the Mauthner cell in hindbrain segment 4 and two other morphologically similar cells (MiD2cm and MiD3cm) in hindbrain segments 5 and 6. Like the Mauthner cells, MiD2cm and MiD3cm have two major dendrites and a commissural axon that extends the length of spinal cord. Much work prior to ours showed that the Mauthner cell is important for initiation of escape turns away from a threatening stimulus.[16,17] The presence of other Mauthner-like neurons (MiD2cm and MiD3cm) raised obvious questions about their functional roles and relationships to the Mauthner cell. It proved difficult, however, to record from these cells with conventional

---

* Color figures follow page 142.

electrophysiological techniques. We studied their activity in escapes by backfilling the cells and imaging them in the brain of living fish in which we elicited escapes by a touch on the head or the tail.

Previous work by Foreman and Eaton suggested that the activity of the set of hindbrain neurons might vary with the form of the escape behavior.[41] Not all escapes are the same. In response to a touch on the tail, the fish make a slower and more shallow turn and move forward away from the stimulus. A touch on the head leads to a faster and large turn, which swivels the fish around so that it swims away from the stimulus. Foreman and Eaton proposed that all three hindbrain neurons might be active to produce the largest and fastest turns to a head stimulus, whereas the Mauthner cell might act alone to produce the response to a tail stimulus.

Our imaging experiments showed that the activity pattern in the hindbrain neurons is exactly like that proposed by Foreman and Eaton.[42] All three neurons (Mauthner, MiD2cm, and MiD3cm) light up during escapes elicited by a head stimulus, whereas only the Mauthner cell responds to a tail stimulus. This is consistent with the idea that the form of the escape is determined in part by the pattern of activity in a serial set of hindbrain neurons. This is an important conclusion because it suggests that the segmentally repeated hindbrain neurons form functional groups. Because all vertebrate hindbrains are segmented, it may be that segmental functional groups are a general feature of the organization of hindbrain.

The optical methods have also proven useful for exploring the types of spinal interneurons active in different movements.[39,43] A spinal neuron can be identified by its dendritic and axonal morphology and then imaged during different movements including swimming, escape, or struggling. Based on previous work in goldfish there was reason to think that spinal interneurons might be shared by escape and swimming circuits. This was difficult to address in a compelling way in goldfish because while fictive swimming could be produced by stimulating midbrain, it was not possible to elicit a full-fledged escape to a sensory stimulus in the fictive preparations. In the intact zebrafish preparation, we could elicit movements more readily by a touch or light stimulus and directly correlate the movements with the cells that showed calcium rises. Our data reveal differences in the activation of the various types of spinal neurons during different behaviors that point to a separation of the functional roles for at least some cell types in spinal cord. For example, some spinal interneurons are active in escape, but not slow-speed swimming movements whereas others are active in swimming, but not escape.[39,43] These optical data from interneurons suggest a greater separation of the behavioral roles of cells than we expected based upon our studies of goldfish and are leading us to reformulate our ideas about the behavioral contributions of interneurons.

With imaging we can monitor groups of identified spinal interneurons as well as individual cells.[44] Although much of our work until now has been directed toward obtaining basic information about the cell types in spinal cord and their activity during different behaviors, we will also be able to examine variations in the activity of populations of neurons during variability in the behaviors. It might be, for example, that there is recruitment of additional interneurons or alterations in the set of cells activated as the strength of escape or swimming is changed, just as the pattern of activation in hindbrain neurons changes with the form of the escape. Such

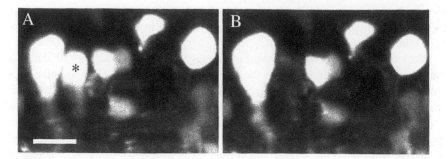

FIGURE 1.2 Specificity of the optical lesioning. (A) Pool of spinal motoneurons in a live fish prior to lesioning. The cell marked by the asterisk was overilluminated to lesion it. An image of the population of neurons immediately after the lesioning is shown in (B). Note that only the targeted cell was affected (only hints of it remain), but immediately adjacent cells are unaffected. Scale bar = 10 μm. (From Liu and Fetcho, *Neuron,* 23, 325, 1999. With permission from Elsevier Science.)

studies of the activity of groups of identified spinal interneurons are nearly impossible with other methods.

1.10 CELL-SPECIFIC PERTURBATION OF ACTIVITY VIA LASER ABLATION

Calcium imaging allows the identification of neurons active in a behavior. The problem remains, however, that it provides just a correlation between activity and behavior. We must establish more causal links between the neurons and the behavior to avoid the trap of the "just so" story. Our initial solution to this problem in zebrafish was to again capitalize on the transparency of the fish and focus a laser onto individual cells in the intact fish to kill the cells.[22] This is possible by focusing the confocal laser at high intensity onto labeled cells in the fish. The labeled cells are killed by the illumination because of the phototoxicity of the indicator dyes. Individual cells can be killed without affecting immediately adjacent cells, as shown in Fig. 1.2. Although our experiments on hindbrain neurons were done in this way, it is also possible to kill unlabeled cells by using a high-intensity pulsed nitrogen laser which can burn a tiny (sub-micron) spot in the nucleus of a cell and kill it. This approach is the one used for years to kill cells in the nervous system of the transparent nematode worm.[26,45] It is quicker and, therefore, more appropriate for removing larger number of cells.

Our imaging data from the hindbrain neurons led to two predictions concerning the effects of ablations. The first was that if we removed all three hindbrain neurons on one side the brain, we would remove the ability of the fish to produce a high speed escape in response to a head or a tail stimulus on that side. The second prediction was that removing only the Mauthner cell would have a greater impact upon escapes in response to tail stimuli than those to head stimuli because the imaging data showed that the Mauthner cell acted without the others in escapes from tail stimuli.

The lesion experiments were done by first labeling the hindbrain neurons by backfilling and then collecting digital images of escapes at 1000 frames/s in response to a squirt of water directed at one or the other side of the head or the tail.[22] These formed a pre-lesion data set. Hindbrain neurons (either all three in the Mauthner array or just the Mauthner cell) were then ablated with the laser and the same fish were tested for escape performance after the ablations. Fish in which all three cells were removed on one side were unable to perform high-speed escape movements in response to a stimulus on the lesioned side, while the performance on the unlesioned side remained strong. In contrast, removal of one Mauthner cell significantly impaired the ability of the fish to perform rapid escape movements in response to a tail stimulus on that side, but had minimal effect on escapes to head stimuli. These results supported the conclusions from the imaging data and provided a more direct link between the cells and the escape behavior. They gave us more confidence that the neurons are indeed contributing to the behavior in the way that the physiological data suggested. It does appear that the pattern of activity in this segmental set in the hindbrain contributes to the form of the behavior produced.

The ability to remove single hindbrain cells specifically allowed for a fairly direct assessment of their contributions to behavior. Without the ability to very specifically perturb these cells, it would seem impossible to move beyond stories based upon correlations between the connectivity and the activity of the cells and the behavior. We are using similar approaches to remove spinal interneurons with a pulsed nitrogen laser. This allows us to target a cell type very specifically, but the larger numbers of neurons of each type in spinal cord make the experiments more difficult. Nevertheless, these perturbations experiments are essential for testing our ideas of spinal interneuron function. Lesion experiments by Buchanan in lampreys, for example, are suggesting important contributions to the swimming rhythm by interneurons with short commissural axons that have not been well studied in prior work.[46,47] These lesion studies may alter in an important way the view of which neurons are central to the mechanism for generating the swimming rhythm.

1.11 WHY GENETIC APPROACHES ARE POTENTIALLY BETTER THAN THOSE USED SO FAR TO STUDY CIRCUITS IN ZEBRAFISH

Even though the approaches we have used to image neuronal activity and laser kill cells in zebrafish are very powerful, they are not without important limitations. The neurons are filled with calcium indicators by injections of the calcium indicator into the central nervous system. The axonal processes of neurons probably must be damaged to get significant uptake of the indicator, which risks disruption of the circuits of interest. This is less of a problem for neurons with long axons where the damage can be confined to a small portion of their more distal processes. It is possible, for example, to backfill the Mauthner and other hindbrain neurons by injections into caudal spinal cord without a substantial effect on the ability of the fish to produce an escape.[22] If the goal is to study local interneurons, however, backfilling will not be very helpful because the circuits in the region of interest will be disrupted. In addition, it would not be possible to study populations of the interneurons without multiple injections which would severely disrupt cord.

We have attempted to overcome the problems of damage by filling the neurons by injecting the indicator into a blastomere in the developing fish, as is done in cell lineage tracing work.[48] The injection labels the progeny of the injected blastomere, so a single cell injected at the four-cell stage produces a larval fish with about 25% of its cells containing indicator. This avoids disruption of processes and the label retains its ability to report calcium rises. The level of indicator is diluted, however, making it difficult to identify spinal neurons and thus of limited usefulness for studies of spinal interneurons. It is easier with this approach to identify neurons in other regions such as the sensory epithelium. Still, what is needed is a method for introducing an indicator into a large number of cells of a particular type without a disruption of the circuits. This may be possible by introducing genes that code for indicator molecules into fish. If the genes are under control of genetic elements that direct their expression to a cell type or a few cell types, they would provide an endogenous molecule for monitoring neuronal activity.

The use of lasers to perturb activity also has two important limitations. First, the lesions are irreversible. Second, if the population of neurons is large, a cell by cell lesioning approach rapidly becomes unwieldy. These problems may also be overcome by genetic methods. If genes that perturb neuronal activity can be introduced into fish under control of genetic elements that allow inducible, cell-specific expression, then it will be possible to reversibly turn off or alter the activity of a cell type. This genetic approach to perturbation would circumvent many of the problems of doing perturbation experiments in systems with many neurons. Such an approach would revolutionize our understanding of the links between neurons and behavior. In the next sections, we assess the prospects for using these approaches in zebrafish and in mammals.

1.12 REVERSE GENETICS IN ZEBRAFISH

In the past few years, the production of transgenic zebrafish has been accomplished and is rapidly becoming routine.[34–36,49] These lines reveal the potential power of the combination of genetic and optical methods. For example, the first stable line of fish expressing green fluorescent protein (GFP) under control of a neuronal specific promoter was a line produced by Higashijima et al., in which a portion of the controlling elements of the Islet-1 gene directs expression of GFP to motoneurons.[35] In these fish, many of the spinal and cranial motoneurons are fluorescent with especially bright labeling in the homozygotes for the transgene. It is possible to resolve the dendrites and follow the axons of the labeled cells in this line, which is making it an important tool for studies visualizing the development of connections between nerves and muscle in living fish. This line, which has now been stable through many generations, shows the feasibility of producing transgenic fish with the stable incorporation of genetically encoded fluorescent markers targeted to a subset of neurons.

Although GFP is useful for morphological and developmental studies, a genetically encoded indicator of activity would offer the possibility of making lines of fish with built-in indicators in particular cell types. Miyawaki et al. have produced such an indicator based upon derivatives of GFP.[50,51] The indicator, called cameleon, consists of a cyan (CFP) and a yellow (YFP) fluorescent protein coupled to each other by calmodulin and a calmodulin binding domain. The indicator depends upon fluorescence resonance energy transfer to signal calcium rises. In the absence of calcium, the CFP is relatively far from the YFP and excitation of the CFP leads to emission at the CFP emission wavelength. Upon binding of calcium, the conformation of the protein changes to bring the CFP close to the YFP. Excitation of the CFP is followed by transfer of the energy to the YFP which then emits at the emission wavelength for YFP. Thus, a rise in calcium leads to a decrease in emission from CFP and an increase from YFP. The ratio of YFP/CFP is used to report calcium levels which can then serve to monitor activity.

In collaboration with Shin-ichi Higashijima and Gail Mandel, we have been developing methods for using cameleon in zebrafish. We have successfully expressed the cameleon transiently by DNA injections into single-celled embryos and have demonstrated that it is possible to record calcium rises in the Rohon-Beard sensory neurons in intact fish after stimulation of the skin.[52] It thus seems feasible to produce fish with genetically encoded calcium indicators and we are working toward that goal. One of the limitations in accomplishing this is the need for cell-specific promoter elements to direct expression in a subset of neurons. Some of these are available, but more will be needed to direct expression to interesting classes of neurons.

1.13 GENETIC PERTURBATION OF ACTIVITY

Genetic expression can be used not only to monitor activity, but also to perturb it. Strategies for accomplishing this have been demonstrated in flies. Synaptic connections of subsets of neurons were eliminated through the expression of a fragment of tetanus toxin which cleaves synaptobrevin, a key component of the synaptic machinery.[53] Genetic ablation of cells has also been accomplished in flies by using a temperature sensitive form of the ricin toxin.[54] At low temperatures the toxicity of the altered ricin is very low, but by raising the temperature the neurons expressing the gene are killed. This approach is feasible in poikilothermic vertebrates, including fish, in which body temperature is controlled externally. Even more subtle perturbations of neurons should be possible with genetics. One could, for example, alter the excitability of a neuron by introducing genes for altered ion channels that clamp the cell at resting potential or make it more excitable. Genes for modified neurotransmitter receptors or for neurotransmitter transporters might also be introduced to alter the strength or transmitter phenotype at the synapses formed by a cell type.[55]

These genetic tools are potentially much more powerful than the backfilling with indicators and laser ablations we have used so far in zebrafish. They will certainly be commonly applied in the future for studies throughout the spinal cord and brain. At this point, two things are limiting studies of this sort. First, there are few genetic elements that target genes to particular classes of vertebrate neurons, although more are becoming available as additional genes and promoters are cloned. If enhancer trap approaches similar to those used in flies can be developed for fish, the ability to express genes in subsets of cells will improve dramatically. The second limitation is that for perturbation experiments it is important that one have both spatial and temporal control of expression. A gene must be turned on to produce the perturbation in only a subset of cells at a particular time after the circuits and behavior have developed. The behavior can then be examined before and immediately after the perturbations. Ideally, the perturbations should be reversible, which should be possible with inducible control over expression of the transgenes. There have been relatively few studies using inducible control of transgene expression in vertebrates, but the number is increasing and there is much active work to perfect inducible systems such as the tetracycline-based system.[56] We can expect that these approaches will become routine as well.

These genetic approaches will provide explicit links between neurons and behavior because alterations in behavior can be studied in the transgenic lines. Again, such work will not eliminate the need for cellular and synaptic studies of the circuits. Cellular studies will always be necessary in both normal and transgenic lines. But, the genetic approaches will allow the tests of neuronal function that have proven so elusive in studies of circuits thus far.

1.14　OPTICAL AND GENETIC APPROACHES ARE POSSIBLE IN MAMMALS AS WELL AS ZEBRAFISH

While the transparency of zebrafish and the relatively small number of neurons in larvae make them especially amenable to optical and genetic studies of neuronal circuits, these approaches are possible in mammals as well. Mouse genetics is, in many ways, currently better than zebrafish. Gene knockouts and transgenic mice are generated routinely. In addition, mice with inducible transgenes have already been produced. The use of inducible lines is still being perfected, but the genetic tools with the potential for altering the activity of a cell type or for introducing genes for indicators of activity are better right now for mice than any other vertebrate.[56] We can anticipate a growth in such studies as inducible transgenic approaches become routine. These approaches may finally move us toward a more concrete idea of the behavioral contributions of neurons in the more complex circuits in the spinal cord or brain of mammals.

One example of such an approach is the recent report of a genetic strategy to remove the inhibitory golgi cells in the cerebellum.[57] The approach was to use a new cell ablation technology called immunotoxin-mediated cell targeting. In this method, a transgenic mouse is generated which expresses the alpha subunit of the human interleukin-2 receptor. The cells expressing the receptor are then killed by introducing into the adult animal a recombinant protein formed by combining a monoclonal antibody against the human interleukin-2 receptor coupled to a toxin (pseudomonas exotoxin- PE38). Spatial control is provided by the controlling elements in the transgene which direct its expression to golgi cells; the temporal control is achieved when the toxin is introduced. This approach allows the demonstration of the contribution of the cerebellar golgi cells to complex motor coordination. This represents just one example of a variety of approaches being developed to control gene expression and alter neuronal circuits with spatial and temporal specificity in mammals.

One of the clear strengths of zebrafish is their transparency, which simplifies optical studies of neuronal activity. It might seem that the possibility to monitor activity in populations of individual cells by using optical methods in mammals would be very difficult because mammals are not transparent. It has been difficult, but the situation is not as dire as it may seem. Recently, two-photon microscopy has allowed the visualization of calcium rises in individual neurons in the intact brain of rats after exposing the brain by removing a portion of the skull.[58] Two-photon microscopy is very effective at imaging in the highly light-scattering nervous tissue of mammals.[59] It should prove especially powerful for future studies of neuronal activity in mammals, particularly small mammals such as rats and mice. There is good reason to expect that the combination of the introduction of genetically encoded indicators into mice with two-photon microscopy will permit the study of population activity in intact mammalian circuits. Thus, the power of optical and genetic approaches to inform us about population activity and the behavioral contribution of neurons extends broadly among vertebrates.

1.15 SUMMARY AND CONCLUSIONS

Years of studies applying patch and sharp electrode recording have identified neurons that participate in spinal circuits and have explored their connectivity and cellular properties. This important work forms a foundation for generating hypotheses about how the neurons work as populations to produce a particular behavior. What has largely been missing, however, is information about the activity in populations of the neurons during behavior as well as experimental studies that perturb the activity in a particular population of neurons to test their behavioral contribution. This is now changing as the tools to study populations of neurons are becoming available. Some of the most powerful tools take advantage of optical and genetic approaches to monitor and perturb activity in populations of neurons. We can expect that studies combining these methods will soon become routine. They will fill the gaps in our understanding of neuronal circuits by providing a much better view of the contributions of neurons to behavior.

ACKNOWLEDGMENTS

Many people have contributed to the work on zebrafish reviewed in this chapter including Don O'Malley, Katharine Liu, Dale Ritter, Dimple Bhatt, Melina Hale, Kingsley Cox, Shin-ichi Higashijima, and Gail Mandel. I thank all of them for being good colleagues and for their substantial contributions to the experiments.

REFERENCES

1. Brodfuehrer, P.D., Debski, E.A., O'Gara, B.A., and Friesen, W.O., Neuronal control of leech swimming, *J. Neurobiol.*, 27, 403, 1995.
2. Stent, G.S., Thompson, W.J., and Calabrese, R.L., Neural control of heartbeat in the leech and in some other invertebrates, *Physiol. Rev.*, 59, 101, 1979.

3. Simmers, J., Meyrand, P., and Moulins, M., Modulation and dynamic specification of motor rhythm-generating circuits in crustacea, *J. Physiol. (Paris)*, 89, 195, 1995.
4. Roberts, A., How does a nervous system produce behaviour? A case study in neurobiology, *Sci. Progr.*, 74, 31, 1990.
5. Grillner, S., Deliagina, T., Ekeberg, O., el Manira, A., Hill, R.H., Lansner, A., Orlovsky, G.N., and Wallen, P., Neural networks that co-ordinate locomotion and body orientation in lamprey, *Trends Neurosci.*, 18, 270, 1995.
6. Norris, B.J., Coleman, M.J., and Nusbaum, M.P., Pyloric motor pattern modification by a newly identified projection neuron in the crab stomatogastric nervous system, *J. Neurophysiol.*, 75, 97, 1996.
7. Buchanan, J.T. and Grillner, S., Newly identified 'Glutamate interneurons' and their role in locomotion in the lamprey spinal cord, *Science*, 236, 312, 1987.
8. Dale, N., Reciprocal inhibitory interneurones in the Xenopus embryo spinal cord, *J. Physiol.*, 363, 61, 1985.
9. Grillner, S. and Matsushima, T., The neural network underlying locomotion in lamprey - synaptic and cellular mechanisms, *Neuron*, 7, 1, 1991.
10. Rovainen, C.M., Identified neurons in the lamprey spinal cord and their roles in fictive swimming, in *Neural Origin of Rhythmic Movements. Symposia of the Society for Experimental Biology No. XXXVII*, A. Roberts and B.L. Robert, Eds., Cambridge University Press, Cambridge, 1983, 305.
11. Fetcho, J.R. and Faber, D.S., Identification of motoneurons and interneurons in the spinal network for escapes initiated by the Mauthner cell in goldfish, *J. Neurosci.*, 8, 4192, 1988.
12. Fetcho, J.R., Morphological variability, segmental relationships, and functional role of a class of commissural interneurons in the spinal cord of Goldfish, *J. Compar. Neurol.*, 299, 283, 1990.
13. Fetcho, J.R., Excitation of motoneurons by the Mauthner axon in goldfish: Complexities in a "simple" reticulospinal pathway, *J. Neurophysiol.*, 67, 1574, 1992.
14. Dale, N., Kinetic characterization of the voltage-gated currents possessed by Xenopus embryo spinal neurons, *J. Physiol. (Lond.)*, 489, 473, 1995.
15. Buchanan, J.T., Identification of interneurons with contralateral, caudal axons in the lamprey spinal cord: synaptic interactions and morphology, *J. Neurophysiol.*, 47, 961, 1982.
16. Zottoli, S.J., Correlation of the startle reflex and Mauthner cell auditory responses in unrestrained goldfish, *J. Exp. Biol.*, 66, 243, 1977.
17. Eaton, R.C. and Hackett, J.T., The role of the Mauthner cell in fast-starts involving escape in teleost fishes, in *Neural Mechanisms of Startle Behavior*, R.C. Eaton, Ed., Plenum Press, New York, 1984, 213.
18. Yasargil, G.M. and Diamond, J., Startle-response in teleost fish: an elementary circuit for neural discrimination, *Nature*, 220, 241, 1968.
19. Eaton, R.C., Lavender, W.A., and Wieland, C.M., Alternative neural pathways initiate fast start responses following lesions of the Mauthner neuron in goldfish, *J. Comp. Physiol.*, 145, 485, 1982.
20. Eaton, R.C., Nissanov, J., and Wieland, C.M., Differential activation of Mauthner and non-Mauthner startle circuits in the zebrafish: Implications for functional substitution, *J. Comp. Physiol.*, 155, 813, 1984.
21. O'Malley, D.M., Kao, Y.H., and Fetcho, J.R., Imaging the functional organization of zebrafish hindbrain segments during escape behaviors, *Neuron*, 17, 1145, 1996.
22. Liu, K.S. and Fetcho, J.R., Laser ablations reveal functional relationships of segmental hindbrain neurons in zebrafish, *Neuron*, 23, 325, 1999.

23. Wallen, P., Ekeberg, O., Lansner, A., Brodin, L., Traven, H., and Grillner, S., A computer-based model for realistic simulations of neural networks. II. The segmental network generating locomotor rhythmicity in the lamprey, *J. Neurophysiol.*, 68, 1939, 1992.

24. Dale, N., Experimentally derived model for the locomotor pattern generator in the Xenopus embryo, *J. Physiol. (Lond.)*, 489, 489, 1995.

25. Windhorst, U., On the role of recurrent inhibitory feedback in motor control, *Progr. Neurobiol.*, 49, 517, 1996.

26. Liu, K.S. and Sternberg, P.W., Sensory regulation of male mating behavior in *Caenorhabditis elegans*, *Neuron*, 14, 79, 1995.

27. Bargmann, C.I. and Horvitz, H.R., Chemosensory neurons with overlapping functions direct chemotaxis to multiple chemicals in *C. elegans, Neuron*, 7, 729, 1991.

28. Selverston, A.I. and Miller, J.P., Mechanisms underlying pattern generation in lobster stomatogastric ganglion as determined by selective inactivation of identified neurons. I. Pyloric system, *J. Neurophysiol.*, 44, 1102, 1980.

29. Sharp, A.A., O'Neil, M.B., Abbott, L.F., and Marder, E., Dynamic clamp: computer-generated conductances in real neurons, *J. Neurophysiol.*, 69, 992, 1993.

30. Myers, P.Z., Eisen, J.S., and Westerfield, M., Development and axonal outgrowth of identified motoneurons in the zebrafish, *J. Neurosci.*, 6, 2278, 1986.

31. Streisinger, G., Walker, C., Dower, N., Knauber, D., and Singer, F., Production of clones of homozygous diploid zebrafish (*Brachidanio rerio*), *Nature*, 291, 293, 1981.

32. Driever, W., Stemple, D., Schier, A., and Solnica-Krezel, L., Zebrafish: genetic tools for studying vertebrate development, *Trends Genet.*, 10, 152, 1995.

33. Granato, M., van Eeden, F.J., Schach, U., Trowe, T., Brand, M., Furutani-Seiki, M., Haffter, P., Hammerschmidt, M., Heisenberg, C.P., Jiang, Y.J., Kane, D.A., Kelsh, R.N., Mullins, M.C., Odenthal, J., and Nusslein-Volhard, C., Genes controlling and mediating locomotion behavior of the zebrafish embryo and larva, *Development*, 123, 399, 1996.

34. Higashijima, S., Okamoto, H., Ueno, N., Hotta, Y., and Eguchi, G., High-frequency generation of transgenic zebrafish which reliably express GFP in whole muscles or the whole body by using promoters of zebrafish origin, *Develop. Biol.*, 192, 289, 1997.

35. Higashijima, S., Hotta, Y., and Okamoto, H., Visualization of cranial motor neurons in live transgenic zebrafish expressing green fluorescent protein under the control of the islet-1 promoter/enhancer, *J. Neurosci.*, 20, 206, 2000.

36. Long, Q., Meng, A., Wang, H., Jessen, J.R., Farrell, M.J., and Lin, S., GATA-1 expression pattern can be recapitulated in living transgenic zebrafish using GFP reporter gene, *Development*, 124, 4105, 1997.

37. O'Donovan, M.J., Ho, S., Sholomenko, G., and Yee, W., Real-time imaging of neurons retrogradely and anterogradely labelled with calcium-sensitive dyes, *J. Neurosci. Meth.*, 46, 91, 1993.

38. Fetcho, J.R. and O'Malley, D.M., Visualization of active neural circuitry in the spinal cord of intact zebrafish, *J. Neurophysiol.*, 73, 399, 1995.

39. Bhatt, D.H., Liu, K.S., and Fetcho, J.R., Identifying spinal interneurons involved in motor behaviors of zebrafish by simultaneous calcium imaging and high speed motion analysis, *Soc. Neurosci. Abstr.*, 26, 1995, 2000.

40. Metcalfe, W.K., Mendelson, B., and Kimmel, C.B., Segmental homologies among reticulospinal neurons in the hindbrain of the zebrafish larva, *J. Comp. Neurol.*, 251, 147, 1986.

41. Foreman, M.B. and Eaton, R.C., The direction change concept for reticulospinal control of goldfish escape, *J. Neurosci.*, 13, 4101, 1993.

42. O'Malley, D.M., Kao, Y.-H., and Fetcho, J.R., Imaging the functional organization of zebrafish hindbrain segments during escape behaviors, *Neuron*, 17, 1145, 1996.

43. Ritter, D. and Fetcho, J.R., Confocal calcium imaging of spinal interneurons during swimming in larval zebrafish, *Soc. Neurosci. Abstr.*, 24, 1667, 1998.

44. Fetcho, J.R. and O'Malley, D.M., Visualization of active neural circuitry in the spinal cord of intact zebrafish, *J. Neurophysiol.*, 73, 399, 1995.

45. Avery, L. and Horvitz, H.R., A cell that dies during wild-type *C. elegans* development can function as a neuron in a ced-3 mutant, *Cell*, 51, 1071, 1987.

46. Buchanan, J.T., Commissural interneurons in rhythm generation and intersegmental coupling in the lamprey spinal cord, *J. Neurophysiol.*, 81, 2037, 1999.

47. Buchanan, J.T. and McPherson, D.R., The neuronal network for locomotion in the lamprey spinal cord: evidence for the involvement of commissural interneurons, *J. Physiol. (Paris)*, 89, 221, 1995.

48. Cox, K.J.A. and Fetcho, J.R., Labeling blastomeres with a calcium indicator: a non-invasive method of visualizing neuronal activity in zebrafish, *J. Neurosci. Meth.*, 68, 185, 1996.

49. Halloran, M.C., Sato-Maeda, M., Warren, J.T., Su, F., Lele, Z., Krone, P.H., Kuwada, J.Y., and Shoji, W., Laser-induced gene expression in specific cells of transgenic zebrafish, *Development*, 127, 1953, 2000.

50. Miyawaki, A., Griesbeck, O., Heim, R., and Tsien, R.Y., Dynamic and quantitative Ca2+ measurements using improved cameleons, *Proc. Natl. Acad. Sci. USA*, 96, 2135, 1999.

51. Miyawaki, A., Llopis, J., Heim, R., McCaffery, J.M., Adams, J.A., Ikura, M., and Tsien, R.Y., Fluorescent indicators of Ca2+ based on green fluorescent proteins and calmodulin, *Nature*, 388, 882, 1997.

52. Higashijima, S., Dallman, J., Mandel, G., and Fetcho, J., Using confocal microscopy and a genetically encoded calcium indicator (cameleon) to monitor neuronal activity in zebrafish, *Soc. Neurosci. Abstr.*, 26, 335, 2000.

53. Sweeny, S.T., Broadie, K., Keane, J., Nieman, H., and O'Kane, C.J., Targeted expression of tetanus toxin light chain in *Drosophila* specifically eliminates synaptic transmission and causes behavioral defects, *Neuron*, 14, 341, 1995.

54. Moffat, K.G., Gould, J.H., Smith, H.K., and O'Kane, C.J., Inducible cell ablation in *Drosophila* by cold-sensitive ricin A chain, *Development*, 114, 681, 1992.

55. Takamori, S., Rhee, J.S., Rosenmund, C., and Jahn, R., Identification of a vesicular glutamate transporter that defines a glutamatergic phenotype in neurons [see comments], *Nature*, 407, 189, 2000.

56. Chen, J., Kelz, M.B., Zeng, G., Sakai, N., Steffen, C., Shockett, P.E., Picciotto, M.R., Duman, R.S., and Nestler, E.J., Transgenic animals with inducible, targeted gene expression in brain, *Mol. Pharmacol.*, 54, 495, 1998.

57. Watanabe, D., Inokawa, H., Hashimoto, K., Suzuki, N., Kano, M., Shigemoto, R., Hirano, T., Toyama, K., Kaneko, S., Yokoi, M., Moriyoshi, K., Suzuki, M., Kobayashi, K., Nagatsu, T., Kreitman, R.J., Pastan, I., and Nakanishi, S., Ablation of cerebellar Golgi cells disrupts synaptic integration involving GABA inhibition and NMDA receptor activation in motor coordination, *Cell*, 95, 17, 1998.

58. Svoboda, K., Denk, W., Kleinfeld, D., and Tank, D.W., *In vivo* dendritic calcium dynamics in neocortical pyramidal neurons, *Nature*, 385, 161, 1997.

59. Denk, W. and Svoboda, K., Photon upmanship: why multiphoton imaging is more than a gimmick, *Neuron*, 18, 351, 1997.

2 Spinal Motoneurons: Synaptic Inputs and Receptor Organization

Robert E. W. Fyffe

CONTENTS

2.1 INTRODUCTION

Spinal motoneurons have long been the focus of studies of synaptic action and membrane properties, and the general firing properties and morphological features of both alpha and gamma motoneurons are well-known.[1] In a variety of mammalian and non-mammalian vertebrate species both types of motoneurons are intermingled in topographically organized elongated columns of cell bodies in lamina IX.[2-6] Whereas motoneuron cell bodies are positioned in circumscribed locations or "pools", their dendritic trees exhibit complex branching architecture. Archetypically, alpha motoneurons innervating hindlimb muscles in the cat have radially organized dendrites, with profuse extensions throughout the ventral horn and adjacent white matter. These dendritic trees are relatively symmetrical, although regions just ventral to or dorsal to the soma have fewer dendritic projections than expected. Dendritic trees of gamma motoneurons innervating the same muscle groups are generally less symmetrical, have fewer branch points and less total membrane area, but have dendrites that can be just as long as those of alpha motoneurons. Notably, alpha motoneuron dendritic morphology deviates from the radially symmetric pattern in a number of motoneuron pools, such as those innervating neck muscles or muscles of respiration, where dorso-medial and dorso-lateral bundles of dendrites are prominent. Detailed quantitative light microscopic descriptions of various alpha and gamma motoneurons are available.[7-22]

Throughout the nervous system, the critical role of the dendrites in neuronal function is emphasized by the fact that they provide more than 95% of the available membrane surface area for reception of synaptic contacts; for alpha motoneurons, this receptive area must accommodate approximately 50,000 synaptic inputs from a variety of segmental and supraspinal sources.[23] Despite broad recognition that neuronal dendrites have active properties (see below), there is consensus that the normal site of action potential initiation is at the axon initial segment or first node of Ranvier on the axon, even though under certain input conditions action potentials can be initiated in the dendrites[24-26] (see also, Reference 27). Ultimately, therefore, cell firing is dependent on the amount of current that reaches the cell soma/initial segment from active synapses that are widely distributed over the dendritic surface.[1,28-31]

Thus, although both presynaptic and postsynaptic factors play critical roles in synaptic efficacy per se, the amount of current delivered to the soma, and hence the overall integrative properties and general excitability of a neuron, is strongly influenced by the interaction of postsynaptic factors such as intrinsic membrane properties and the distribution and density of receptors and ion channels over the somato-dendritic membrane as well as by the spatial distribution of the synapses on the complex branching dendritic tree. From an historical perspective the study of motoneuron dendrites has been particularly influential in promoting these concepts and this chapter will review some issues of continuing relevance to neuronal integration, with particular focus on spinal motoneurons that innervate skeletal muscles.

2.2 SYNAPTIC TERMINALS ON MOTONEURONS

The synaptic terminals that are present on the motoneuron soma (and dendrites) can be classified into a relatively small number of categories based on ultrastructural criteria such as the size of the terminal, the shape of the synaptic vesicles contained in the bouton, and the disposition of the postsynaptic densities at the synaptic junction.[32–34] In general, four main types (S-, F-, C-, and M-type boutons; see Figure 2 in Reference 33) of boutons are described on alpha motoneurons, although modifications to the classification scheme have been introduced by subsequent authors[23,35] (see also, Figure 3.4 in Reference 1), in part because contemporary labeling techniques used to visualize identified motoneurons or boutons may obscure some of the defining features in the pre- or postsynaptic elements of the synapse. Because postsynaptic structural elements can be obscured in this way, synaptic vesicle shape (and distribution of vesicles within the terminal) and bouton size were used as the main classification factors in intracellular staining studies, resulting in use of a tripartite system encompassing F-type (which contain pleomorphic synaptic vesicles) and two categories of S-type (small and large boutons with spherical synaptic vesicles) boutons. An additional bouton type, the P bouton, makes presynaptic connections with some of the other bouton types in contact with the motoneuron surface and may form triadic arrangements.[33,36]

Detailed synaptological studies have attempted to determine the frequency of each bouton type on different areas of the surface membrane, and where possible, their origin. The task of systematically surveying the complete motoneuron surface is daunting and unrealistic, if not impossible, because the surface area of an alpha motoneuron often exceeds 5×10^5 μm^2, most of which is dendritic membrane, and total dendritic lengths exceed 10^5 μm. Electron microscopic studies can only sample a very small fraction of that area, and typically, a detailed study can only be expected to sample from at most a few neurons. Quite justifiably, quantitative electron microscopic studies of bouton frequency and packing density have focused on the somatic membrane, and to a lesser extent on selected dendritic regions at various distances from the soma. Estimates of overall bouton frequency and total number of synapses are then based on extrapolation of data from these sampled regions.

Identification of motoneuron somata for the purposes of ultrastructural analysis may be based on intracellular labeling, on the transport of markers from the periphery, or on soma size and location in the ventral horn. Although primary dendrites are easily recognized as they emerge from the soma, ultrastructural analysis of identified thin distal dendrites requires the use of intracellular staining strategies and subsequent light–electron microscopic correlation of selected labeled profiles. Coupled with 3-dimensional reconstruction of dendritic paths, this approach provides an accurate measurement of distance from the soma. Even if labeled dendritic profiles are not rigorously connected to a full reconstruction of an individual neuron their approximate position can be estimated if their diameter is known, because of the fairly consistent relationship between dendrite diameter and distance that has been revealed by quantitative light microscopic studies of neurons reconstructed in three dimensions.[37] Surprisingly, in view of the inherent technical difficulties and the uncertainties about conclusions drawn from "small" samples (which may actually represent thousands of electron micrographs and measurements), there is a growing consensus from quantitative ultrastructural studies that spinal alpha motoneurons receive approximately 50,000 synaptic boutons over their total somatic and dendritic surface membrane.[23] Other recent studies have placed the number of synapses in the range of 50,000 to 140,000 on alpha motoneurons.[37] In the following discussions it is tacitly assumed that the value is closer to the lower end of that range, i.e., approximately 50,000 synapses per motoneuron. Although it is difficult to define accurately the area of the soma surface,[11] various quantitative electron microscopic studies provide estimates of around 10 to 12 synapses per 100 μm^2 of somatic membrane, thus suggesting that there may be around 500 to 1000 synapses on each alpha motoneuron cell body. This represents only 1 to 2% of the total number of synaptic inputs on each motoneuron.

Despite the well-recognized problems associated with sampling and classifying bouton types, elegant quantitative ultrastructural analyses have also reached a relatively strong consensus regarding the frequency of boutons on the soma surface and on the proportion of surface membrane occupied by the various synaptic types. For cat and primate alpha motoneurons, the percentage of somatic membrane covered by bouton profiles is usually around 50% (range 40 to 60%)[23,33,34,38–41] but may be as high as 70% in neck motoneurons.[35] In contrast, gamma motoneurons exhibit fewer somatic synapses and a lower (20 to 40%) level of membrane coverage.[40,42,43,45] In alpha motoneurons, the percentage of proximal dendritic membrane in contact with axon terminals is generally about the same, or slightly higher, than for the soma. However, dendritic membrane coverage declines markedly at greater distances from the soma, to levels around 20 to 30% or less.[23,35] The frequency of occurrence of different bouton types also varies from cell to cell and in different regions of the dendritic tree, as discussed in the following sections.

2.2.1 F-TYPE BOUTONS

F-type boutons are the most numerous type of synapse on the somatic surface of alpha motoneurons, comprising more than half (usually 50 to 60%) of the contacts at the soma, and accounting for a similar proportion of the synaptic membrane coverage. F-type bouton frequency remains relatively high, comparable to somatic levels, on the proximal dendrites but declines on more distal dendrites. F-type boutons contain pleomorphic (elongate or irregular shape) synaptic vesicles, usually form symmetric synaptic junctions, and are generally assumed to represent inhibitory terminals. In keeping with this assumption, boutons of this class arising from identified inhibitory interneurons,[44] and F-type boutons in contact with the somata or dendrites of presumed motoneurons,[37,40,46] are enriched with glycine-like immunoreactivity.

2.2.1.1 Colocalization of Glycine and GABA at Ventral Horn Synapses

Glycine and GABA are the two major inhibitory amino acid transmitters in the spinal cord and are involved in a variety of inhibitory actions on motoneurons. A number of specific antibodies that were developed to reveal the presence of GABA, glycine, and their respective receptors and vesicular transporters, have been used extensively in investigations of inhibitory inputs to motoneurons in cat and rat spinal cord.[37,39,46–53] These studies substantiate the link between F-type bouton morphology and an inhibitory role for this type of synapse, and importantly, have helped to consolidate the idea that classical amino acid neurotransmitters may coexist and act in concert at fast central synapses. It is now clear that motoneurons receive inputs from glycine, GABA, and mixed glycine and GABA synapses in various proportions.

One commonly used marker of presumed inhibitory synapses is gephyrin, which is a peripheral membrane/cytosolic protein involved in the clustering and/or stabilization of postsynaptic receptors at glycinergic and GABAergic synaptic sites.[54,55] On motoneuron cell bodies the vast majority (approx. 90%) of synapses formed by F-boutons exhibit postsynaptic gephyrin immunoreactivity.[52] Interestingly, in Renshaw cell interneurons a very high proportion (around 90%, compared to 50 to 60% on alpha motoneurons) of all somatic synapses are formed by F-boutons, and virtually all of these synapses (96%) are immunopositive for gephyrin.[52]

Although initially discovered in association with glycine receptors, and known to be tightly associated with membrane-spanning subunits of the glycine receptor in spinal cord synapses, especially in the ventral horn,[48,56–58] gephyrin is also involved in the clustering and/or stabilization of $GABA_A$ receptors in many brain regions, including the spinal cord.[57,59,60] A major challenge in recent years has been to untangle the intricate relationships between the molecular components that underlie inhibitory transmission mediated by glycine and GABA in the ventral horn of the spinal cord; in this effort, the detailed studies from the laboratories of F.J. Alvarez, A.J. Todd, and A. Triller have been particularly illuminating.[57,58,61–63] Related studies of retinal synapses have provided similar findings.[64] Cumulatively, the studies of motoneurons and Renshaw cells indicate that

1. Immunoreactivity for glycine receptors and certain $GABA_A$ receptors is colocalized with gephyrin at synaptic specializations in the spinal cord.
2. Virtually all (90 to 98%) of the gephyrin-immunoreactive postsynaptic sites are associated with glycine-enriched presynaptic terminals; a significant minority (around 30 to 35%) of the terminals also contain GABA (this proportion is much higher on Renshaw cells); very few (around 2%) of the presynaptic boutons contain only GABA.
3. Glycine receptors and $GABA_A$ receptors are colocalized in at least two thirds of the gephyrin-labeled synapses; of the remainder, the majority have glycine receptors exclusively, and only 2 to 3% have GABA receptors exclusively.
4. There are many synapses on motoneurons and Renshaw cells at which both glycine and GABA are enriched presynaptically, and at which both glycine and $GABA_A$ receptors (and gephyrin) are present postsynaptically.

Although interpretation of these results is complicated (for example, they suggest the existence of some synapses at which $GABA_A$ receptors are present postsynaptically, but GABA is not in the apposed presynaptic bouton), the significance of mixed glycine–GABA synapses is emphasized by functional confirmation that corelease of GABA and glycine occurs at synapses of spinal neurons.[65]

2.2.2 C-Terminals

Another well-recognized class of bouton is the C-terminal,[32] although its defining feature, i.e., the presence of a sub-synaptic cistern adjacent to the postsynaptic membrane, can be obscured easily by histochemical or intracellular staining of the motoneuron (note that in recent publications these boutons, along with M-type boutons, may be referred to as a subtype of the large S-type of synapse). C-type boutons comprise less than 10% of the population of synapses, but because of their large size (typically > 4 μm in diameter; see Color Figure 2*), they contribute about 20% of the total synaptic coverage on the motoneuron somatic membrane. C-terminals are occasionally present on the proximal dendrites but are essentially absent from more distal locations; indeed the total number of large S-type boutons in contact with distal dendrites represents less than 5% of all distal synapses. C-terminals have been shown to be cholinergic in nature,[66,67] and postsynaptic muscarinic (m2) acetylcholine receptors appear to be present at these synapses.[68] Interestingly, activation of m2 receptors may decrease motoneuron excitability, and this receptor is present in alpha motoneurons but is absent or present only at low levels in gamma motoneurons.[69] Detailed ultrastructural studies of gamma motoneurons have shown that these neurons lack C-terminals entirely.[42,43,45] Light microscopic studies also suggest that C-terminals are unique to alpha motoneurons in the ventral horn. Studies in which cholinergic terminals are labeled by antibodies against the vesicular acetylcholine transporter (VAChT) reveal that although Renshaw cells receive powerful cholinergic input from motor axon recurrent collaterals and express a variety of cholinergic receptors, they do not receive any close appositions from boutons in the size range of C-terminals. Renshaw cell interneurons do, however, display numerous close appositions (up to about 400 to 500 contacts per Renshaw cell) from small- to medium-sized cholinergic boutons. Interestingly, these inputs are almost exclusively made on the dendrites of the Renshaw cells.[70]

Unfortunately, and despite their conspicuous appearance, the significance and origin of the large cholinergic C-terminals on motoneurons remain unknown. The C-terminals contain a range of nerve terminal proteins consistent with the mechanisms necessary for fast transmitter release, and by comparison of the complement of proteins present in cholinergic terminals in the Renshaw cell area, are unlikely to originate from motoneurons themselves.[71] Additional clues to their functional role may come from observations that gap junction proteins (connexins) are associated with the postsynaptic subsurface cisterns that characterize these synapses.[72]

2.2.3 S-Type Boutons

The remaining (approximately 20 to 30%) of somatic synapses are generally of the smaller S-type, and of variable size (0.5 to 3.0 μm in diameter). S-type bouton frequency remains about 30% on the proximal dendrites, and rises to more than 60% on the distal dendrites.[23,35] This type of bouton is usually associated with asymmetric synaptic junctions and is considered to be excitatory in nature. In keeping with this idea, all glutamate immunopositive boutons in one detailed study were

---

* Color figures follow page 142.

classified as S-type,[37] and the same study showed that more than a third of the boutons apposing motoneuron dendrites were glutamatergic. A rather small percentage (~6%) of S-type boutons do not appear labeled for glutamate (or GABA or glycine). Identified Ia afferent fiber terminals in contact with motoneurons have the ultrastructural characteristics of S-type boutons.[36,73]

2.2.3.1 Synapses Formed by Aminergic and Peptidergic Terminals on the Soma of Motoneurons

Immuno-electron microscopic studies of glycine-, GABA- and glutamate-containing terminals in the ventral horn suggest that almost all F- and S-type boutons, which together form the vast majority of somatic synapses, are associated with inhibitory or excitatory amino acid neurotransmitters;[37,53] however, motoneurons also receive innervation from aminergic, cholinergic, and peptidergic systems.[74] Indeed, the strong serotoninergic innervation of alpha motoneurons is in part conveyed by a prominent plexus of terminals that is closely wrapped around the cell body,[75] although the vast majority of the numerous appositions formed by 5-HT axons are distributed on the dendrites.[75] Ultrastructurally, 5-HT immunoreactive terminals that make contact with identified motoneuron dendrites contain spherical vesicles, and some dense core vesicles[75] (and would thus be classified as a form of S-type bouton). It, thus, may appear surprising that virtually all somatic S-type boutons can be accounted for by their content of amino acids; however, it is also possible that amines, acetylcholine, and neuropeptides are colocalized with amino acid neurotransmitters such as glutamate.[37] It is also known that a proportion of serotoninergic terminals, perhaps up to 30% in the cat ventral horn, do not form conventional synaptic junctions or are separated from the postsynaptic membrane by thin glial sheaths.[75,76] However, quantitative ultrastructural studies do not reveal a significant number of non-synaptic terminals in close apposition to the motoneuron soma.

2.2.4 Summary

A range of studies using quantitative approaches, including immunohistochemistry, have provided quite consistent data on the packing density and relative frequency of different bouton types over the motoneuron surface. At the soma and proximal dendrites, F-type (GABA/glycine) boutons outnumber S-type (glutamatergic/aminergic/cholinergic) boutons by a factor of about 3:1, whereas on more distal dendrites, where there is also a lower packing density, the S-type boutons generally outnumber the F-type. Importantly, different populations of motoneurons likely exhibit variations on this theme, reflecting the different sources of inputs to these populations. For example, phrenic motoneurons display approximately equal proportions of S- and F-boutons on their cell bodies and dendrites. A consensus value of about 50,000 synapses per motoneuron has emerged from these studies, and this value can now serve as a useful gauge with which to interpret the relative weight of afferent inputs for which the number of synapses can be determined by selective labeling with intracellular tracers or immunohistochemistry (see below).

2.3 DIVERSITY OF SYNAPTIC TERMINAL STRUCTURE: FUNCTIONAL IMPLICATIONS

At central synapses, structural features such as the size of the synaptic cleft (and the kinetics of transmitter clearance), the number, density, and spatial organization (and sensitivity and kinetics) of postsynaptic receptor/ion channels, and the number and size of transmitter release sites per presynaptic bouton (which likely relates to vesicle release probability) contribute critically to the nature of the postsynaptic conductance change elicited at the synapse.[29] The presence of multiple synaptic specializations at central synapses is common in a variety of CNS regions, and it is likely that these multiple active zones correspond to independent transmitter release sites in each bouton.[29,77] At synapses on motoneurons, most attention has been directed to determining the number and size of synaptic specializations (active zones) established by single presynaptic boutons, and to defining the incidence of P-type bouton contacts upon direct inputs to the motoneurons. These parameters can only be accurately assessed by serial electron microscopy and 3-dimensional reconstruction of individual boutons (but see below).

Within each bouton category there is considerable variability in terms of bouton size and synaptic configuration. The observed ultrastructural synaptic diversity is not simply due to sampling of boutons from different input sources because differences are apparent between synapses arising from a single, functionally identified and intracellularly labeled, presynaptic fiber and are observed even between adjacent boutons of a single preterminal axonal branch.[36,73,78–81] The excitatory S-type boutons formed by Ia afferent fibers on the soma and dendrites of alpha motoneurons provide clear examples of variability in terms of bouton size (volume), number/area of active zones, and incidence of presynaptic contacts.[36,73,81] Further specialization of bouton/synapse structure emerges when Ia boutons in other laminae of the spinal cord or at other segmental levels are analyzed, particularly the giant boutons in Clarke's column,[77–80,82] providing further indication that the characteristics of synaptic connections are very dependent on the nature of the postsynaptic target.

Differential presynaptic control of transmitter release from afferent fiber boutons is also likely based on observations that the frequency and positioning of P-type boutons vary across different parts of the same preterminal arborization, between different arborizations formed in different target regions by a single afferent, and between Ia and Ib afferents.[36,79,80,83]

In the specific case of synapses revealed by postsynaptic gephyrin immunofluorescence, the number and size of active zones in a presynaptic terminal can be revealed with light microscopic techniques because of the extremely close match between active zone and apposed postsynaptic receptor cluster configurations (determined by electron microscopy).[48] Analysis of gephyrin clusters has demonstrated that sequential *en passent* boutons arising from the axons of Ia inhibitory interneurons (which mediate reciprocal inhibition and form F-type glycinergic contacts[44,48]) vary considerably from each other in terms of active zone number and area.[48]

2.3.1 Relationships between Ultrastructural Features at Central Synapses

Quantitative ultrastructural studies not only reveal the enormous diversity referred to above, but have revealed striking correlations between many of the measurable parameters, particularly for factors that likely underlie the functional strength or efficacy of the synapse.

At excitatory Ia afferent synapses in lamina IX, elegant studies revealed strong (positive) correlation between the volume (size) of the bouton and the number of vesicles, active zone area, and number of active zones of each bouton.[81,84] The scaling of these factors with bouton volume might represent an ultrastructural size principle that may be a general feature of diverse types of synaptic contacts.[84] The functional implications of scaling and structural variability between synapses are underscored by mounting evidence, from combined electrophysiological and immunohistochemical staining studies, that larger postsynaptic currents are associated with larger postsynaptic receptor clusters.[85,86] These results thus broaden support for the notion that large boutons are likely to generate stronger postsynaptic effects than those produced at small synapses.[29,48,81,84,87]

The functional implications of variability, or scaling, of synaptic size (or other relevant parameter) have to take into account the extensive branching nature of the postsynaptic dendrites upon which the synapses are located. Spinal motoneurons particularly illustrate this problem because they have dendrites that can extend 1000 to 1500 μm from the cell body, and all regions of the dendritic surface membrane, including the most distal, can receive synaptic inputs. Thus, as demonstrated repeatedly, the electrical signals elicited at distal synapses will be subject to attenuation and filtering as they move toward the cell body. Yet, electrophysiological studies of Ia inputs to motoneurons,[88] and more recently of synapses in hippocampal pyramidal neurons,[89] indicate that distal synapses contribute signals that on average are as powerful, when they reach the cell body, as those that are generated nearby on the proximal dendrites. Several possible mechanisms could account for the boosting of distal synaptic inputs, including, for example, activation of voltage-gated ion channels in the dendrites or soma, or alterations in postsynaptic receptor density or number at distal vs. proximal synapses. Although voltage-gated ion channels are indeed present in dendrites (see below), recent studies suggest that these active conductances are more concerned with modulation of temporal and kinetic properties of synaptic responses than with amplification of their amplitude,[90,91] at least in pyramidal cells of the hippocampus. On the other hand, Magee and Cook[89] have presented evidence of a progressive increase with distance of the synaptic conductance produced by excitatory inputs to the apical dendrites of CA1 pyramidal neurons (up to about 325 μm from the soma) that could well be due to an increase in the number of postsynaptic receptors at the more distal sites (it is not yet known whether the same trend continues out to the ends of the apical dendrites). This finding is consistent with the explanation previously proposed to account for the observed amplitudes of excitatory postsynaptic potentials generated at distally located Ia afferent synapses on motoneurons.[92] Although other mechanisms, including the influence of local membrane passive properties and dendrite diameter, may still have a role in shaping synaptic potentials, recent immunohistochemical evidence on receptor expression supports the idea that postsynaptic receptor cluster size is scaled according to location within the dendritic tree, and could indeed help to compensate for the electrotonic attenuation imposed by cell geometry and membrane properties.[29,48]

However, it is important to note that the scaling of cluster size represents the *average* measurements of populations distributed over the dendrites; individual synapses at comparable distances actually exhibit considerable variability. Such site to site variability could account for the variability in electrophysiological measurements of postsynaptic potentials or currents at different synapses.

2.4 PASSIVE AND ACTIVE PROPERTIES OF DENDRITES

The importance of dendritic structure in influencing synaptic responses was emphasized by the seminal work of Wilfrid Rall, who used cable theory and mathematical modelling approaches to change our view of the passive and active properties, and thus the role, of branching dendrites.[93] Although the passive membrane properties of dendrites are complex, knowledge of the electrotonic (passive) structure of a neuron, in conjunction with the cell's detailed morphology, remains a prerequisite for understanding the spread of electrical signals within the cell and for developing models of dendritic neurons.[93–101] Many of the assumptions and limitations relating to understanding the specific membrane properties are discussed elsewhere.[1,94] Evidence from both alpha and gamma motoneurons suggests that these cells exhibit spatially nonuniform R_m, which may affect membrane responses to voltage perturbations.[97] Several factors may contribute to nonuniformity including cell membrane damage during recording different levels of synaptic activity on the dendrites and soma, and activity of voltage-gated ion channels. Recent studies suggest, for example, that voltage-dependent potassium channels may contribute to the somatic shunt in neck motoneurons.[102] On the other hand, the use of two-electrode whole cell recording of motoneuron properties in *in vitro* slices of rat spinal cord, in conjunction with reconstruction of the dendritic structure of the recorded cell, indicate that membrane resistivity may be fairly uniform; however, in this study the value for membrane capacitance was about twice that which is commonly assumed for neuronal membranes.[103] Nevertheless, if there is nonuniformity of physiological origin, it is clear that even in the passive case, any such nonuniformity of membrane conductances will have major implications for the input–output functions of neurons.[97,100,102–108]

It is also important to note that the electrotonic (passive) structure of neurons is quite dynamic and that the profile of the membrane properties can be reconfigured by synaptic activity.[109,110] For example, using geometrically realistic models of spinal motoneurons, it has been suggested that under conditions mimicking intense synaptic bombardment (i.e., low R_m values) the efficiency of transferring current to the soma is reduced markedly, with the result that the distal dendrites become functionally disconnected from the soma.[110] Dynamic physical changes in dendritic tree size are also observed in the context of dendritic expansion during development and changes following axotomy. The latter procedure produces conflicting results ranging from dendritic tree expansion,[112] to shrinkage,[111,113] possibly reflecting experimental and analytical differences in the respective studies.

2.4.1 VOLTAGE-DEPENDENT CHANNELS IN DENDRITES

Recent work has confirmed earlier indications that the dendrites of central neurons express a variety of voltage- and calcium-dependent membrane conductances that are superimposed on the linear passive properties of the dendrites. These conductances may also act to shape the spread of electrical signals in dendrites.[28,90,114,115] Backpropagating action potentials in dendrites, first described years ago in axotomized motoneurons undergoing chromatolysis,[116,117] have been shown to affect integration of synaptic inputs; conversely, spike backpropagation can be strongly modulated by the presence of inhibitory synaptic potentials.[118] Importantly, when appropriately timed, backpropagating action potentials can produce long-term modifications of synaptic strength, including "Hebbian-like" plasticity.[107,119] Unfortunately, there is little information about dendritic action potentials in intact motoneurons[120] although dendrites of presumed motoneurons in culture appear to support action potentials and calcium conductances.[121]

Although there is considerable information about the repertoire of voltage-dependent ionic conductances expressed by motoneurons, and the roles of the various currents in determining motoneuron firing characteristics[28,74,102,122–125] (see also, Chapter 4 by Heckman and Lee, this volume), detailed study of the distribution and density of voltage-gated ion channels in dendrites is in its infancy and has so far focused mainly on patch clamp recordings of currents in the apical dendrites of hippocampal and neocortical pyramidal neurons which can be visualized *in vitro*.[90,114,126,129] In these types of pyramidal cells, some striking results have been obtained recently regarding the distribution of K^+ currents that act to shape action potentials and modulate action potential propagation in dendrites. Using various configurations of the patch clamp recording technique, it has been shown that the density of voltage-gated K^+ channels underlying A-type K^+ currents increases with distance from the soma in CA1 pyramidal cells.[90] There is a similar, but much less steep, current density gradient in large layer-5 neocortical pyramidal neurons;[126] indeed, in a related study, a slight decrease in total K^+ current density was observed at increasing distances.[127] In both cell types, delayed rectifier-type potassium channel density appears to be relatively uniform, or may even decrease in the distal dendrites. The differences[128] that have emerged in these initial elegant studies caution against generalizing results from one cell type to another, and point to the multitude of potential functional roles that any channel may subserve. These results also point to the need for systematic analysis of a range of different functional classes of cells, including motoneurons. The use of specific antibodies against channel subunits to determine subcellular distribution of channels will be a valuable adjunct to the electrophysiological analyses.

In summary, passive and voltage-dependent conductances appear to be nonuniformly distributed over the cell surface, and there is evidence of systematic gradients in channel density, at least for some voltage-dependent potassium channels. However, there is little information concerning such channels in mammalian motoneurons *in situ*.

2.5 DISTRIBUTION OF SYNAPTIC INPUTS

Specific types of synaptic input to motoneurons have been identified anatomically by their neurochemical profile (as defined by transmitter or receptor immunohistochemistry) and/or by intracellular or anterograde staining of defined presynaptic input systems.

2.5.1 Ia AFFERENT FIBERS

The most intensively studied input to alpha motoneurons is that generated by muscle spindle primary (Ia) afferent fibers. Intra-axonal staining with horseradish peroxidase of physiologically identified hindlimb, neck, and tail muscle Ia afferents revealed unprecedented details of the morphology of the intraspinal collaterals of these fibers and their terminations in the intermediate region and ventral horn and other regions of the spinal cord including Clarke's column.[12,130–136] Terminal branches in lamina IX intersect with and form excitatory contacts with the dendrites of alpha motoneurons.[12,30,131,132,137] Electrophysiological and immunohistochemical data suggest that Ia afferents form glutamatergic synapses in the spinal cord, most probably acting at non-NMDA type glutamate receptors.[138–142] Ia afferent synapses are formed by *en passent* or terminal S-type boutons, and these boutons are frequently postsynaptic to P-type boutons,[36,73] some of which are enriched with GABA immunoreactivity.[142]

The synapses formed by Ia afferents on alpha motoneurons are widespread over the dendritic surface, with few (less than 5% of the total) in contact with the soma.[12,131,132,137] Electrophysiological analyses also indicate that Ia afferents make synaptic connections over a wide range of electrotonic locations.[94,143,144] Elegant studies in which both the electrophysiological and anatomical characteristics of connections between a single Ia fiber and a motoneuron were obtained revealed a good match between the time course of the postsynaptic potential and the anatomical location of the input synapses; these studies also revealed a good match between the quantal components of the EPSP and the observed number of boutons in the connection.[137] However, interpretation of these observations is subject to uncertainty because of assumptions made in the electrophysiological analyses and also in light of the variability of synaptic structure and number of release sites per bouton.[29,77]

The collaterals of each Ia afferent fiber can supply multiple contacts to each target motoneuron (with a range of 1 to 35 and an average of about 10 contacts from each afferent fiber).[132] The total number of Ia afferent boutons on a cat lumbosacral motoneuron is probably in the range of 1000 to 2000 (95% of which are on the dendrites), based on the number of muscle spindle afferents in a particular muscle, their connectivity with homonymous and heteronymous motoneurons, and the number of contacts per Ia/motoneuron pair.

2.5.1.2 Distribution of Glutamate Receptors

As reviewed elsewhere,[74] motoneurons express a variety of ionotropic and metabotropic glutamate receptors, some which are presumably associated with Ia afferent synapses. Among the AMPA type receptor subunits, relatively high levels of GluR2/3 and GluR4 are evident, along with low levels of GluR1.[145] Expression of these subunits is differentially affected by motoneuron axotomy and/or deafferentation (see Chapter 12). The subcellular localization of specific GluR subunits is not yet definitively established. Likewise, motoneurons express high levels of certain metabotropic glutamate receptors such as mGluR1a, and low levels of others (i.e., mGluR5);[146] again, mGluR expression is selectively reduced after axotomy.[147] Ultrastructurally, mGluR immunoreactivity is mainly extrasynaptic although it is found concentrated in some perisomatic regions.[146]

2.5.2 CORTICOSPINAL AXONS

Combined intraaxonal and intracellular staining to visualize identified corticomotoneuronal axons and motoneurons in the primate cervical spinal cord indicated that each axon establishes very few direct contacts on each target neuron, and that the contacts that are formed are primarily on mid-order dendrites (40 to 750 μm from the soma).[148] The paucity of contacts appears to be consistent with the small amplitude EPSPs generated in forelimb and hand motoneurons by impulses in single corticospinal axons.

2.5.3 VESTIBULOSPINAL AXONS

Vestibulospinal axons make direct connections with neck motoneurons, as revealed by anterograde transport of the tracer PHA-L.[149] These connections appear to be primarily on dendrites of selected orientation, namely, those oriented rostrocaudally rather than on those oriented dorsomedially or dorsolaterally. The number of contacts from vestibulospinal axons may be relatively small, but until the number of contributing axons is established, the relative strength of this input remains uncertain.

2.5.4 INHIBITORY INPUTS FROM RENSHAW CELLS AND Ia INHIBITORY INTERNEURONS

Based on the effects of intrasomatic current injection on recurrent and reciprocal IPSPs in motoneurons, it was suggested that synapses from Ia inhibitory interneurons (mediating reciprocal inhibition) were located on or near the soma and that synapses from Renshaw cells (mediating recurrent inhibition) were located somewhat more distally.[150] This conclusion has been amply substantiated and elaborated by subsequent anatomical and electrophysiological analyses, in particular by the direct confirmation of the predominantly dendritic location of Renshaw cell synapses.[44] Each Renshaw cell makes an average of about 3 synaptic contacts (range 1 to 9) on each motoneuron, at locations ranging from about 50 to 700 μm from the soma. The relatively few contacts from each Renshaw cell axon are consistent with the small amplitude IPSPs generated by activation of a single Renshaw cell.[151] IPSPs generated by Ia inhibitory interneurons appear to be located juxtasomatically,[152] as supported by direct anatomical observations on the axon collaterals of these interneurons (R.E.W. Fyffe, unpublished results).

The dendritic distribution of Renshaw cell synapses was further supported by electrophysiological analysis of the impedance changes generated when recurrent inhibitory synapses were activated (T.M. Hamm et al., personal communication). Indeed, both anatomical[44] and electrophysiological (T.M. Hamm, personal communication) studies arrived at remarkably similar predictions of the electrotonic (and physical) location of these synapses. Further, recurrent inhibition within a motoneuron pool is topographically constrained, with the strongest inhibitory inputs coming from Renshaw cells located near to the target motoneuron.[153] This finding is consistent with the overall distribution of motor axon recurrent collaterals (which provide excitatory input to the Renshaw cells) and the axonal trajectory and distribution of boutons from the Renshaw cells.

Both Renshaw cell and Ia inhibitory interneuron axons form F-type boutons,[154,155] at least some of which are enriched for glycine immunoreactivity[155] and associated with postsynaptic gephyrin clusters.[48] However, given the new insights regarding colocalization of GABA and glycine (see above), the nature of the transmitter(s) released by these interneurons remains unresolved.[139,156]

2.5.4.1 Distribution of Receptors for GABA and Glycine

As discussed in 2.2.1.1, the molecular constituents of glycine and $GABA_A$ receptors have been investigated using receptor subunit specific antibodies and antibodies against receptor-associated clustering/stabilizing proteins such as gephyrin. Spinal motoneurons express glycine and GABA receptors throughout development and maturation; however, changes in receptor subunit composition can impart differing functional properties to the receptor/channel, and as the postsynaptic effect of $GABA_A$ or glycine receptor activation is dependent on intracellular chloride concentration (which is differentially regulated during development), these transmitters have depolarizing, rather than hyperpolarizing, effects on most neonatal neurons.

Receptors for both amino acids are localized in somatic and dendritic membrane, including distal dendritic locations. *In vivo*, glycine receptor labeling in early postnatal as well as adult motoneurons is specifically associated with synaptic sites; however, in embryonic neurons some receptors may be present in extrasynaptic membrane.[56,157] It is clear that the distribution and clustering of glycine receptors vary dependent on cell type, and that within a single cell the size of the clusters may vary over an order of magnitude.[48] In most cell types, the size of postsynaptic glycine receptor clusters increases with distance from the soma (see above), although on the most distal dendrites, the dimensions of the dendrite itself limit the size of the clusters that can be established.

Postsynaptic $GABA_A$ receptors are complicated by virtue of the heterogeneity of receptor subunits that make up the functional receptor/channel. Motoneurons appear to express α_5, $\beta_{2/3}$, and γ_2 subunits at relatively high levels (but no α_1 subunits; α_2, and α_3, subunits appear to be cytoplasmically localized and difficult to interpret; F.J. Alvarez et al., personal communication). $GABA_A$ subunits associated with gephyrin are predominantly localized in postsynaptic patches, generally apposed to glycinergic or mixed GABA/glycine terminals. However, motoneurons also exhibit significant extrasynaptic membrane labeling, extending out into the dendrites.[47]

2.5.5 SEROTONINERGIC INPUTS

Combined immunohistochemistry and intracellular staining of motoneurons indicate that alpha motoneurons receive numerous direct contacts from descending serotoninergic axons.[75,158] The serotoninergic input is widely distributed over the entire dendritic tree, at an overall density of about one contact per 100 μm^2 of surface membrane; the 5-HT appositions are distributed more or less uniformly with distance from the soma, ranging out to the most distal dendrites at distances greater than 1000 μm.[75] The total number of 5-HT appositions on alpha motoneurons may be as high as 2000 or more and the vast majority are on the dendrites (there is an average of 52 somatic appositions per motoneuron). Interestingly, a similar packing density (just under 1 per 100 μm^2 of surface membrane) is reported for 5-HT appositions on the dendrites of gamma motoneurons, in which the density of somatic contacts is slightly higher than for the dendritic contacts and considerably higher than for alpha motoneurons.[159] Not all 5-HT appositions detected with these staining techniques actually form synaptic specializations, and where synapses are indeed formed, the specializations were small with indistinct postsynaptic densities. Overall, only about one third of the appositions in one study conclusively formed conventional synaptic junctions, and in a number (approximately 15%) of appositions predicted by light microscopic criteria, the presynaptic 5-HT bouton was separated from the motoneuron dendrite membrane by thin glial protrusions.[75] A related study[159] of noradrenergic innervation of gamma motoneurons suggests a lower density of noradrenergic inputs compared to the 5-HT input, but this has not yet been systematically studied in alpha motoneurons.

2.5.5.1 Distribution of 5-HT Receptors

Motoneurons express high levels of the 5-HT$_3$ receptor subtype (uniquely among 5-HT receptors, this subtype acts as a ligand-gated ion channel and generally enhances motoneuron excitability), with membranous localization extending over the somatic and proximal dendritic surface.[160] Interestingly, 5-HT$_{1A}$ receptors (member of the G-protein coupled receptor superfamily) appear to be localized primarily at the axon hillock in primate motoneurons.[161] Other members of the family (e.g., 5-HT$_{1B}$, 5-HT$_{2C}$, and 5-HT$_{2A}$) are present, like 5-HT$_3$ receptors, in somatodendritic regions.[162] Given the important role of 5-HT in controlling motoneuron firing, and the enormous diversity of 5-HT receptor subunits, much additional immunolocalization information is still required.

2.5.6 ARE SYNAPTIC INPUTS COMPARTMENTALIZED?

The functional significance of the diffuse and widespread distribution of motoneuron dendrites has been debated for many years, particularly with respect to the possible targeting of specific inputs to selected regions of the dendritic tree, for example, to dendrites of different orientation, or to proximal vs. distal locations. It should be noted that not all motoneurons display the same form when their 3-dimensional structure is considered. Hindlimb alpha motoneurons have marked radial symmetry, although zones dorsal and ventral to the soma display fewer dendritic profiles than expected.[7] Gamma motoneurons are generally less radially symmetrical than alpha motoneurons and have less profuse branching patterns as well as less surface area.[21] Phrenic motoneurons[16-18] and dorsal neck motoneurons[9,10,163] have extensive and more polarized dendrites that project into distinct terminal fields, and the neck motoneurons in particular have prominent rostrocaudal dendrites. In sacral and thoracic segments where dendrites are strongly polarized, the dendrites of neighboring motoneurons may form bundles where groups of dendrites come in intimate contact with each other. The projection of dendrites into different terminal fields makes it possible for them to receive inputs from different sets of presynaptic sources depending on their spatial location in the cord.

With respect to lumbosacral motoneurons, Sprague speculated that the dorsally directed component of the dendritic tree primarily receives dorsal root fiber input whereas dendrites that are directed ventrally or laterally primarily receive propriospinal input.[164] Part of this speculation has been refined by detailed analysis of Ia-motoneuron connections by Burke and his colleagues who showed that dendrites oriented in the dorsolateral and ventromedial axes had relatively few (< 8%) of the total contacts whereas rostrocaudally oriented dendrites had more than 60% of the contacts (as noted above, less than 5% of Ia inputs are located on the motoneuron soma surface).[132] Overall, the terminals of Ia afferent collaterals occupy a 3-dimensional zone that is only partly congruent with the radially organized dendrites of the motoneurons. Within this region of afferent/dendrite overlap (including the dendrites that have predominantly rostrocaudal trajectories) contacts occur more or less randomly.[132]

Vestibulospinal inputs are also predicated on dendritic orientation, and preferentially contact the prominent rostrocaudal dendrites of dorsal neck motoneurons.[149] In this case, the connectivity appears to be very selective because the trajectory and terminal arborizations of individual vestibulospinal axons present them with opportunity to contact other parts of the dendritic tree.

In contrast to these selective patterns of connectivity, the spatial distribution of 5-HT contacts on alpha motoneurons does not appear to be determined by dendritic orientation or path length from the soma.[75] The serotoninergic fibers that innervate the lumbosacral ventral horn generate a dense plexus of 5-HT varicosities, so that the dendritic and presynaptic axonal arborizations are completely overlapping. In keeping with this degree of overlap, and although some segments of dendrite appeared to lack 5-HT inputs, the 5-HT inputs are distributed quite uniformly over the whole motoneuron surface, at a density of about one bouton per 100 μm^2 of surface membrane.

The inhibitory inputs from Renshaw cells and Ia inhibitory interneurons appear to be differentially distributed, with the former being predominantly on the dendrites and the latter contributing inputs to the soma and proximal dendrites. There is insufficient information to determine any orientation selectivity for Renshaw cell synapses on the dendrites. Finally, one type of cholinergic input, represented by the conspicuous C-terminals, is only found on the motoneuron soma or on the base of the primary dendrites.

A complex picture thus emerges even though the above results represent only a small fraction of the total synaptic input to motoneurons. In some cases (i.e., Ia, vestibulospinal) the inputs are widespread, but on a subset of dendrites. As a result of this selectivity, some dendrites do not "see" these synaptic actions directly. Other inputs (i.e., Ia inhibitory interneuron synapses, cholinergic C-terminals) are preferentially targeted to the soma and proximal dendrites, which may have strategic advantages as far as influencing the effects of more distant synapses. Fast inhibition is not restricted to juxtasomatic locations, because the inhibitory input from Renshaw cells displays a widespread dendritic distribution. Finally, 5-HT terminals are fairly uniformly distributed over the motoneuron surface. These arrangements provide opportunity for selective interactions between different inputs, perhaps to the extent of allowing each dendrite, or segment of dendrite, to integrate inputs independently of other dendrites. The widespread distribution of inhibitory and modulatory inputs emphasizes the importance of local dendritic interactions and control mechanisms.

ACKNOWLEDGMENT

Work from the author's laboratory is supported by the NIH (NS 25547).

REFERENCES

1. Burke, R.E., Spinal cord: ventral horn, in *The Synaptic Organization of the Brain*, G.M. Sheperd, Ed., Oxford University Press, 1998, 77.
2. Romanes, G.J., The motor cell columns of the lumbo-sacral spinal cord of the cat, *J. Comp. Neurol.*, 94, 313, 1951.
3. Nicolopoulos-Stournaras, S. and Iles, J.F., Motor neuron columns in the lumbar spinal cord of the rat, *J. Comp. Neurol.*, 217, 75, 1983.
4. Burke, R.E., Strick, P.L., Kanda, K., Kim, C.C., and Walmsley, B., Anatomy of medial gastrocnemius and soleus motor nuclei in cat spinal cord, *J. Neurophysiol.*, 40, 667, 1977.
5. Fetcho, J.R., A review of the organization and evolution of motoneurons innervating the axial musculative of vertebrates, *Brain Res. Rev.*, 12, 243, 1987.
6. Vanderhorst, V.G. and Hostege, G., Organization of lumbosacral motoneuronal cell groups innervating hindlimb, pelvic floot, and axial muscles in the cat, *J. Comp. Neurol.*, 382, 46, 1997.
7. Cullheim, S., Fleshman, J.W., Glenn, L.L., and Burke, R.E., Three-dimensional architecture of dendritic trees in type-identified α-motoneurons, *J. Comp. Neurol.*, 255, 82, 1987.
8. Cullheim, S., Fleshman, J.W., Glenn, L.L., and Burke, R.E., Membrane area and dendritic structure in type-identified triceps surae alpha motoneurons, *J. Comp. Neurol.*, 255, 68, 1987.
9. Rose, P.K., Distribution of dendrites from biventer cervicis and complexus motoneurons stained intracellularly with horseradish peroxidase in the adult cat, *J. Comp. Neurol.*, 197, 395, 1981.
10. Rose, P.K., Branching structure of motoneuron stem dendrites: a study of neck muscle motoneurons intracellularly stained with horseradish peroxidase in the cat, *J. Neuroscience*, 2, 1596, 1982.

11. Rose, P.K., Keirstead, S.A., and Vanner, S.J., A quantitative analysis of the geometry of cat motoneurons innervating neck and shoulder muscles, *J. Comp. Neurol.*, 239, 89, 1985.

12. Brown, A.G. and Fyffe, R.E.W., Direct observations on the contacts made between Ia afferent fibers and α-motoneurones in the cat's lumbosacral spinal cord, *J. Physiol.*, 313, 121, 1981.

13. Ulfhake, B. and Kellerth J.-O, Electrophysiological and morphological measurements in cat gastrocnemius and soleus α-motoneurones, *Brain Res.*, 307, 167, 1984.

14. Ulfhake, B. and Kellerth, J.-O., A quantitative light microscopic study of the dendrites of cat spinal α-motoneurons after intracellular staining with horseradish peroxidase, *J. Comp. Neurol.*, 202, 571, 1981.

15. Ulfhake, B. and Kellerth, J.-O., A quantitative morphological study of HRP-labelled cat α-motoneurones supplying different hindlimb muscles, *Brain Res.*, 264, 1, 1983.

16. Cameron, W.E., Averill, D.B., and Berger, A.J., (1985) Quantitative analysis of the dendrites of cat phrenic motoneurons stained intracellularly with horseradish peroxidase, *J. Comp. Neurol.*, 230, 91, 1985.

17. Lipski, J., Fyffe, R.E.W., and Jodkowski, J., Recurrent inhibition of phrenic motoneurons, *J. Neurosci.*, 5, 1545, 1985.

18. Lipski, J. and Martin-Body, R.L., Morphological properties of respiratory intercostal motoneurons in cats as revealed by intracellular injection of horseradish peroxidase, *J. Comp. Neurol.*, 260, 423, 1987.

19. Chen, X.Y. and Wolpaw, J., Triceps surae motoneuron morphology in the rat: a quantitative light microscopic study, *J. Comp. Neurol.*, 343, 143, 1994.

20. Lindsay, A.D., Greer, J.J., and Feldman, J.L., Phrenic motoneuron morphology in the neonatal rat, *J. Comp. Neurol.*, 308, 169, 1991.

21. Moschovakis, A.K., Burke, R.E., and Fyffe, R.E.W., The size and dendritic structure of HRP-labeled gamma motoneurons in the cat spinal cord, *J. Comp. Neurol.*, 311, 531, 1991.

22. Burke, R.E., Dum, R.P., Fleshman, J.W., Glenn, L.L., Lev-Tov, A., O'Donovan, M.J., and Pinter, M.J., An HRP study of the relation between cell size and motor unit type in cat ankle extensor motoneurons, *J. Comp. Neurol.*, 209, 17, 1982.

23. Brännström, T., Quantitative synaptology of functionally different types of cat medial gastrocnemius α-motoneurons, *J. Comp. Neurol.*, 330, 439, 1993.

24. Colbert, C.M. and Johnston, D., Axonal action-potential initiation and Na+ channel densities in the soma and axon initial segment of subicular pyramidal neurons, *J. Neurosci.*, 16, 6676, 1996.

25. Stuart, G., Schiller, J., and Sakmann, B., Action potential initiation and propagation in rat neocortical pyramidal neurons, *J. Physiol.*, 505, 617, 1997.

26. Martina, M., Vida, I., and Jonas, P., Distal initiation and active propagation of action potentials in interneuron dendrites, *Science*, 287, 295, 2000.

27. Coombs, J.S., Curtis, D.R., and Eccles, J.D., The generation of impulses in motoneurones, *J. Physiol.*, 139, 232, 1957.

28. Binder, M.D., Heckman, C.J., and Powers, R.K., The physiological control of motoneuron activity in *Handbook of Physiology, Exercise: Regulation and Integration of Multiple Systems*, Rowell, L.B. and Shepherd J.T., Eds., American Physiological Soc., New York, 1996, 3.

29. Walmsley, B., Alvarez, F.J., and Fyffe, R.E.W., Diversity of structure and function at mammalian central synapses, *TINS.*, 21, 81, 1998.

30. Segev, I., Fleshman, J.W. Jr., and Burke, R.E., Computer simulation of Group Ia EPSPs using morphologically realistic models of cat α-motoneurons, *J. Neurophysiol.*, 64, 648, 1990.

31. Segev, I. and Burke, R.E., Compartmental models of complex neurons, in *Methods in Neuronal Modeling*, Koch, D. and Segev, I., Eds., MIT Press, Cambridge, Massachusetts, 1998, 93.

32. Conradi, S., Ultrastructure and distribution of neuronal and glial elements on the motoneuron surface in the lumbosacral spinal cord of the adult cat, *Acta. Physiol. Scand. Suppl.*, 332, 5, 1996.

33. Conradi, S., Kellerth, J.-O., and Berthold, C.-H., Electron microscopic studies of serially sectioned cat spinal α-motoneurons. II. A method for the description of architecture and synaptology of the cell body and proximal dendritic segments, *J. Comp. Neurol.*, 184, 741, 1979.

34. Conradi, S., Kellerth, J.-O., Berthold, C.-H., and Hammarberg, C., Electron microscopic studies of serially sectioned cat spinal α-motoneurons. IV. Motoneurons innervating slow-twitch (type S) units of the soleus muscle, *J. Comp. Neurol.*, 184, 769, 1979.

35. Rose, P.K. and Neuber-Hess, M., Morphology and frequency of axon terminals on the somata, proximal dendrites and distal dendrites of dorsal neck motoneurons in the cat, *J. Comp. Neurol.*, 307, 259, 1991.

36. Fyffe, R.E.W. and Light, A.R., The ultrastructure of group Ia afferent fiber synapses in the lumbosacral spinal cord of the cat, *Brain Res.*, 300, 201, 1984.

37. Örnung, G., Ottersen, O.P., Cullheim, S., and Ulfhake, B., Distribution of glutamate-, glycine- and GABA-immunoreactive nerve terminals on dendrites in the cat spinal motor nucleus, *Exp. Brain Res.*, 118, 517, 1998.

38. Kellerth, J.-O., Berthold, C.-H., and Conradi, S., Electron microscopic studies of serially sectioned cat spinal α-motoneurons. III. Motoneurons innervating fast-twitch (type FR) units of the gastrocnemius muscle, *J. Comp. Neurol.*, 184, 755, 1979.

39. Destombes, J., Horcholle-Bossavit, G., and Thiesson, D., Distribution of glycinergic terminals on lumbar motoneurons of the adult cat: an ultrastructural study, *Brain Res.*, 599, 353, 1992.

40. Destombes, J., Horcholle-Bossavit, G., Thiesson, D., and Jami, L., Alpha and gamma motoneurons in the peroneal nuclei of the cat spinal cord: an ultrastructural study, *J. Comp. Neurol.*, 317, 79, 1992.

41. Starr, K.A. and Wolpaw, J.R., Synaptic terminal coverage of primate triceps surae motoneurons, *J. Comp. Neurol.*, 345, 345, 1994.

42. Lagerbäck, P-Å, An ultrastructural study of cat lumbosacral γ-motoneurons after retrograde labelling with horseradish peroxidase, *J. Comp. Neurol.*, 240, 256, 1983.

43. Lagerbäck, P-Å, Cullheim, S., and Ulfhake, B., Electron microscopic observations on the synaptology of cat sciatic γ-motoneurons after intracellular staining with horseradish peroxidase, *Neurosci. Lett.*, 70, 23, 1986.

44. Fyffe, R.E.W., Spatial distribution of recurrent inhibitory synapses on spinal motoneurons in the cat, *J. Neurophys.*, 65, 1134, 1991.

45. Johnson, I.P., A quantitative ultrastructural comparison of alpha and gamma motoneurons in the thoracic region of the spinal cord of the adult cat, *J. Anat.*, 147, 55, 1986.

46. Örnung, G., Shupliakov, O., Lindå, H., Ottersen, O.P., Storm-Mathisen, J., Ulfhake, B., and Cullheim, S., Qualitative and quantitative analysis of glycine- and GABA-immunoreactive nerve terminals on motoneuron cell bodies in the cat spinal cord: a postembedding electron microscopic study, *J. Comp. Neurol.*, 365, 413, 1996.

47. Alvarez, F.J., Taylor-Blake, B., Fyffe, R.E.W., De Blas, A.L., and Light, A.R., Distribution of immunoractivity for the β3 subunits of the GABA$_A$ receptor in the mammalian spinal cord, *J. Comp. Neurol.*, 365, 392, 1996.

48. Alvarez, F.J., Dewey, D.E., Harrington, D.A., and Fyffe, R.E.W., Cell-type specific organization of glycine receptor clusters in the mammalian spinal cord, *J. Comp. Neurol.*, 379, 150, 1997.

49. Shupliakov, O., Örnung, G., Brodin, L., Ulfhake, B., Ottersen, O.P., Storm-Mathisen, J., and Cullheim, S., Immunocytochemical localization of amino acid neurotransmitter candidates in the ventral horn of the cat spinal cord, *Exp. Brain Res.*, 96, 404, 1993.

50. Örnung, G., Shupliakov, O., Ottersen, O.P., Storm-Mathisen, J., and Cullheim, S., Immunohistochemical evidence for coexistence of glycine and GABA in nerve terminals on cat spinal motoneurones: an ultrastructural study, *NeuroReport*, 5, 889, 1994.

51. Holstege, J.C. and Calkoen, F., The distribution of GABA in lumbar motoneuronal cell groups. A quantitative ultrastructural study in rat, *Brain Res.*, 530, 130, 1990.

52. Harrington, D.A., Alvarez, F.J., and Fyffe, R.E.W., Somatic membrane covering by glycinergic terminals and glycine receptors of α-motoneurons and Renshaw cells in cat spinal cord, *Soc. Neurosci. Abst.*, 20, 1588, 1994.

53. Murphy, S.M., Pilowsky, P.M., and Llewellyn-Smith, I.J., Vesicle shape and amino acids in synaptic inputs to phrenic motoneurons: Do all inputs contain either glutamate or GABA?, *J. Comp. Neurol.*, 373, 200, 1996.

54. Kirsch, J. and Betz, H., Glycine receptor activation is required for receptor clustering in spinal neurons, *Nature*, 392, 717, 1998.

55. Betz, H., Gephyrin, a major player in GABAergic postsynaptic membrane assembly? *Nature Neurosci.*, 7, 541, 1998.

56. Geiman, E.J., Knox, M.C., and Alvarez, F.J., Postnatal maturation of gephyrin/glycine receptor clusters on developing Renshaw cells, *J. Comp. Neurol.*, 426, 130, 2000.

57. Todd, A.J., Watt, C., Spike, R.C., and Sieghart, W., Colocalization of GABA, glycine, and their receptors at synapses in the rat spinal cord, *J. Neurosci.*, 16, 974, 1996.

58. Todd, A.J., Spike, R.C., Chong, D., and Neilson, M., The relationship between glycine and gephyrin in synapses of the rat spinal cord, *Eur. J. Neurosci.*, 7, 1, 1995.

59. Kneussel, M., Brandstä, J.H., Laube, B., Stahl, S., Muller, U., and Betz, H., Loss of postsynaptic GABA$_A$ receptor clustering in gephyrin-deficient mice, *J. Neurosci.*, 19, 9289, 1999.

60. Dumoulin, A., Levi, S., Riveau, B., Gasnier, B., and Triller, A., Formation of mixed glycine and GABAergic synapses in cultured spinal cord neurons, *Eur. J. Neurosci.*, 12, 3883, 2000.

61. Todd, A.J. and Sullivan, A.C., Light microscope study of the coexistance of GABA-like and glycine-like immunoreactivities in the spinal cord of the rat, *J. Comp. Neurol.*, 296, 496, 1990.

62. Zheng, W., Geiman, E.J., Fritschy, J-M, Pearson, J.C., and Alvarez, F.J., Quantitative analysis of GABA, glycine and their receptors in inhibitory synapses on spinal cord Renshaw cells, *Soc. Neurosci. Abst.*, 26, 692, 2000.

63. Triller, A., Cluzeaud, F., and Korn, H., Gamma-aminobutyric acid containing terminals can be apposed to glycine receptors at central synapses, *J. Cell. Biol.*, 104, 947, 1987.

64. Sassoe-Pognetto, M., Kirsch, J., Grunert, U., Greferath, U., Fritschy, J.M., Mohler, H., Betz, H., and Wassle, H., Colocalization of gephyrin and GABA$_A$-receptor subunits in the rat retina, *J. Comp. Neurol.*, 357, 1, 1995.

65. Jonas, P., Bischofberger, J., and Sandkuler, J., Corelease of two fast neurotransmitters at a central synapse, *Science,* 281, 419, 1998.
66. Nagy, J.I., Yamamoto, T., and Jordan, L.M., Evidence for the cholinergic nature of C-terminals associated with subsurface cisterns in α-motoneurons of rat, *Synapse,* 15, 17, 1993.
67. Li, W., Ochalski, P.A.Y., Brimijoin, S., Jordan, L.M., and Nagy, J.I., C-terminals on motoneurons: electron microscope localization of cholinergic markers in adult rats and antibody-induced depletion in neonates, *Neuroscience,* 65, 879, 1995.
68. Skinner, J.C., Alvarez, F.J., and Fyffe, R.E.W., C-terminals are associated with postsynaptic muscarinic (m2) acetylocholine receptors in α-motoneurons in the rat spinal cord, *Soc. Neurosci. Abst.,* 25, 1917, 1999.
69. Welton, J., Stewart, W., Kerr, R., and Maxwell, D.J., Differential expression of the muscarinic m2 acetylcholine receptor by small and large motoneurons of the rat spinal cord, *Brain Res.,* 817, 215, 1999.
70. Alvarez, F.J., Dewey, D.E., McMillin, P., and Fyffe, R.E.W., Distribution of cholinergic contacts on Renshaw cells in the rat spinal cord: a light microscopic study, *J. Physiol.,* 515, 787, 1999.
71. Hellström, J., Arvidsson, U., Elde, R., Cullheim, S., and Meister, B., Differential expression of nerve terminal protein isoforms in VAChT-containing varicosities of the spinal cord ventral horn, *J. Comp. Neurol.,* 411, 578, 1999.
72. Yamamoto, T., Hertzberg, E.L., and Nagy J.I., Subsurface cisterns in α-motoneurons of the rat and cat: immunohistochemical detection with antibodies against connexin32, *Synapse,* 8, 119, 1991.
73. Conradi, S., Cullheim, S., Gollvik, L., and Kellerth, J.-O., Electron microscopic observations on the synaptic contacts of group Ia muscle spindle afferents in the cat lumbosacral spinal cord, *Brain Res.,* 265, 31, 1983.
74. Rekling, J.C., Funk, G.D., Bayliss, D.A., Dong, X.-W., and Feldman, J.L., Synaptic control of motoneuronal excitability, *Physiol. Rev.,* 80, 767, 2000.
75. Alvarez, F.J., Pearson, J.C., Harrington, D., Dewey, D., Torbeck, L., and Fyffe, R.E.W., Distribution of 5-hydroxytryptamine-immunoreactive boutons on α-motoneurons in the lumbar spinal cord of adult cats, *J. Comp. Neurol.,* 393, 69, 1998.
76. Ulfhake, B., Arvidsson, U., Cullheim, S., Hokfelt, T., Brodin, E., Verhofstad, A.A.J., and Visser, T., An ultrastructural study of 5-hydroxytryptamine-, thyrotropin-releasing hormone- and substance P-immunoreactive axonal boutons in the motor nucleus of spinal cord segments L7-S1 in the adult cat, *Neuroscience,* 23, 917, 1987.
77. Walmsley, B., Central synaptic transmission: Studies at the connection between primary afferent fibers and dorsal spinocerebellar tract neurons in Clarke's column of the spinal cord, *Prog. Neurobiol.,* 36, 391, 1991.
78. Walmsley, B., Wieniawa-Narkiewicz, E., and Nicol, M.J., The ultrastructural basis for synaptic transmission between primary muscle afferents and neurons in Clarke's column of cat, *J. Neurosci.,* 5, 2095, 1985.
79. Walmsley, B., Wieniawa-Narkiewicz, E., and Nicol, M.J., Ultrastructural evidence related to presynaptic inhibition of primary muscle afferents in Clark's column of cat, *J. Neurosci.,* 7, 236, 1987.
80. Walmsley, B., Graham, B., and Nicol, M.J., Serial E-M and simulation study of presynaptic inhibition along a group 1a collateral in the spinal cord, *J. Neurophysiol.,* 74, 616, 1995.
81. Pierce, J.P. and Mendell, L.M., Quantitative ultrastructure of Ia boutons in the ventral horn: scaling and positional relationships, *J. Neurosci.,* 13, 4748, 1993.

82. Tracey, D.J. and Walmsley, B., Synaptic input from identified muscle afferents to neurones of the dorsal spinocerebellar tract in the cat, *J. Physiol.*, 350, 599, 1984.

83. Alvarez, F.J., Ultrastructural basis for presynaptic inhibition, in *Presynaptic Inhibition and Neural Control Mechanisms,* Rudomin, P., Romo, R., and Mendell, L., Eds., Oxford University Press, New York, 1998, 13.

84. Pierce, J.P. and Lewin, G.R., An ultrastructural size principle, *Neuroscience*, 58(3), 441, 1994.

85. Lim, R., Alvarez, F.J., and Walmsley, B., Quantal size is correlated with receptor cluster area at glycinergic synapses in the rat brainstem, *J. Physiol.*, 516(2), 505, 1999.

86. Oleskevich, S.O., Alvarez, F.J., and Walmsley, B., Glycinergic miniature synaptic currents and receptor cluster sizes differ in spinal cord interneurons, *J. Neurophys.*, 82, 312, 1999.

87. Schikorski, T. and Stevens, C.F., Quantitative ultrastructural analysis of hippocampal excitatory synapses, *J. Neurosci.*, 17(15), 5858, 1997.

88. Iansek, R. and Redman, S.J., The amplitude, time course and charge of unitary excitatory post-synaptic potentials evoked in spinal motoneurone dendrites, *J. Physiol.*, 234, 665, 1973.

89. Magee, J.C. and Cook, E.P., Somatic EPSP amplitude is independent of synapse location in hippocampal pyramidal neurons, *Nature Neurosci.*, 3, 895, 2000.

90. Hoffman, D.A., Magee, J.C., Colbert, C.M., and Johnston, D., K^+ channel regulation of signal propagation in dendrites of hippocampal payramidal neurons, *Nature*, 387, 869, 1997.

91. Magee, J.C., Dendritic I_h normalizes temporal summation in hippocampal CA1 neurons, *Nature Neurosci.*, 2, 508, 1999.

92. Redman, S. and Walmsley, B., The synaptic basis of the monosynaptic stretch reflex, *Trends Neurosci.*, 4, 248, 1981.

93. Segev, I., Rinzel, J., and Shepherd, G.M., *The Theoretical Foundations of Dendritic Function,* MIT Press, Cambridge Massachusetts, 1995.

94. Rall, W., Burke, R.E., Holmes, W.R., Jack, J.J.B., Redman, S.J., and Segev, I., Matching dendritic neuron models to experimental data, *Physiol. Rev.*, 72(4), S159, 1992.

95. Rall, W. and Agmon-Sir, H., Cable theory for dendritic neurons, in *Methods in Neuronal Modeling*, Koch, C. and Segev, I., Eds., MIT Press, Cambridge, Massachusetts, 1998, 27.

96. Spruston, N., Jaffe, D.B., and Johnston, D., Dendrite attenuation of synaptic potentials and currents: the role of passive membrane properties, *TINS*, 17, 161, 1994.

97. Burke, R.E., Fyffe, R.E.W., and Moschovakis, A.K., Electrotonic architecture of cat gamma motoneurons, *J. Neurophysiol.*, 72, 1, 1994.

98. Koch, C. and Segev, I., *Methods in Neuronal Modeling*, MIT Press, Cambridge, Massachusetts, 1998.

99. Zador, A.M., Agmon-Sir, H., and Segev, I., The morphoelectrotonic transform: a graphical approach to dendritic function, *J. Neurosci.*, 15, 1669, 1995.

100. London, M., Meunier, C., and Segev, I., Signal transfer in passive dendrites with nonuniform membrane conductance, *J. Neurosci.*, 19, 8219, 1999.

101. Chitwood, R.A., Hubbard, A., and Jaffe, D.B., Passive electrotonic properties of rat hippocampal CA3 interneurones, *J. Physiol.*, 515, 743, 1999.

102. Campbell, D.M. and Rose, P.K., Contribution of voltage-dependent potassium channels to the somatic shunt in neck motoneurons of the cat, *J. Neurophysiol.*, 77, 1470, 1997.

103. Thurbon, D., Lüscher, H.-R., Hofstetter, T., and Redman, S.J., Passive electrical properties of ventral horn neurons in rat spinal cord slices, *J. Neurophysiol.*, 79, 2485, 1998.

104. Clements, J.D. and Redman S.J., Cable properties of cat spinal motoneurones measured by combining voltage clamp, current clamp and intracellular staining, *J. Physiol.*, 409, 63, 1989.

105. Fleshman, J.W., Segev, I., and Burke, R.E., Electrotonic architecture of type-identified α-motoneurons in the cat spinal cord, *J. Neurophysiol.*, 60, 60, 1988.

106. Rose, P.K. and Dagum, A., Non-equivalent cylinder models of neurons — interpretation of voltage transients generated by somatic current injection, *J. Neurophysiol.*, 60, 125, 1988.

107. Magee, J.C. and Johnston, D., A synaptically controlled, associative signal for Hebbian plasticity in hippocampal neurons, *Science*, 275, 209, 1997.

108. Segev, I. and Rall, W., Excitable dendrites and spines: earlier theoretical insights elucidate recent direct observations, *TINS*, 21, 453, 1998.

109. Bernander, O., Douglas, R.J., Martin, K.A.C., and Koch, C., Synaptic background activity influences spatiotemporal integration in single pyramidal cells, *Proc. Natl. Acad. Sci.*, 88, 11569, 1991.

110. Korogod, S.M., Kulagina, I.B., Horcholle-Bossavit, G., Gogan, P., and Tyc-Dumont, S., Activity-dependent reconfiguration of the effective dendritic field of motoneurons, *J. Comp. Neurol.*, 422, 18, 2000.

111. Lindå, H., Cullheim, S., and Risling, M., A light and electron microscopic study of intracellularly HRP-labeled lumbar motoneurons after intramedullary axotomy in the adult cat, *J. Comp. Neurol.*, 318, 188, 1992.

112. Rose, P.K. and Odlozinski, M., Expansion of the dendritic tree of motoneurons innervating neck muscles of the adult cat after permanent axotomy, *J. Comp. Neurol.*, 390, 392, 1998.

113. Brännström, T., Havton, L., and Kellerth, J.-O., Changes in size and dendritic arborization patterns of adult cat spinal α-motoneurons following permanent axotomy, *J. Comp. Neurol.*, 318, 439, 1992.

114. Johnston, D., Magee, J.C., Colbert, C.M., and Christie, B.R., Active properties of neuronal dendrites, *Ann. Rev. Neurosci.*, 19, 165, 1996.

115. Stuart, G., Spruston, N., and Hausser, M., *Dendrites*, Oxford University Press, Oxford, 1999.

116. Eccles, J.C., Libet, B., and Young, R.R., The behaviour of chromatolysed motoneurones studied by intracellular recording, *J. Physiol.*, 143, 11, 1958.

117. Kuno, M., and Llinas, R., Enhancement of synaptic transmission by dendrite potentials in chromatolysed motoneurones of the cat, *J. Physiol.*, 210, 807, 1970.

118. Tsubokawa, H. and Ross, W.N., IPSPs modulate spike backpropagation and associated $[Ca^{2+}]_i$ changes in the dendrites of hippocampal CA1 pyramidal neurons, *J. Neurophysiol.*, 76, 2896, 1996.

119. Markram, H., Lubke, J., Frotscher, M., and Sakmann, B., Regulation of synaptic efficacy by coincidence of postsynaptic APs and EPSPs, *Science*, 275, 213, 1997.

120. Fujita, Y., Dendrite spikes in normal spinal motoneurons of cats, *Neurosci. Res.*, 6, 299, 1989.

121. Larkum, M.E., Rioult, M.G., and Luscher, H., Propagation of action potentials in the dendrites of neurons from rat spinal cord slice cultures, *J. Neurophysiol.*, 75, 154, 1996.

122. Schwindt, P.C. and Crill, W.E., Factors influencing motoneuron rhythmic firing: results from a voltage-clamp study, *J. Neurophysiol.*, 48, 875, 1982.

123. Berger, A.J. and Takahashi, T., Serotonin enhances a low-voltage-activated calcium current in rat spinal motoneurons, *J. Neurosci.,* 10, 1922, 1990.
124. Safronov, B.V. and Vogel, W., Single voltage-activated Na$^+$ and K$^+$ channels in the somata of rat motoneurones, *J. Physiol.,* 487(1), 91, 1995.
125. Hille, B., *Ionic Channels of Excitable Membranes,* Sinauer Assoc. Suderland Massachussetts, 1992.
126. Bekkers, J.M., Distribution and activation of voltage-gated potassium channels in cell-attached and outside-out patches from large layer 5 cortical pyramidal neurons of the rat, *J. Physiol.,* 525, 611, 2000.
127. Korngren, A. and Sakmann, B., Voltage-gated K$^+$ channels in layer 5 neocortical pyramidal neurons from young rats: subtypes and gradients, *J. Physiol.,* 525, 621, 2000.
128. Storm, J.F., K$^+$ channels and their distribution in large cortical pyramidal neurones, *J. Physiol.,* 525, 565, 2000.
129. Stuart, G.J. and Sakmann, B., Active propagation of somatic action potentials into neocortical pyramidal cell dendrites, *Nature,* 367, 69, 1994.
130. Brown, A.G. and Fyffe, R.E.W., The morphology of group Ia afferent fiber collaterals in the spinal cord of the cat, *J. Physiol.,* 274, 111, 1978.
131. Burke, R.E., Walmsley, B., and Hodgson, J.A., HRP anatomy of group Ia afferent contacts on alpha motoneurones, *Brain Res.,* 160, 347, 1979.
132. Burke, R.E. and Glenn, L.L., Horseradish peroxidase study of the spatial and electrotonic distribution of group Ia synapses on type-identified ankle extensor motoneurons in the cat, *J. Comp. Neurol.,* 372, 465, 1996.
133. Hongo, T., Kudo, N., Sasaki, S., Yamashita, M., Yoshida, K., Ishizuka, N., and Mannen, H., Trajectory of group Ia and Ib fibers from the hind-limb muscles at the L3 and L4 segments of the spinal cord of the cat, *J. Comp. Neurol.,* 262, 159, 1987.
134. Ishizuka, N., Mannen, H., Hongo, T., and Sasaki, S., Trajectory of group Ia afferent fibers stained with horseradish peroxidase in the lumbosacral spinal cord of the cat: three dimensional reconstructions from serial sections, *J. Comp. Neurol.,* 186, 189, 1979.
135. Keirstead, S.A. and Rose, P.K., Structure of the intraspinal projections of single, identified muscle spindle afferents from neck muscles of the cat, *J. Neurosci.,* 8, 3413, 1988.
136. Ritz, L.A., Bailey, S.M., Carter, R.L., Sparkes, M.L., Masson R.L., and Rhoton, E.L., Crossed and uncrossed projections to cat sacrocaudal spinal cord: II. Axons from muscle spindle primary endings, *J. Comp. Neurol.,* 304, 316, 1991.
137. Redman, S. and Walmsley, B., The time course of synaptic potentials evoked in cat spinal motoneurones at identified group Ia synapses, *J. Physiol.,* 343, 117, 1983.
138. Jake, C.E. and Yoshioka, K., Ia afferent excitation of motoneurons in the *in vitro* new-born rat spinal cord is selectively antagonized by kynurenate, *J. Physiol.,* 370, 515, 1986.
139. Schneider. S.P. and Fyffe, R.E.W., Involvement of GABA and glycine in recurrent inhibition of spinal motoneurons, *J. Neurophysiol.,* 36, 397, 1992.
140. Walmsley, B. and Bolton, P.S., An *in vitro* pharmacological study of single group Ia fiber contacts with motoneurones in the cat spinal cord, *J. Physiol.,* 481, 731, 1994.
141. Pinco, M. and Lev-Tov, A., Synaptic excitation of alpha-motoneurons by dorsal root afferents in the neonatal rat spinal cord, *J. Neurophysiol.,* 70, 406, 1993.
142. Maxwell, D.J., Christie, W.M., Short, A.D., and Brown, A.G., Direct observations of synapses between GABA-immunoreactive boutons and muscle afferent terminals in lamina VI of the cat's spinal cord, *Brain Res.,* 530, 215, 1990.

143. Jack, J.J.B., Miller, S., Porter, R., and Redman, S.J., The time course of minimal excitatory post-synaptic potentials evoked in spinal motoneurons by group Ia afferent fibers, *J. Physiol.*, 215, 353, 1971.
144. Rall, W., Burke, R.E., Nelson, P.G., Smith, T.G., and Frank, K., The dendritic location of synapses and possible mechanisms for the monosynaptic EPSP in motoneurons, *J. Neurophysiol.*, 30, 1169, 1967.
145. Alvarez, F.J., Fyffe, R.E.W., Dewey, D.E., Haftel, V.K., and Cope, T.C., Factors regulating AMPA-type glutamate receptor subunit changes induced by sciatic nerve injury in rats, *J. Comp. Neurol.*, 426, 229, 2000.
146. Alvarez, F.J., Villalba, R.M., Carr, P.A., Grandes, P., and Somohano, P.M., Differential distribution of metabotropic glutamate receptors 1a, 1b, and 5 in the rat spinal cord, *J. Comp. Neurol.*, 422, 464, 2000.
147. Alvarez, F.J., Dewey, D.E., Carr, P.A., Cope, T.C., and Fyffe, R.E.W., Downregulation of metabotropic glutamate receptor 1a in motoneurons after axotomy, *NeuroReport*, 8, 1711, 1997.
148. Lawrence, D.G., Porter, R., and Redman S.J., Corticomotoneuronal synapses in the monkey: light microscopic localization upon motoneurons of intrinsic muscles of the hand, *J. Comp. Neurol.*, 232, 499, 1985.
149. Rose, P.K., Jones, T., Nirula, R., and Corneil, T., Innervation of motoneurons based on dendritic orientation, *J. Neurophysiol.*, 73, 1319, 1995.
150. Burke, R.E., Fedina, L., and Lundberg, A., Spatial synaptic distribution of recurrent and group Ia inhibitory systems in cat spinal motoneurones, *J. Physiol.*, 214, 350, 1971.
151. Van Keulen, L., Autogenetic recurrent inhibition of individual spinal motoneurones of the cat, *Neurosci. Lett.*, 21, 297, 1981.
152. Stuart, G.J. and Redman, S.J., Voltage dependence of Ia reciprocal inhibitory currents in cat spinal motoneurones, *J. Physiol.*, 420, 111, 1990.
153. McCurdy, M.L. and Hamm, T.M., Spatial and temporal features of recurrent facilitation among motoneurons innervating synergistic muscles of the cat, *J. Neurophys.*, 72, 227, 1994.
154. Rastad, J., Ultrastructural morphology of axon terminals of an inhibitory spinal interneurone in the cat, *Brain Res.*, 223, 397, 1981.
155. Fyffe, R.E.W., Glycine-like immunoreactivity in synaptic terminals of identified inhibitory interneurons in the cat's spinal cord, *Brain Res.*, 547, 175, 1991.
156. Cullheim, S. and Kellerth, J.-O., Two kinds of recurrent inhibition of cat spinal alpha-motoneurones as differentiated pharmacologically, *J. Physiol.*, 312, 209, 1981.
157. Colin, I., Rostaing, P., Augustin, A., and Triller, A., Localization of components of glycinergic synapses during rat spinal cord development, *J. Comp. Neurol.*, 398, 359, 1998.
158. Pilowsky, P.M., de Castro, D., Llewellyn-Smith, I., Lipski, J., and Voss, M.D., Serotonin immunoreactive boutons make synapses with feline phrenic motoneurons, *J. Neurosci.*, 10, 1091, 1990.
159. Gladden, M.H., Maxwell, D.J., Sahal, A., and Jankowska, E., Coupling between serotoninergic and noradrenergic neurons and α-motoneurons in the cat, *J. Physiol.*, 527, 213, 2000.
160. Morales, M., Battenberg, E., and Bloom, F.E., Distribution of neurons expressing immunoreactivity for the 5HT3 receptor subtype in the rat brain and spinal cord, *J. Comp. Neurol.*, 385, 385, 1998.
161. Kheck, N.M., Gannon, P.J., and Azmitia, E.C., 5-HT1A receptor localization on the axon hillock of cervical spinal motoneurons in primates, *J. Comp. Neurol.*, 355, 211, 1995.

162. Ridet, J.L., Tamir, H., and Privat A., Direct immunocytochemical localization of 5-hydrotryptamine receptors in the adult rat spinal cord: a light and electron microscopic study using an anti-idiotypic antiserum, *J. Neurosci. Res.,* 38, 109, 1994.

163. Keirstead, S.A. and Rose, P.K., Dendritic distribution of splenius motoneurons in the cat: comparison of motoneurons innervating different regions of the muscle, *J. Comp. Neurol.,* 219, 273, 1983.

164. Romanes, G.J., The motor pools of the spinal cord, *Prog. Brain Res.,* 12, 93, 1964.

3 5-HT Receptors and the Neuromodulatory Control of Spinal Cord Function

*Shawn Hochman, Sandra M. Garraway,
David W. Machacek, and Barbara L. Shay*

CONTENTS

ABSTRACT   The purpose of this chapter is to present some recent experimental
data obtained in our laboratory that provide new insights and suggest new hypotheses
on the organization of serotonergic systems within the mammalian spinal cord. Our
proposed conceptual framework for understanding 5-hydroxytryptamine (5-HT;
serotonin) function incorporates the existence of multiple descending serotonergic
systems and multiple spinal serotonin receptor subtypes.

3.1 OVERVIEW

Investigations on the spinal actions of 5-HT can be partitioned into three areas:
sensory mechanisms, motor control, and autonomic function. While there is clearly
a strong descending serotonergic control of spinal autonomic function,[1,2] this will
not be explored here. Studies on 5-HT and sensory mechanisms have focused on
the modulation of nociception, demonstrating the actions of 5-HT and 5-HT receptor-
selective ligands on dorsal horn neurons and on nocisponsive reflexes.[3–7] Studies of
5-HT in motor control have focused on the modifiability of motoneuron function,
particularly with respect to the activation of persistent inward currents,[8–10] as well

as those concerned with the initiation and modulation of motor behaviors such as locomotion.[11-17] Motoneurons are relatively easy to target experimentally, and consequently have provided important information on the actions of 5-HT at the cellular level within the spinal cord.[18-21] However, spinal motoneurons comprise a very small fraction of the neurons within the spinal cord, and the spinal networks that receive descending commands and coordinate sensorimotor activities are pre-motoneuronal. For example, in rats, 5-HT can activate the spinal locomotor circuitry, yet the mechanism by which 5-HT is capable of recruiting the locomotor central pattern generator (CPG) is almost completely unknown. Clearly, further insight on 5-HT function requires study of the actions of 5-HT on spinal neurons engaged in the control of both segmental and ascending sensorimotor information processing. In this regard, we can particularly thank the efforts of Jankowska's[22,23] and Willis' groups[24-26] for undertaking such studies on identified neuronal populations *in vivo*.

Physiologically, the spinal actions of 5-HT have been segregated into a modulatory depression of sensory input and a facilitation of motor output. These effects and the activity patterns of serotonergic neurons during various sensory and motor behaviors have resulted in a heuristic hypothesis on 5-HT and motor control forwarded by Jacobs and Fornal.[27] They hypothesized that

> the primary function of 5-HT neurons is to facilitate motor output ... In an ancillary manner, the system acts to inhibit sensory information processing ... When the 5-HT system is inactivated, these relationships are reversed: motor output is disfacilitated and sensory information processing is disinhibited.

The appeal of this hypothesis is in its attempt to address the breadth of CNS behaviors whose activities are related to 5-HT. Accordingly, serotonergic systems have been shown to exert profound modulatory actions in spinal cord by inhibiting sensory systems and facilitating motor systems.[28,29] In support of this, descending serotonergic activity can powerfully inhibit nociceptive information in neurons by activation of serotonergic 5-HT$_1$ and 5-HT$_3$ receptors.[30-32] Conversely, with respect to motor control, 5-HT is released in spinal cord during locomotion,[14,17] and activation of spinal cord serotonergic receptors have been reported to initiate and modulate locomotor patterns[11-13,15,16] and increase motoneuron excitability.[18,19,33]

However, it is now clear that 5-HT can have actions that oppose the general hypothesis forwarded by Jacobs and Fornal,[27] as stimulation of the nucleus reticularis gigantocellularis has pronociceptive actions that involve serotonergic activity.[34,35] These studies demonstrate that while particular serotonergic systems originating in the brainstem are responsible for the pro-motor, anti-sensory modulatory responses, other serotonergic systems perform outside the aforementioned general hypothesis on 5-HT function.

Given the multiple serotonergic bulbospinal projections described below (3.2.2) and the many 5-HT receptor subtypes found in the spinal cord (3.2.3 below), it is likely that no simple hypothesis on the actions of 5-HT in the spinal cord can account for all the behaviors modulated by 5-HT. Rather, the actions of 5-HT must be addressed in the context of: (i) the several brainstem regions that project descending serotonergic fibers to the spinal cord, (ii) the several 5-HT metabotropic receptor subtypes with differing actions on signal transduction, and (iii) the different topographic distributions of both distinct serotonergic systems and receptor subtypes.

In order to account for the plethora of bulbospinal serotonergic systems and receptor subtypes, we suggest an alternate perspective on the spinal actions of 5-HT. The viewpoint taken is that the spinal cord functions in several distinct behavioral modulatory states. Motor states would include those associated with locomotion, reflex activity, and posture. Sensory states would include normal, suppressed, and amplified sensory input states. We propose that each state is regulated by a distinct bulbospinal modulatory system, and that each serotonergic system exerts a broad influence on spinal cord function by targeting specific metabotropic receptor subtypes that alter cellular signal transduction pathways throughout a broad spinal projection territory. Hence, just as there are several brainstem regions with descending serotonergic projections (see 3.2.2 below), so are there several different modulatory states that 5-HT can regulate in the spinal cord. We forward the following hypothesis:

> **Hypothesis #1.** *Behaviourally relevant sensory and motor acts are modulated by brainstem centers that recruit bulbospinal aminergic systems. Distinct serotonergic systems in the brainstem reconfigure spinal neural networks into various functional states. Part of their ability to control separate functional systems is based on the postsynaptic properties of 5-HT receptor subtypes.*

Evidence supporting the existence of 5-HT receptor subtype-selective control of separate spinal cord sensory and motor states is provided below in 3.3.

Receptor- and voltage-gated channels are dynamically modulated through the phosphorylation and dephosphorylation reactions initiated via signal transduction pathways.[36] 5-HT interacts with these systems via numerous metabotropic receptor subtypes and presumably modifies many membrane channels so that the entire physiological performance of a cell, as well as its network interactions, can be reconfigured.[36–38] As distinct metabotropic receptor subtypes alter activity in signal transduction pathways differently, activation of distinct 5-HT receptors should have different physiological consequences on spinal cord function.

> **Hypothesis #2.** *Metabotropic receptor subtypes that increase phosphorylation reactions ($5\text{-}HT_2$, $5\text{-}HT_{4,6,7}$) are net excitatory and would be found on specific cellular and synaptic locations that favor facilitated activity while receptor subtypes which inhibit phosphorylation reactions ($5\text{-}HT_1$) are net inhibitory and would be located at synaptic and cellular regions targeted for depression (see Table 3.1). Distinct metabotropic receptor subtypes are involved in the control of different spinal cord states.*

This hypothesis is broadly consistent with the numerous actions of 5-HT in the CNS[39] and represents a logical extension of the trend observed by Aghajanian et al.[40] regarding the actions of $5\text{-}HT_1$ and $5\text{-}HT_2$ receptor subtypes. The notion that different 5-HT receptor subtypes control different behavioral states is not new and has a rich history in relation to a variety of brain disorders. For example, the $5\text{-}HT_1$ family of receptors have been implicated in depression ($5\text{-}HT_{1A}$) and migraine ($5\text{-}HT_{1B}$ and $5\text{-}HT_{1D}$), the $5\text{-}HT_2$ receptors in psychosis ($5\text{-}HT_{2A}$), anxiety, feeding, and seizures ($5\text{-}HT_{2C}$), and the $5\text{-}HT_3$ receptors in emesis. We assert that a similar dissection of 5-HT receptor subtype with distinct functions occurs in the spinal cord.

TABLE 3.1
Monoamine Receptor Subtypes and Their Effects
on Signal Transduction Pathways

Effector Coupling	↑cAMP	↑IP3/DAG	↓cAMP	Ionotropic
Serotonin	$5\text{-}HT_{4,6,7}$	$5\text{-}HT_{2A-C}$	$5\text{-}HT_{1A,B,D,E,F}$	$5\text{-}HT_3$
Noradrenaline	β_{1-3}	$\alpha_{1A,B,D}$	α_{2A-D}	
Dopamine	$D_{1,5}$		D_{2-4}	

Note: The $5\text{-}HT_{2C}$ receptor was previously referred to as the $5\text{-}HT_{1C}$ receptor.

The primary purpose of this chapter is to provide new experimental data obtained in our laboratory that support the aforementioned hypotheses (3.3). However, in order to permit a broad appreciation of the serotonergic systems in the spinal cord, we first provide a general review of the bulbospinal serotonergic descending systems (3.2.1) and the 5-HT receptor subtypes found in the spinal cord (3.2.2).

3.2 BACKGROUND

3.2.1 BRAINSTEM SEROTONERGIC NEURONAL POPULATIONS WITH PROJECTIONS TO SPINAL CORD

It has been known since the landmark studies of Dahlström and Fuxe[42,43] that the brainstem contains serotonergic nuclei that project to the spinal cord. These projections are diffuse and originate from several brainstem monoaminergic nuclei.[42,44] Steinbusch[45] demonstrated that serotonergic fibers extensively innervate the spinal cord of the rat, with the highest density of innervation found in the ventral horn and high to medium density found at all levels of the dorsal horn. Similarly, Marlier et al.[46] reported high to intermediate concentrations of serotonergic fibers innervating the spinal cord dorsal horn of the rat. Simply stated, serotonergic fibers project throughout the spinal cord gray matter.

The absence of distinct boundaries between 5-HT-containing neurons within raphe nuclei and those found in the surrounding reticular formation has led to an alphanumeric classification of brainstem 5-HT-containing neurons into 9 groups (B1–B9).[47] B1–B4 cell groups differentiate embryologically from a single caudal group, while B5–B9 neurons develop from a rostral cell cluster.[48] In rat, 5-HT-containing neurons of the B1–B4 cell groups possess descending projections to the spinal cord and contain the following cytoarchitectural regions: raphe pallidus (B1), caudal ventrolateral medulla (B1), raphe obscurus (B2), raphe magnus (B3), rostral ventrolateral medulla (B3), lateral paragigantocellularis reticularis (B3), and the central gray of the medulla oblongata (B4).[47] In addition, it appears that 5-HT-containing neurons from the B5–B9 cell group have descending projections to the cervical spinal cord.[49] Thus, the brainstem contains numerous distinct topographic populations of serotonergic neurons with projections to spinal cord.

TABLE 3.2
Development and Projections of Nuclei with Serotonin-Containing Neurons

Nucleus	Group	Projection	Predominant Termination Sites	Arrival of Fibers in Spinal Cord	Refs.
Subnucleus reticularis dorsalis	B1	Ipsilateral dorsolateral funiculus	Laminae V–VII, X	?	180, 251
Raphe pallidus	B1	Predominantly ventro- and ventrolateral funiculi	Ventral horn and intermediolateral cell column	Cervical at E14 Sacral at E16–17	47, 252
Raphe obscurus	B2	Bilateral ventral funiculus	Ventral horn	Cervical at E14 Sacral at E16–17	47, 252
Raphe magnus	B3	Ipsilateral dorsolateral funiculus	Bilaterally mainly in ventral horn, superficial dorsal horn, and some intermediolateral column	Cervical at E14 Sacral at E16–17	47, 252
Reticularis paragiganto-cellularis	B3	Bilateral dorsolateral and ventral funiculi	Bilateral intermediate gray, ventral horn and intermediolateral cell column	Thoracic at E16	47, 252
Rostral ventrolateral medulla	B3	Ipsilateral dorsolateral funiculus	Intermediolateral column	?	48

Developmentally, serotonin-containing neurons are among the first CNS neurons to develop and are generated between embryonic days (E)11–15.[50] Table 3.2 summarizes the development of projections from several serotonergic nuclei to the spinal cord. Descending serotonergic fibers are found in the spinal cord as early as E14. At birth, serotonin immunoreactivity is found in the gray matter at all spinal cord levels, particularly in the ventral horn. Thereafter, staining density increases, peaking at postnatal day (P)7 in cervical and P14 in lumbar cord, then labeling density is reduced to achieve an adult density pattern at P21.[51,52] Despite the early anatomical presence of descending serotonergic projections, there is some ambiguity over whether functional actions are observed. Fitzgerald and Koltzenburg[53] reported that stimulation of the dorsolateral funiculus (DLF) was incapable of producing inhibition of sensory responses in the dorsal horn until P10–12 and was not fully expressed until P19. However, several other studies provide evidence for the existence of descending inhibition much earlier than P10.[54-58] Though none of these other studies directly investigated the DLF or the descending monoaminergic systems, Wallis et al.[55] showed that in the P1 rat the strong descending inhibition of the monosynaptic reflex elicited by stimulating the ventrolateral funiculus (VLF) is mediated by serotonin. It is likely that the observed absence of DLF stimulation-evoked inhibition of C-fiber input in the newborn rat, reported by Fitzgerald and Koltzenburg,[53] is due to the late development of C-fiber projections into the deep dorsal horn[59] rather than a lack of maturity or functional actions in descending serotonergic projections.

Based on the different projection sites of distinct bulbospinal serotonergic pathways, it is reasonable to assume that 5-HT exerts a neuromodulatory role on spinal cord function that can at least partly be partitioned into topographical locations (see Table 3.2). These include the superficial dorsal horn with fibers originating from raphe magnus, the ventral horn excluding motor nuclei (laminae VII–VIII) with fibers originating from the subnucleus reticularis dorsalis, and the motor nuclei (lamina IX) with fibers originating from the raphe (magnus, pallidus, and obscurus) and reticularis paragigantocellularis nuclei. In addition to different projection sites the separate descending systems can differ cytochemically[60] and ultrastructurally.[61] For example, 5-HT colocalizes with thyrotropin-releasing hormone and substance P in somatic motoneurons whereas 5-HT predominantly colocalizes only with thyrotropin-releasing hormone on parasympathetic preganglionic motoneurons.[62] More generally, raphespinal serotonergic neurons located in the more rostral medulla tend to lack neuropeptides and project to the dorsal horn while more caudal raphespinal neurons co-contain neuropeptides and project to the ventral horn.[63] Also, particularly in the dorsal horn, many 5-HT varicosities end blindly and do not form conventional synapses, and in this regard have been suggested to modulate spinal activity via volume transmission.[61,64]

3.2.2   5-HT Receptors Found in the Spinal Cord

The same as different serotonergic nuclei have different projection sites and properties within the spinal cord, the distribution of 5-HT receptor subtypes is also heterogeneous.

1. $5-HT_1$ receptors dominate in the dorsal horn.
2. $5-HT_2$ receptors are more abundant in the ventral horn, particularly on motoneurons.
3. $5-HT_3$ receptors appear to be rather exclusively associated with nociceptive processing.
4. Preliminary evidence suggests that $5-HT_7$ receptors appear to be strongest in the intermediate regions of the spinal cord.

A detailed description is provided in 3.3.4 below.

Currently, there are seven families of 5-HT receptors ($5-HT_{1-7}$), comprising at least 14 distinct receptor subtypes.[66,67] Several of these receptors have been identified in the spinal cord (see below). With the exception of the ionotropic $5-HT_3$ receptor, all serotonergic receptors are G-protein-coupled metabotropic receptors. Metabotropic receptors are capable of exerting a broad modulatory influence on cell and network behavior. This is because most, if not all, ligand- and voltage-gated channels can be modulated by 5-HT.[39,67] Table 3.1 summarizes the 5-HT receptor subtypes (as well as the other descending monoamine transmitters, dopamine (DA) and noradrenaline (NA)) and their coupling to signal transduction pathways.

TABLE 3.3
Relative Affinities of Various 5-HT Receptor Ligands

	5-HT$_{1A}$ ↓AC	5-HT$_{1B}$ ↓AC	5-HT$_{2A}$ ↑PLC	5-HT$_{2C}$ ↑PLC	5-HT$_4$ ↑AC	5-HT$_6$ ↑AC	5-HT$_7$ ↑AC
Agonists							
	5-HT(4 nM)	5-HT(12 nM)	5-HT(13,000 nM)	5-HT(24 nM)	5-HT(100 nM)	5-HT(56 nM)	5-HT(1.8 nM)
	8-OH-DPAT(6.3 nM)	8-OH-DPAT(1,260 nM)	8-OH-DPAT(<100,000 nM)	8-OH-DPAT(<100,000)	8-OH-DPAT(inactive)		8-OH-DPAT(35 nM)
	5-CT(2.5 nM)	5-CT(12.6 nM)	5-CT(~1,000 nM)	5-CT(~1,000 nM)	5-CT(3000 nM)	5-CT(250 nM)	5-CT(0.3 nM)
	CGS-12066B(300 nM)	CGS-12066B(25 nM)		CGS-12066B(79,000)			CGS-12066B(?)
	DOI(6,938 nM)	DOI(2,041 nM)	DOI(208 nM)	DOI(100 nM)			DOI(2,500 nM)
Antagonists							
	GR 113808(<1000 nM)	GR 113808(<1000 nM)	GR 113808(<1000 nM)	GR 113808(<1000 nM)	GR 113808(0.2 nM)		
	methiothepin(79 nM)	methiothepin(50 nM)	methiothepin(1 nM)	methiothepin(3-27 nM)	methiothepin(inactive)	methiothepin(1.8 nM)	methiothepin(.01 nM)
	(-)pindolol(21 nM)	(-)pindolol(45 nM)	(-)pindolol(3,100 nM)	(-)pindolol(34,000 nM)		pindolol(<10,000 nM)	pindolol(<1,000 nM)
	Way-100635(1 nM)		WAY-100635(<125 nM)	WAY-100635(125 nM)	WAY-100635(<125 nM)		
	NAN-190(1.3 nM)	NAN-190(616 nM)	NAN-190(218 nM)	NAN-190(602 nM)		NAN-190(<10,000 nM)	NAN-190(144 nM)
	clozapine(1,800 nM)			clozapine(110 nM)		clozapine(13.0 nM)	clozapine(13.5 nM)
			normethyl-clozapine(19.4 nM)	normethyl-clozapine(7.1 nM)			
	spiperone(63 nM)	spiperone(5,011 nM)	spiperone(1 nM)	spiperone(5,011 nM)	spiperone(inactive)		spiperone(5,011 nM)
	cyproheptadine(~300 nM)	cyproheptadine(840 nM)	cyproheptadine(3.2 nM)	cyproheptadine(~10 nM)	cyproheptadine(13 nM)	cyproheptadine(134 nM)	cyproheptadine(66 nM)
	ketanserin(>1,000 nM)	ketanserin(1,910 nM)	ketanserin(~1 nM)	ketanserin(~50 nM)	ketanserin(inactive)	ketanserin(>10,000 nM)	ketanserin(43 nM)
	ritanserin(3,570 nM)	ritanserin(1,737 nM)	ritanserin(1.5 nM)	ritanserin(0.7 nM)		ritanserin(44 nM)	ritanserin(22 nM)

Note: Approximate affinity values (EC$_{50}$ and IC$_{50}$) for some ligands at 5-HT$_{1A}$, 5-HT$_{1B}$, 5-HT$_{2A}$, 5-HT$_{2C}$, 5-HT$_4$, 5-HT$_6$, and & 5-HT$_7$, receptors. Ligand affinity values were derived from the following References 66, 68, 222, 253, and 254.

Prior to reviewing our knowledge of the properties of individual 5-HT receptors in the spinal cord, it is important to emphasize that most of our understanding of 5-HT receptors in the spinal cord is based on receptor binding and pharmacological approaches. Both approaches rely on the specificity of a given drug for one receptor subtype over another. As there can be considerable overlap between binding affinities of a specific ligand for various receptor subtypes (see Table 3.3), it is clear that great caution must be taken when trying to ascribe results to one particular receptor subtype over another. For example, [3H]8-hydroxy-2-(di-n-propylamino) tetralin (8-OH-DPAT) was used in binding studies to determine the distribution of 5-HT$_{1A}$ receptors, yet the more recently cloned 5-HT$_7$ receptor has similar high affinity for 8-OH-DPAT[68] thereby questioning the reliability of the observations arising from earlier work. Similar problems of interpretation have occurred with respect to pharmacological actions.[69] New studies employing *in situ* hybridization and receptor-specific immunocytochemistry are required to more reliably map 5-HT receptors in the spinal cord.

3.2.2.1   5-HT$_1$ Receptors

3.2.2.1.1   Anatomy

5-HT$_{1A}$ and 5-HT$_{1B}$ receptors account for 27 and 18% of high affinity 5-HT binding sites in the rat spinal cord, respectively.[70] These receptors are present on primary afferent terminals and dorsal horn neurons[71–75] and may constitute dominant receptor subtypes in the dorsal horn.[73] As in other regions of the CNS, the 5-HT$_{1B}$ receptor appears to function as an autoreceptor on descending serotonergic terminals.[76,77] Also, some 5-HT$_1$ receptors are found on capsaicin sensitive C-fibers that project to the superficial dorsal horn.[71] Interestingly, Huang and Peroutka[70] reported that at least 33% of the total 5-HT binding sites in the rat spinal cord are distinct from 5-HT$_{1A}$, 5-HT$_{1B}$, or 5-HT$_{2C}$. 5-HT$_{1D}$ and 5-HT$_{1F}$ receptors are present in spinal cord dorsal horn of humans[78] and 5-HT$_{1D}$ receptors are present in the dorsal horn of the cat.[79] Though not yet tested, 5-HT$_{1D}$ and 5-HT$_{1F}$ receptors may also contribute to the widespread depressant action of 5-HT in the dorsal horn (described below). These aforementioned results, however, cannot be accepted definitively as the majority used binding studies with ligands whose specificity is not absolute.

3.2.2.1.2   Pharmacology

5-HT$_1$ receptors are predominantly associated with a depression in spinal cord sensory responsiveness. It is thought that the 5-HT-evoked depression of sensory input to dorsal horn neurons[6] is partly attributable to postsynaptic actions on the N-methyl-D-aspartate (NMDA) receptor. This occurs via a 5-carboxamidotryptamine (5-CT) sensitive, presumably 5-HT$_1$ receptor-dependent, mechanism.[80] Stimulation of the raphe magnus also inhibits activity in dorsal horn neurons presumably via spinal 5-HT$_1$ receptors.[81] In addition, following raphe magnus stimulation, there is evidence for a selective depression of group II muscle afferent input,[82] an action mimicked by 5-HT$_{1A}$ receptor agonists.[83,84] In frog, 5-HT can also depress primary afferent depolarization (PAD) mediated by γ-aminobutyric acid (GABA) presumably via 5-HT$_{1A}$ receptor actions directly on primary afferent terminals (tetrodotoxin insensitive).[85]

While the 5-HT$_{1B}$ receptor appears to have antinociceptive actions,[3,86,87] the 5-HT$_{1A}$ receptor has been implicated in pronociceptive[86,88] and antinociceptive effects.[3,87,89] Part of the conflicting reports on the actions of 5-HT$_{1A}$ receptors on nociception may be due to the ligand chosen. Some studies used 8-OH-DPAT as a selective 5-HT$_{1A}$ receptor agonist, but 8-OH-DPAT has since been shown to also have high affinity for the 5-HT$_7$ receptor (see Table 3.3). It is possible that antinociceptive actions were due to a dominant activation of the 5-HT$_{1A}$ receptor while pronociceptive actions were due to a dominating activation of the 5-HT$_7$ receptor.

5-HT$_1$ receptor activation also depresses short-latency reflexes. Wu, Wang, and Dun[90] recorded from motoneurons in slice to demonstrate that dorsal root-evoked synaptic responses were depressed by 5-HT$_1$ receptor agonists, presumably via presynaptic mechanisms. Similarly, Wallis and Wu[91] used the isolated neonatal rat spinal cord and examined low- and high-threshold afferent-evoked reflexes and found that only the monosynaptic reflex was depressed by 5-HT$_{1like}$ receptor agonists. Clarke, Ogilvie, and Houghton[92] demonstrated that, in the decerebrate rabbit, 5-HT$_1$ receptor agonists depressed reflexes recorded in medial gastrocnemius following low-threshold electrical stimulation of the sural nerve.

There is conflicting information on the actions of 5-HT$_1$ receptors on motoneuron properties. Holohean, Hackman, and Davidoff[93] used pharmacological studies in frog to demonstrate that membrane hyperpolarizations were via 5-HT$_1$ receptor activation. The opposite actions were observed in cat spinal motoneurons[94] and in large spinal neurons in primary culture.[95]

3.2.2.2 5-HT$_2$ Receptors

3.2.2.2.1 Anatomy

5-HT$_2$ receptor subtypes have been identified in the spinal cord using binding studies,[73,96,97] immunocytochemistry,[74,98,99] and *in situ* hybridization.[100–102] With respect to *in situ* hybridization, 5-HT$_{2A,B\&C}$ receptors have been found in the spinal cord of rat, monkey, and humans, but only 5-HT$_{2A}$ and 5-HT$_{2B}$ are seen in the cat.[100] In comparison, in the rat, an *in situ* hybridization study found high levels of 5-HT$_{2A}$ receptors in the spinal cord ventral horn and 5-HT$_{2C}$ receptors in the whole gray matter of the spinal cord, but found no evidence of 5-HT$_{2B}$ receptor mRNA expression.[102] Binding studies suggest that there is substantial 5-HT$_{2C}$ receptor labeling in rat spinal cord[96] and another *in situ* study reports the 5-HT$_{2C}$ receptor distribution to be strongest in laminae V and VII.[101] Studies using 5,7-dihydroxytryptamine to deplete 5-HT fibers in the spinal cord suggest that the 5-HT$_2$ receptors are not autoreceptors,[103] and therefore, are located on non-serotonergic neuronal sites.[104] There is a relatively small percentage of 5-HT$_{2A/2C}$ receptors present in the rat dorsal horn.[98,99,102]

3.2.2.2.2 Pharmacology

While there are some reports of 5-HT$_2$ receptors having inhibitory actions in spinal cord,[55,94,105,106] the majority of studies demonstrate 5-HT$_2$ receptor-mediated increases in spinal cord excitability at many levels. For example, 5-HT$_2$ receptors mediate a long-lasting facilitation of miniature EPSCs in superficial dorsal horn neurons,[107] depolarize dorsal horn neurons in frog,[108] and facilitate focal stimulation-induced synaptic activity in ventral horn cells.[109] Intrathecal administration of 5-HT$_2$ agonists induces back muscle contractions and wet dog shakes,[110–112] and a dose-dependent behavioral syndrome consisting of biting and licking directed toward caudal body parts and reciprocal hindlimb scratching.[113,114] These behaviors are blocked by 5-HT$_2$ receptor antagonists.[110,111] 5-HT$_2$ receptor agonists increase the activity of motoneurons and also facilitate mono- and polysynaptic reflexes.[115–118] 5-HT$_2$ receptors depolarize[19,93] and increase glutamate-evoked firing in motoneurons.[119] Notably, cyproheptadine, a 5-HT$_2$ receptor antagonist controls spasticity in humans.[120] Pharmacological studies in the frog suggest that 5-HT$_2$ receptors depolarize primary afferents[121] and depress GABA-mediated PAD[85] at least partially via actions on interneurons. Last, Zhuo and Gebhart[122] stimulated the reticularis gigantocellularis and gigantocellularis pars α to demonstrate facilitation of the tail-flick reflex which is blocked by methysergide. While these actions were reported to be mediated by 5-HT$_1$ receptors, the current receptor reclassification of 5-HT$_{1C}$ as 5-HT$_{2C}$ and the high affinity of methysergide for 5-HT$_2$ receptors strongly suggest that these actions were mediated by 5-HT$_2$ receptor activation.

3.2.2.3   5-HT$_3$ Receptors

3.2.2.3.1   Anatomy
Unlike the metabotropic 5-HT receptors, the 5-HT$_3$ receptor is ionotropic and leads to the opening of a monovalent cation permeable channel. Binding studies in rat demonstrate 5-HT$_3$ receptors in the superficial dorsal horn that are markedly reduced following dorsal rhizotomy and capsaicin-induced degeneration of nociceptors, but unchanged after 5,7-dihydroxytryptamine chemical lesioning of descending serotonergic fibers.[72,123–126] There are also 5-HT$_3$ receptor binding sites in the most superficial layer (lamina I) of the human spinal cord.[127] Antibodies selective for the 5-HT$_{3A-S}$ subunit had predominant staining in the dorsal horn that at the electron microscopic level was associated with terminals and axonal profiles.[128] *In situ* hybridization and immunohistochemical studies have confirmed that 5-HT$_3$ receptors are found densely in the superficial dorsal horn that is markedly decreased following rhizotomy.[129,130] Thus, 5-HT$_3$ receptors are found on the terminals of dorsal root ganglia as well as on intrinsic neurons of the spinal cord. Some of the intrinsic spinal neurons containing 5-HT$_3$ receptors are enkephalinergic[131] and GABAergic.[132] Motoneurons are also immunolabeled for 5-HT$_3$ receptors and the 5-HT$_{3\alpha}$ subunit decreases following sciatic nerve crush and axotomy.[133]

3.2.2.3.2   Pharmacology
Since the majority of 5-HT$_3$ receptors present in the spinal cord dorsal horn are found on primary afferent terminals where they can mediate PAD[5], synaptic depression via presynaptic inhibitory mechanisms is expected. Reports from previous studies on the events mediated by 5-HT$_3$ receptor activation are conflicting; for instance, in relation to nociception, both pronociceptive[89] and antinociceptive effects[30,134–139] have been reported. In frog, 2-Me-5-HT, a 5-HT$_3$ receptor agonist, depresses polysynaptic reflexes without affecting motoneuron membrane potential,[140] while many dorsal horn neurons are depolarized by 5-HT$_3$ receptor agonists.[108] Gao and Ziskind-Conhaim[141] observed that 5-HT$_3$ receptor agonists depolarized motoneurons in embryonic rat. Importantly,

pharmacological studies on 5-HT$_3$ receptor function should be interpreted cautiously as many 5-HT$_3$ receptor ligands have a high affinity for a glycine binding site and also potentiate glycine-evoked Cl⁻ currents.[142,143]

3.2.2.4 5-HT$_{4-7}$ Receptors

While no binding, immunocytochemical, or *in situ* hybridization studies have examined whether 5-HT$_4$ receptors are found in the spinal cord, pharmacological studies have failed to provide evidence of 5-HT$_4$ receptors in spinal cord.[144,145] The possible roles of 5-HT$_5$ receptors in the CNS are also poorly understood at this time.[68] 5-HT$_6$ receptors have been identified in spinal cord using both immunocytochemistry and *in situ* hybridization.[146] A study using 5,7-dihydroxytryptamine indicates that the 5-HT$_6$ receptor is not an autoreceptor,[147] but its actions are yet to be determined. While there is pharmacological evidence suggestive of the presence of 5-HT$_7$ receptors in the spinal cord,[69,92,148,149] there are currently no reported labeling studies that definitively document their presence in the spinal cord. However, preliminary studies undertaken in our laboratory demonstrate pharmacological and immunocytochemical evidence for the presence of 5-HT$_7$ receptors in the spinal cord (see 3.3.4.2). In addition, previous studies that have observed actions consistent with 5-HT$_7$ receptor activation are described below.

3.2.2.4.1   5-HT Effects Possibly Mediated by 5-HT$_7$
Receptor Activation

Takahashi and Berger[18] recorded from neonatal rat motoneurons in slice and suggested that the observed 5-HT-induced depolarization was via activation of an inward rectifier, presumably due to 5-HT$_{1A}$ receptor activation. Connell and Wallis[150] undertook an extensive pharmacological assay of the 5-HT-induced depolarization of motoneurons in neonatal rats but could not ascribe function to an identifiable receptor subtype. At the time of these studies, the 5-HT$_7$ receptor was not known, but the receptor antagonists that blocked the depolarization in these studies are now consistent with an action at 5-HT$_7$ receptors.[66] Additionally, Roberts et al.[151] demonstrated that nucleus raphe obscurus stimulation depolarized motoneurons with a receptor pharmacology inconsistent with any 5-HT receptor subtype known at the time but would be consistent with the current knowledge for activation of the 5-HT$_7$ receptor. Clarke et al.[92] demonstrated in the decerebrate rabbit that sural stimulation-evoked high-threshold reflexes in the ankle extensor medial gastrocnemius muscle nerve were facilitated by ritanserin-sensitive receptors that are, in the face of other data, likely to be 5-HT$_7$ receptor mediated.

3.3 5-HT RECEPTOR SUBTYPE-SELECTIVE EFFECTS
ON SPINAL CORD FUNCTION: NEW FINDINGS

Our laboratory uses several *in vitro* neonatal rat spinal cords preparations (Fig. 3.1). The *in vitro* preparation is a powerful model system to study the actions of 5-HT receptor ligands on spinal cord function because receptor ligands can be applied at known concentrations without worry of penetration through the blood–brain barrier.

A   Spinal cord slice

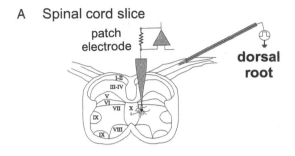

B   Intact spinal cord

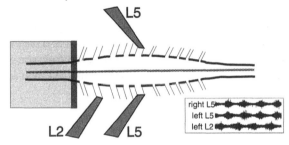

C   Hemisected spinal cord

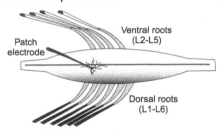

FIGURE 3.1 *In vitro* spinal cord preparations. (A) Spinal cord slice. Whole-cell blind patch recordings are obtained from neurons within visually identifiable regions. Dorsal roots are stimulated electrically to study afferent-evoked synaptic responses. (B) Intact spinal cord. Suction electrodes are attached to identified ventral roots to record motor activity following the addition of various neurochemicals. In some instances, a Vaseline™ wall is constructed at the L1–L2 junction to allow for application of neurochemicals in the rostral spinal cord regions of the spinal cord without directly affecting motoneuron properties at L2 and L5. (C) Hemisected spinal cord preparation. Suction electrodes attached to dorsal and ventral roots are used for stimulation and recording, respectively. In addition, whole-cell blind patch clamp recordings are obtained from neurons within visually identifiably spinal cord regions.

A limitation on the use of bath-applied drugs is their lack of ability to selectively activate only subsets of neurons directly targeted by bulbospinal pathways releasing the endogenous transmitter. However, in the case of neuromodulatory transmitters like 5-HT, typically having diffuse projections throughout the spinal cord, and often signaling by volume transmission, bath application may in fact reasonably reproduce modulatory states activated by descending commands. Additionally, prospective pharmacotherapeutic approaches using neuroactive drugs of clinical relevance will work in a mechanistically similar manner, by diffusing in a non-selective manner throughout the spinal cord.[152]

3.3.1   5-HT$_{1A}$ AND 5-HT$_7$ RECEPTOR SUBTYPES MODULATE SENSORY TRANSMISSION IN DEEP DORSAL HORN NEURONS

3.3.1.1   Background

We used the spinal cord slice preparation and whole-cell patch recordings of sensory synaptic input onto deep dorsal horn (DDH) neurons (Fig. 3.1A) to characterize the modulatory actions of 5-HT and receptor-selective ligands on primary afferent-evoked synaptic responses. Although several investigators have examined the actions of 5-HT receptor ligands on the control of spinal cord function *in vivo,* e.g., References 69, 117, and 153, only a few studies have examined their actions at the spinal cellular level *in vitro.*[5,6,80]

3.3.1.2   Experimental Observations

As stated above, *in vitro* studies offer the advantage of applying multiple ligands at known concentrations.[154] In addition, intracellular recordings permit a cellular characterization of neuromodulatory mechanisms of action. We examined dorsal root-evoked synaptic responses on deep dorsal horn neurons in two age groups of neonatal rats: P3–6 and P10–14. In agreement with other intracellular studies,[5,6] 5-HT depressed evoked excitatory postsynaptic potentials (EPSPs) in the majority of DDH neurons (Fig. 3.2A). Selective activation of 5-HT$_{1A}$ and 5-HT$_{1B}$ receptors also depressed evoked responses (Fig. 3.2B) suggesting that these receptors contribute to the depressant action produced by 5-HT. However, other receptors must also contribute as 5-HT can produce additional synaptic depression even in the presence of 5-HT$_{1A}$ and 5-HT$_{1B}$ receptor agonists and antagonists (Fig. 3.2B bottom). It is highly likely that 5-HT$_3$ receptor activation at least partly contributes to the additional synaptic depression[5] (see 3.2.2.3 above). Other candidate subtypes currently untested include 5-HT$_{1D}$ and 5-HT$_{1F}$ receptors (see 3.2.2.1 above).

Although 5-HT predominantly depresses evoked synaptic responses, presumed selective activation of 5-HT$_7$ receptors facilitated evoked EPSPs in the majority of neurons studied (Fig. 3.2C). Activation of 5-HT$_2$ receptors could also facilitate evoked responses in some neurons (Fig. 3.2B) but were without effect in the majority of neurons tested. In summary, primary afferent synapses are modulated by several 5-HT receptor subtypes and most evoked responses can be depressed using 5-HT$_1$ receptor agonists and facilitated with 5-HT$_7$ receptor agonists (see Fig. 3.2). Thus, the depressive effect of 5-HT typically observed in DDH neurons is due to dominating actions at receptors evoking depression (i.e., 5-HT$_{1A}$ and 5-HT$_{1B}$) compared to those producing facilitation (i.e., 5-HT$_2$ and 5-HT$_7$). These actions were largely independent of age range examined.[149]

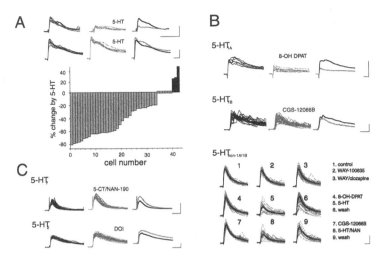

FIGURE 3.2 5-HT receptor pharmacology of evoked responses in DDH neurons. (A) While 5-HT can depress or facilitate evoked responses, the predominant action is depressant. (A(top)) Raw EPSP waveforms overlapped before and after application of 5-HT in two different cells demonstrate the ability of 5-HT to depress or facilitate evoked responses. In all panels A–C, average evoked responses are presented at right overlapped to aid comparison of action. (A(bottom)) Histogram summarizing the actions of 5-HT in 42 deep dorsal horn neurons. Note the extent to which depression dominates 5-HT's modulatory actions. (B) 5-HT$_{1A}$ (top) and 5-HT$_{1B}$ (middle) receptor agonists depress evoked responses. In several cells, the depressive actions of 5-HT could not be accounted for by actions at 5-HT$_{1A}$ and 5-HT$_{1B}$ receptors, demonstrating that 5-HT can evoke synaptic depression by other receptor subtypes (see Table 3.3 for relative affinities of the ligands applied in this figure). (C) 5-HT$_7$ and 5-HT$_2$ receptor activation using selective agonists facilitates evoked responses. Scale bars are 10 mV, 100 ms.

In the absence of applied agonists, 5-HT$_{1A}$ receptor antagonists usually facilitated evoked EPSPs (Fig. 3.3A) suggesting that there is an endogenous release of 5-HT that tonically depresses EPSPs via 5-HT$_{1A}$ receptor activation.[55] 5-HT has very high affinity for the 5-HT$_{1A}$ receptor (Table 3.2) and Hadjiconstantinou et al.[155] demonstrated that endogenous spinal 5-HT persists for over a week after transection. It is possible that low levels of endogenously released 5-HT serve to tonically regulate synaptic gain of primary afferent input. 5-HT also has a very high affinity for the 5-HT$_7$ receptor, and in a few cases we observed that application of NAN-190 alone produced a depression of the evoked response (Fig. 3.3B). We presume this action is mediated by blockade of the 5-HT$_7$ receptor, which binds NAN-190 with moderate affinity (see Table 3.3). Unlike the 5-HT$_{1A/7}$ receptors (Fig. 3.3B), there was no evidence to support tonic activation of the 5-HT$_{2A/2C}$ receptor, since ketanserin applied alone had no effect on naïve synaptic responses (Fig. 3.3C). These results are consistent with the higher affinity of 5-HT for 5-HT$_{1A}$ and 5-HT$_7$ receptors over 5-HT$_2$ receptors (see Table 3.3) and also the low expression of 5-HT$_{2A/2C}$ receptors in the dorsal horn (see 3.2.2.2).

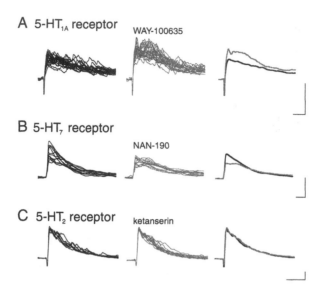

FIGURE 3.3 Evidence for a 5-HT-induced tonic modulation of evoked synaptic responses. (A) Application of the 5-HT$_{1A}$ receptor antagonist WAY-100635 facilitates evoked response, suggesting that 5-HT$_{1A}$ receptors were tonically activated in this neuron. (B) Application of the selective 5-HT$_{1A/7}$ receptor antagonist NAN-190 results in a depression in EPSP amplitude, suggesting that 5-HT$_{7}$ receptors were tonically activated in this neuron. (C) The 5-HT$_{2}$ receptor antagonist ketanserin is ineffective at modulating EPSP amplitude, suggesting that 5-HT$_{2}$ receptors are not tonically activated. In all panels, average values are presented overlaid to the right for comparison. Scale bars are 10 mV, 100 ms.

3.3.2 5-HT$_{1A/1B}$ RECEPTORS FACILITATE THE INDUCTION OF LONG-TERM DEPRESSION

3.3.2.1 Background

Spinal neurons are sensitized following stimuli that activate nociceptive fibers. This *central sensitization* has been experimentally characterized by an increased excitability in response to sensory inputs, a prolonged afterdischarge to repeated stimulation (termed wind-up), and expanded peripheral receptive fields.[156] Interestingly, repetitive activation of nociceptors can also induce maintained alterations in synaptic strength observed either as long-term synaptic potentiation (LTP) or depression (LTD). LTP and LTD have been observed in the dorsal and ventral horns of the spinal cord following repetitive stimulation of primary afferents.[157–164]

The induction of synaptic plasticity in the spinal cord could represent a physiological mechanism for controlling the gain in sensory signaling. Interestingly, descending systems appear to be able to control both the induction and direction of the evoked synaptic plasticity, usually favoring depression. For example, Sandkühler and Liu[165] demonstrated that natural activation of nociceptors in skin induced LTP of C-fiber-evoked field potentials in dorsal horn, but only following spinalization, suggesting a potent inhibitory control from descending systems.[161] Thus, it is reasonable to assume that synaptic plasticity can participate in the physiological encoding of altered sensory states and that in the absence of descending inhibitory controls, sensory input preferentially produces LTP. The preferential increase in sensory gain in the absence of descending inhibition would be consistent with the observations of hyperreflexia, hyperalgesia, and allodynia that follow spinal cord injury.[166–170]

3.3.2.2 Experimental Observations

5-HT is released in spinal cord by descending systems that modulate spinal sensory integration. As demonstrated in 3.3.1 above, 5-HT can potently depress primary afferent-evoked synaptic responses in DDH neurons (Fig. 3.2A). Since primary afferent activity-induced LTP may contribute to the central sensitization of nociception, we studied the effects of 5-HT on the expression of LTP and LTD in DDH neurons in the spinal slice preparation. We compared the actions of 5-HT on afferent-evoked EPSPs before, during, or after high frequency conditioning stimulation. Even though 5-HT caused a depression of the naïve synaptic response (Color Figure 3A*), conditioning stimulation in the presence of 5-HT was not only still capable of inducing LTD (Color Figure 3C), but also significantly increased its incidence from 54% in controls to 88% (Color Figure 3D). 5-HT also potently depressed post-conditioning synaptic responses, regardless of whether the induced plasticity was LTP or LTD (Color Figure 3B). Activation of ligands selective for 5-HT_1, but not 5-HT_2 or 5-HT_3 receptors, best reproduced these actions (Color Figure 3E). These results demonstrate that in addition to depressing EPSP amplitude, 5-HT can also control the direction of its long-term modifiability, favoring the expression of LTD. These findings suggest cellular mechanisms that contribute to the descending serotonergic control over plasticity in sensory gain.

3.3.3 5-HT_{2C} Receptors Induce a Long-Lasting Facilitation of Spinal Reflexes

3.3.3.1 Background

Descending systems control the strength of flexion reflexes; for example, in rat and cat, spinalization results in increased flexion reflexes characterized by reduced thresholds and larger receptive fields.[169,171,172] Descending systems also modulate plasticity in spinal reflex pathways in an activity-dependent manner. Hence, although flexor reflexes can be enhanced for hours following conditioning C-fiber stimulation in the spinal rat,[173] identical stimuli evoke a long-lasting inhibition in the intact anesthetized rat,[17] highlighting the importance of intact descending inhibitory controls. Indeed, many studies have shown that descending bulbospinal systems exert an inhibitory control of spinal nociceptive systems.[175–180] Interestingly, more recent studies have also demonstrated the existence of bulbospinal systems that facilitate spinal nociceptive systems.[34,181,182]

The spinal flexion reflex can undergo LTP in mammals, including cat[183] and rat.[163] In the rat, stimulation of C-fibers evokes a plasticity in the induced flexor

---

* Color figures follow page 142.

reflex,[184] with activation of fibers in joint and muscle being more effective than skin.[173,185] These actions appear to be NMDA receptor dependent.[162,163,186,187] Group I metabotropic glutamate receptors (mGluR1/mGluR5) are implicated in central sensitization,[188] perhaps facilitating LTP via a protein kinase C (PKC)-dependent potentiation of NMDA receptors.[189,190] Group I metabotropic glutamate receptors couple G_q to phospholipase C thereby increasing the activity of PKC and IP_3. Several studies have demonstrated a PKC dependence of central sensitization.[191–193] Like group I metabotropic glutamate receptors, the 5-HT_2 class of serotonin receptors also activate PKC (Table 3.2). 5-HT_2 receptor activation with the selective agonist 1-(2,5-dimethoxy-4-iodophenyl)-2-amino-propane (DOI) can produce a long-lasting facilitation of glutamatergic transmission in some dorsal horn neurons.[107] Maintained increases in motoneuronal excitability[109] and stretch reflexes[194] have also been reported with DOI. Thus, 5-HT_2 receptors may recruit the same cell-signaling pathways as group I metabotropic receptors, and hence contribute to central sensitization and flexion reflex LTP. Since central sensitization and reflex LTP have similar methods of induction, time course, NMDA receptor dependence, and reductions in threshold for recruitment, it is likely that these phenomenon share common interneurons.[195] However, this remains unexplored. We have taken advantage of the *in vitro* spinal cord preparations (Fig. 3.1) to discover and then characterize a 5-HT receptor activation-induced plasticity in spinal sensory systems as described below.

3.3.3.2 Experimental Observations

3.3.3.2.1 5-HT-Induced Long-Lasting Reflex Facilitation

We have used the intact or hemisected isolated spinal cord from neonatal rats ranging in age from P2–P14 to demonstrate that 5-HT produces a long-lasting facilitation of spinal reflexes.[196] Fig. 3.4A presents an example of evoked reflex responses prior to, during, and following washout of 5-HT. Bath superfusion of 5-HT-depressed reflex responses has been described by others.[33] However, following 5-HT washout, reflex amplitude was increased. In order to appreciate the magnitude and duration of reflex facilitation, reflexes were rectified and integrated to allow for quantitative comparisons of reflex amplitude. Fig. 3.4B clearly demonstrates that a long-lasting reflex facilitation (LLRF) was observed following 5-HT washout and this facilitation could be maintained for several hours. The threshold for evoking reflexes was also reduced (Fig. 3.2B). In order to link LLRF to an essential requirement for 5-HT receptor activation, pharmacological analyses demonstrated that a selective 5-HT_{2C} receptor antagonist prevented the induction of LLRF (Fig. 3.4C), while a selective 5-HT_2 receptor agonist alone was sufficient to induce LLRF (Fig. 3.4D). In comparison, 5-HT_1 receptor antagonists did not block LLRF (not shown). The observation that 5-HT itself induces LLRF only following washout demonstrates the strong depressant actions of other activated 5-HT receptors on the recruitment of spinal reflexes. Presumably, the 5-HT_2 receptor-mediated effects remain following washout due to their uniquely long-lasting, PKC-mediated, actions. 5-HT-induced LLRF was statistically significant following electrical stimulation of both low- and high-threshold afferents, though high threshold afferents are facilitated to a much greater degree.

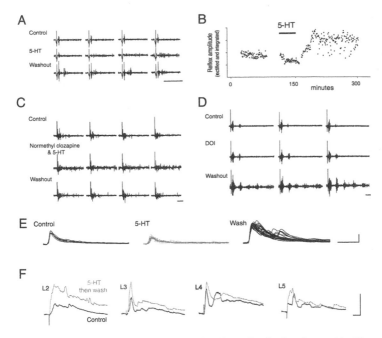

FIGURE 3.4 5-HT induces a long-lasting facilitation of spinal reflexes (A–D) as well as EPSP amplitude in spinal neurons (E). (A) Raw sample of reflexes recorded in a ventral root following dorsal root stimulation. Reflexes recorded under control conditions (top row) were strongly depressed in the presence of 5-HT (middle row). Note also that 5-HT increased spontaneous activity due to its direct excitatory actions on motoneurons. Following washout of 5-HT (bottom row) reflexes were facilitated beyond control values. The reflex facilitation following 5-HT washout was long lasting. (B) Quantification of reflex facilitation over time. Values obtained from the calculated integral of rectified short-latency reflexes (7–67 ms after the stimulus artefact) clearly demonstrate reflex depression during 5-HT application followed by a long-lasting facilitation after drug washout. (C) Application of 5-HT in the presence of the 5-HT$_{2C}$ receptor antagonist normethyl clozapine prevented the expression of reflex facilitation following washout (compare top and bottom rows). (D) The 5-HT$_2$ receptor agonist DOI alone facilitated reflex responses (middle row). Reflex facilitation persisted and became progressively greater even following washout of DOI (bottom row). In panels A–D, constant current electrical stimuli were delivered at intensities between 100 and 500 μA and 100 and 500 μs and at a frequency of 0.02 Hz. (E) Whole-cell patch recording from a neuron within the spinal cord deep dorsal horn reveals long-lasting increases in dorsal root stimulation-evoked synaptic responses following 5-HT washout. Records are of overlapped raw EPSPs before (left), during (middle), and after (right) 5-HT application. Similar effects were observed in many neurons sampled from this region. (F) 5-HT also induces a long-lasting increase in EPSP amplitude following stimulation of dorsal roots from several adjacent spinal segments. In this L4-segment spinal neuron, afferent input from stimulation of several roots was facilitated following 5-HT washout. Responses are presented overlaid as average evoked responses for control (black) and following 5-HT washout (gray). Scale bars are 10 mV and 100 ms.

3.3.3.2.2   5-HT-Induced Long-Lasting Facilitation of Synaptic
Strength in Spinal Neurons

Laminae IV–VII spinal neurons also underwent a 5-HT-induced long-lasting facilitation of their primary afferent-evoked input (Fig. 3.4E) suggesting that interneurons may contribute to LLRF. In addition, in preliminary work in the isolated hemisected spinal cord, we have demonstrated that 5-HT can produce a long-lasting increase in dorsal root stimulation-evoked EPSP amplitude, from several adjacent spinal segments, onto a subpopulation of laminae IV–VII neurons (Fig. 3.4F). The observed increased EPSP amplitudes in spinal neurons from distant spinal segments would support an increased receptive field size. These characteristics of increased EPSP amplitudes with an increase in the strength of multisegmental convergence compare favorably with observations of central sensitization following tissue injury.

3.3.4   5-HT$_7$ RECEPTOR ACTIVATION MAY BE ESSENTIAL
FOR 5-HT-INDUCED LOCOMOTOR RHYTHMOGENESIS

3.3.4.1   Background

Surprisingly little is known about the locomotor CPG's pattern generating circuitry[16,197–204] or underlying intrinsic cellular properties.[205–209] In writing a review on spinal locomotor rhythm generation in 1991, Gossard and Hultborn[199] concluded "the mammalian CPG could still be considered as a virtual black box, even after decades of research." At that stage, *in vivo* experiments in cat had been at the forefront of investigations on mammalian spinal motor systems for the past century. However, since that time, many labs have studied mammalian spinal locomotor mechanisms using the *in vitro* neonatal rat spinal cord preparation.[210,211] In particular, pharmacological, lesioning, and activity-dependent labeling studies have complemented observations in the cat and rabbit[212–215] that hindlimb CPG elements are dominant in segments more rostral than the majority of hindlimb motor nuclei, and that critical neurons are located in the medial intermediate gray matter.[16,57,200,202,216–218] However, to date no studies have clearly recorded from interneurons that form part of the rhythm- and/or pattern-generating circuitry.[205–207] As Hultborn et al.[203] concedes: "There is no doubt of the importance of investigating the spinal mechanisms of locomotion in mammals, including primates and man, the critical question here is whether/how that can be done at the level of identified networks and neurons." Since 5-HT is released in the spinal cord during locomotion,[14,17] and activation of spinal cord serotonergic receptors has been reported to initiate and modulate locomotor patterns,[11–13,15,16] we have undertaken additional studies to determine the importance of 5-HT receptors in 5-HT-induced locomotion in the isolated neonatal rat spinal cord.[11–13,15,16,219,220]

Previous studies have not clearly identified the 5-HT receptor subtype(s) responsible for locomotor rhythmogenesis in rat. Moreover, attempts to activate the locomotor circuitry using 5-HT receptor agonists in chronic spinal cats have failed.[221] In these studies, the 5-HT receptor agonists used (quizapine and 5-MeODMT) have strong to moderate affinities on 5-HT$_{1A,1B,\&2C}$ receptors with unknown affinities at 5-HT$_{4,6,\&7}$ receptors,[222] suggesting that one cannot yet eliminate 5-HT receptors as

important to cat locomotor rhythmogenesis. Indeed, the substantial overlap in receptor affinities of selective ligands between adrenergic and serotonergic receptor
subtypes[223] implies that the observation of clonidine, an α_2-adrenergic agonist,
effectively initiating locomotion in spinal cats, must be interpreted cautiously,[221]
particularly since the actual concentration of drug seen by spinal neurons *in vivo* is
unknown. Knowledge of the 5-HT receptor subtype(s) responsible for locomotion
in rat would clearly guide pharmacotherapeutic strategies that seek to activate the
locomotor CPG.

5-HT receptor activation is critical to locomotor rhythmogenesis in the adult
spinal rat.[14,224–226] Presumably, released 5-HT activates receptors in spinal cord normally controlled by bulbospinal serotonergic fibers in the intact animal. That pharmacological approaches or transplantation of serotonergic cells can activate the
locomotor CPG in the spinal rat supports a potent facilitatory role for 5-HT in
locomotor rhythmogenesis. The ability of serotonin (5-HT) to induce rhythmogenesis has also been widely described for hindlimb locomotion in the neonatal
rat.[13,15,227,228] One such study, attempting to identify receptor subtypes underlying
5-HT-evoked locomotion, concluded that both 5-HT$_1$ and 5-HT$_2$ receptors are essential for locomotion.[13] However, receptor ligands were applied at concentrations (i.e.,
50 to 75 µM) which exceed their subtype specificity to identify a site of pharmacological action.[29,222,229] A more recent study by Nistri's group used more appropriate
concentrations of 5-HT receptor ligands to demonstrate that 5-HT$_{1A}$ and 5-HT$_{1B/D}$
receptors contribute to a slowing of the NMDA-induced locomotor rhythm by
5-HT.[230] Another study by this group concluded that 5-HT$_2$ receptors are necessary
for 5-HT-induced locomotor rhythm based on blockade with 1 µM ritanserin.[231]
However, ritanserin and other arylpiperidine derivatives previously used as selective
5-HT$_2$ receptor antagonists (i.e., ketanserin and cyproheptadine) have now been
shown to have a similar antagonist affinity for the 5-HT$_7$ receptor (see Table 3.3).
Similarly, in the mudpuppy *Necturus*, the 5-HT-induced increase in burst amplitude
and cycle duration during NMDA-evoked locomotion was interpreted as acting via
5-HT$_1$/5-HT$_2$ receptor mechanisms due to its block with methiothepin.[232] However,
methiothepin also has very high affinity for 5-HT$_6$ and 5-HT$_7$ receptors (Table 3.3).
Our goal is to characterize the role of 5-HT receptor subtypes on locomotor rhythmogenesis by undertaking a detailed pharmacological dissection of 5-HT receptor
subtypes that increase neuronal excitability, particularly of the receptor subtypes that
remain untested in spinal cord (i.e., 5-HT$_6$ and 5-HT$_7$).

3.3.4.2 Experimental Observations

3.3.4.2.1 5-HT$_7$ Receptor Pharmacology and Locomotion

Figure 3.5 presents some preliminary results presented at the 1998 SFN meeting.[148]
Contrary to the report of Cazalets et al.,[13] 5-HT$_{1A}$ receptors do not appear to be
required for locomotor activity (Fig. 3.5A). In fact, activation of these receptors with
the selective agonist 8-OH-DPAT (0.1 µM) very effectively blocked locomotion, as
did selective activation of 5-HT$_{1B}$ receptors (Fig. 3.5B). Our findings are consistent
with a 5-HT$_1$ receptor-induced slowing of the NMDA-evoked locomotor rhythm.[230]
At the time, we identified the absence of investigations on 5-HT$_{6\&7}$ receptors, cloned

A　5-HT$_{1A}$ receptor ligands

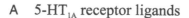
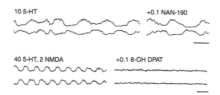

B　5-HT$_{1B}$ receptor agonist

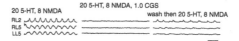

C　5-HT$_2$ receptor ligands

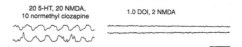

D　5-HT$_7$ receptor ligands

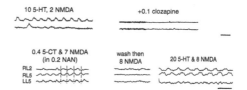

FIGURE 3.5 Locomotor receptor pharmacology. (A) The 5-HT$_{1A}$ receptor agonist 8-OH-DPAT blocks 5-HT-evoked alternating locomotor-like activity (bottom). The 5-HT$_{1A}$ receptor antagonist NAN-190 does not block 5-HT-evoked locomotion (top). (B) The 5-HT$_{1B}$ receptor agonist 7-trifluoromethyl-4-(4-methyl-1-piperazinyl)-pyrrolo[1,2-a]quinoxaline maleate (CGS) does not increase motor activity, may depress motor activity, and prevents the induction of 5-HT-induced locomotion. (C) The high affinity 5-HT$_{2C}$ receptor antagonist normethyl clozapine cannot block 5-HT-evoked locomotion (left). The selective 5-HT$_2$ receptor agonist DOI increases ENG activity (right: note rectified/integrated traces are elevated vertically), but cannot activate alternating locomotor-like activity. (D) The 5-HT$_7$ receptor antagonist clozapine blocks locomotor-like activity (top). The 5-HT$_{7/1A}$ receptor agonist 5-CT is capable of producing weak locomotor-like activity (bottom). All drug concentrations are expressed in μM. Unless otherwise stated, waveforms represent activity in right and left L2 or L5 ventral roots. These roots monitor rhythmic motor activity in flexors and extensors, respectively (Cazalets et al. 1995). Waveforms are presented as rectified and low-pass filtered (1 Hz) to better visualize rhythmical activity. Scale bars are 10 s. RL, right lumbar segment; LL, left lumbar segment.

in 1993,[233] on spinal locomotor function. Importantly, these receptors positively couple to adenylate cyclase, and so should have a net excitatory action. The lack of specific commercially available receptor ligands for these receptors, however, makes electropharmacological characterization complex. Nonetheless, based on the observation that the selective 5-HT$_2$ receptor agonist DOI could not evoke locomotion, while normethyl-clozapine, a specific 5-HT$_{2C}$ receptor antagonist, could not block 5-HT-induced locomotion, even at high concentrations (Fig. 3.5C), we considered the possibility that 5-HT$_{6\ and/or\ 7}$ receptors were involved in locomotor rhythmogenesis. Clozapine (at 100 nm), which blocks these receptors with high affinity, was able to block evoked locomotion (Fig. 3.5D). Moreover, 5-CT, an agonist with very high affinity for the 5-HT$_7$ but not the 5-HT$_6$ receptor, supported alternating locomotor-like activity, albeit weakly (Fig. 3.5D). We assume that 5-CT generates only weak activity because it also potently activates 5-HT$_{1A}$ receptors that oppose locomotor activation. More studies are clearly required. Nonetheless, our preliminary data implicate the 5-HT$_7$ receptor as critical for CPG activation.

3.3.4.2.2   5-HT$_7$ Receptor Immunolabeling and the Locomotor CPG

A clear advance in our understanding of the spinal locomotor CPG would be made if CPG neurons were identifiable with a discrete marker. Accordingly, we have used a recently synthesized antibody to the 5-HT$_7$ receptor and identified strong somatic labeling in a discrete neuronal distribution, consistent with a contribution to locomotor pattern generation (Fig. 3.7). These neurons are observed precisely where lesioning studies have localized the dominant components of the locomotor CPG:[200] the intermediate gray matter of caudal thoracic-rostral lumbar spinal cord segments (compare Fig. 3.6A to Fig. 3.6B). In another experiment, we combined locomotor activity-dependent labeling with 5-HT$_7$ immunostaining. Dramatically, in the T10-L2 spinal segments, 37% of locomotor activity-dependent sulforhodamine-labeled neurons were intensely 5-HT$_7$ immunoreactive, compared to only 9% in more caudal segments L3-S1 (Fig. 3.6C). This is a particularly strong correspondence considering as few as 0.1% of neurons are activity-labeled during locomotion in the spinal cord.[218]

3.4 COMPARISON OF 5-HT ACTIONS TO OTHER MONOAMINES

3.4.1 Evidence that Brainstem Monoamine Transmitters have Common Cellular Neuromodulatory Actions

3.4.1.1 Background

As serotonergic, noradrenergic, and dopaminergic systems have a similarly diffuse distribution in the spinal cord[46,234–239] and their monoamine transmitters frequently exert similar actions,[135,240–242] it is possible that these transmitter systems act at similar spinal sites and by similar mechanisms. However, as there are many bulbospinal

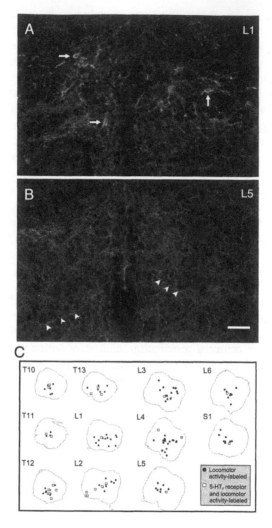

FIGURE 3.6 5-HT$_7$ receptor immunolabeling and locomotor activity-labeled neurons. (A and B) 5-HT$_7$ receptor immunolabeling in the spinal cord central gray matter at L1 (A) and L5 (B) spinal segments. (A) In the rostral lumbar spinal cord, this region is dominated by strong staining of neuronal somata (arrows). (B) This region in the lumbar enlargement is characterized by weaker labeling of somata but obvious punctate labeling, presumably of dendritic processes (arrowheads). (C) A large number of locomotor activity-labeled neurons express intense somatic 5-HT$_7$ receptor immunolabeling. This figure presents a serial reconstruction of neurons labeled with sulforhodamine in an activity-dependent manner during 5-HT-induced locomotion in the isolated spinal cord. Spinal segments T10 through S1 were mapped for activity-dependent labeling as marked. Neurons that were also 5-HT$_{7+}$ (i.e., double-labeled) are presented as red squares. Note that lower-thoracic, rostral-lumbar segments contain the greatest number of double-labeled neurons, consistent with other studies implicating this region in locomotor rhythmogenesis. Each reconstructed spinal segment presents only three 10 μm sections, spaced 300 μm apart, overlaid. Scale bar = 50 μm.

monoaminergic systems and a variety of spinal monoamine metabotropic receptor subtypes,[70,73,243,244] neuromodulation in the spinal cord must be a highly differentiated process. Indeed, different noradrenergic or serotonergic nuclei can exert opposing spinal modulatory actions,[34,181,182] and the actions of 5-HT and NA on the afferent-evoked recruitment of functionally identified spinal neurons can differ considerably.[23,245–246]

Although numerous studies have compared the actions of the monoamine transmitters on the modulation of sensory input onto spinal neurons,[23,186,240–242,245–248] only modifications in extracellular spiking or field potentials were recorded, and transmitters were applied by iontophoresis.[245] Thus, the effects of monoamines on intrinsic cellular properties and synaptic potentials in individual neurons were not studied. We used a more direct examination of the actions of the monoamines with intracellular recordings to provide additional insight into monoamine transmitter function.[5,6,80,249]

3.4.1.2   Experimental Observations

Recordings from DDH neurons in the spinal slice preparation were used to compare the actions of 5-HT, NA, DA, and acetylcholine (ACh) on dorsal root stimulation-evoked EPSPs and on membrane cellular properties. In most cells, evoked EPSPs were depressed by the bulbospinal transmitters 5-HT, NA, and DA, while ACh generally facilitated evoked responses (Fig. 3.7A). Although none of the transmitters modified neuronal passive membrane properties, the monoamines increased the number of spikes in most neurons that originally fired phasically in response to depolarizing current steps (Fig. 3.7B). These results demonstrate that even though the deep dorsal horn contains many functionally distinct subpopulations of neurons, the bulbospinal monoamine transmitters can act at both synaptic and cellular sites to alter neuronal sensory integrative properties in a rather predictable manner.

3.5   CONCLUDING REMARKS

We hope that our recent experimental findings help highlight the diversity of modulatory spinal actions produced by 5-HT via actions at different receptor subtypes. However, because several of the selective 5-HT receptor ligands have actions at more that one receptor subtype, both earlier (3.2.2) and our current pharmacological studies (3.3) must be interpreted cautiously. We have interpreted our findings in relation to the aforementioned Hypothesis #2 so that, for example, the facilitatory actions of the $5\text{-HT}_{1/7}$ agonist 8-OH-DPAT were interpreted as acting via 5-HT_7 receptor activation ($\uparrow$cAMP) while the depressant actions of the $5\text{-HT}_{1/7}$ agonist 5-CT were interpreted as acting via 5-HT_1 receptor activation ($\downarrow$cAMP). Additional work using more selective ligands is required to determine whether these interpretations are valid. Moreover, the minority of previous pharmacological studies that observed actions that oppose Hypothesis #2 must also be re-examined before the generality of this hypothesis can be considered disproved.

Last, important future studies are required to (i) better determine the distribution of spinal 5-HT receptor subtypes using receptor-selective immunolabeling and *in situ* hybridization, (ii) identify the links between distinct bulbospinal serotonergic

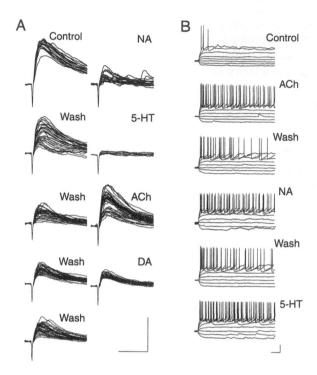

FIGURE 3.7 Comparing the actions of monoamine transmitters in individual neurons. (A) NA, 5-HT and DA reversibly depress primary afferent-evoked EPSPs while ACh facilitated evoked responses. These actions were common in many of the neurons recorded from the deep dorsal horn. (B) The monoamines convert neuronal firing properties from phasic to repetitive in response to current injection. Current steps were delivered at 20 pA increments and voltage responses are presented superimposed. Figures are presented as raw waveforms overlaid. Scale bars are 20 mV, 200 ms.

systems and the control of different spinal modulatory states, and (iii) determine whether there is a link between distinct bulbospinal systems and actions at specific 5-HT receptor subtypes. Clearly, many more studies are required before we can obtain a satisfactory understanding of the descending serotonergic control of spinal cord function.

ACKNOWLEDGMENTS

We would like to thank Carolyn Gibbs and Michael Sawchuk for providing expert technical assistance. Support for these studies was provided by grants from the Manitoba Health Research Council, the Medical Research Council of Canada, the National Science and Engineering Research Council of Canada (NSERC), the Christopher Reeve Paralysis Foundation, and the National Institutes of Health (NINDS). S.G. received studentship funding from the Manitoba Neurotrauma Initiative, D.M. from NSERC, and B.S. from the Physiotherapy Foundation of Canada.

ABBREVIATIONS

5-CT: 5-carboxamidotryptamine
5-HT: 5-hydroxytryptamine; serotonin
8-OH-DPAT: 8-hydroxy-2-(di-n-propylamino)tetralin
ACh: acetylcholine
CGS: 7-trifluoromethyl-4-(4-methyl-1-piperazinyl)-pyrrolo[1,2-a]quinoxaline maleate
CPG: central pattern generator
DA: dopamine
DDH: deep dorsal horn
DLF: dorsolateral funiculus
DOI: 1-(2,5-dimethoxy-4-iodophenyl)-2-amino-propane
E: embryonic day
EPSP: excitatory postsynaptic potential
GABA: γ-aminobutyric acid
LLRF: long-lasting reflex facilitation
LTD: long-term depression
LTP: long-term potentiation
NA: noradrenaline
NMDA: N-methyl-D-aspartate
P: postnatal day
PAD: primary afferent depolarization
PKC: protein kinase C
VLF: ventrolateral funiculus

REFERENCES

1. Korner, P.I., Head, G.A., Badoer, E., Bobik, A., and Angus, J.A., Role of brain amine transmitters and some neuromodulators in blood pressure, heart rate, and baroreflex control, *J. Cardiovasc. Pharmacol.*, 10 (Suppl. 12), S26, 1987.
2. Urban, M.O., Coutinho, S.V., and Gebhart, G.F., Biphasic modulation of visceral nociception by neurotensin in rat rostral ventromedial medulla, *J. Pharmacol. Exp. Ther.*, 290, 207, 1999.
3. Eide, P.K., Joly, N.M., and Hole, K., The role of spinal cord 5-HT$_{1A}$ and 5-HT$_{1B}$ receptors in the modulation of a spinal nociceptive reflex, *Brain Res.*, 536, 195, 1990.
4. Gjerstad, J., Tjolsen, A., and Hole, K., The effect of 5-HT$_{1A}$ receptor stimulation on nociceptive dorsal horn neurones in rats, *Eur. J. Pharmacol.*, 318, 315, 1996.
5. Khasabov, S.G., Lopez-Garcia, J.A., Asghar, A.U., and King, A.E., Modulation of afferent-evoked neurotransmission by 5-HT3 receptors in young rat dorsal horn neurones *in vitro*: a putative mechanism of 5-HT3 induced anti-nociception, *Br. J. Pharmacol.*, 127 843, 1999.
6. Lopez-Garcia, J.A. and King, A.E., Pre- and post-synaptic actions of 5-hydroxytryptamine in the rat lumbar dorsal horn *in vitro*: Implications for somatosensory transmission, *Eur. J. Neurosci.*, 8, 2188, 1996.
7. Tjolsen, A., Berge, O.-G., and Hole, K., Lesions of bulbo-spinal serotonergic or noradrenergic pathways reduce nociception as measured by the formalin test, *Acta Physiol. Scand.*, 142, 229, 1991.

8. Hounsgaard, J. and Kiehn, O., Serotonin-induced bistability of turtle motoneurones caused by a nifedipine-sensitive calcium plateau potential, *J. Physiol. (Lond.)*, 414, 265, 1989.

9. Hounsgaard, J., Hultborn, H., Jespersen, B., and Kiehn, O., Bistability of alpha-motoneurones in the decerebrate cat and in the acute spinal cat after intravenous 5-hydroxytryptophan, *J. Physiol. (Lond.)*, 405, 345, 1988.

10. Hsiao, C.F., Del Negro, C.A., Trueblood, P.R., and Chandler, S.H., Ionic basis for serotonin-induced bistable membrane properties in guinea pig trigeminal motoneurons, *J. Neurophysiol.*, 79, 2847, 1998.

11. Viala, D. and Buser, P., The effects of dopa and 5-HTP on rhythmic efferent discharges in hind limb nerves in the rabbit, *Brain Res.*, 12, 437, 1969.

12. Barbeau, H. and Rossignol, S., Initiation and modulation of the locomotor pattern in the adult chronic spinal cat by noradrenergic, serotonergic and dopaminergic drugs, *Brain Res.*, 546, 250, 1991.

13. Cazalets, J.R., Sqalli-Houssaini, Y., and Clarac, F., Activation of the central pattern generators for locomotion by serotonin and excitatory amino acids in neonatal rat, *J. Physiol. (Lond.)*, 455, 187, 1992.

14. Gerin, C., Becquet, D., and Privat, A., Direct evidence for the link between monoaminergic descending pathways and motor activity. 1. A study with microdialysis probes implanted in the ventral funiculus of the spinal cord, *Brain Res.*, 704, 191, 1995.

15. Kiehn, O. and Kjaerulff, O., Spatiotemporal characteristics of 5-HT and dopamine-induced rhythmic hindlimb activity in the *in vitro* neonatal rat, *J. Neurophysiol.*, 75, 1472, 1996.

16. Cowley, K.C. and Schmidt, B.J., Regional distribution of the locomotor pattern-generating network in the neonatal rat spinal cord, *J. Neurophys.*, 77, 247, 1997.

17. Fyda, D. and Jordan, L.M. Role of spinal monoaminergic systems in brainstem-evoked locomotion in the neonatal rat. *Soc. Neurosci. Abst.*, 25, 1916, 1999.

18. Takahashi, T. and Berger, A.J., Direct excitation of rat spinal motoneurones by serotonin, *J. Physiol. (Lond.)*, 423, 63, 1990.

19. Wang, M.Y. and Dun, N.J., 5-Hydroxytryptamine responses in neonate rat motoneurones *in vitro*, *J. Physiol. (Lond.)*, 430, 87, 1990.

20. Sillar, K.T. and Simmers, A.J., 5-HT induces NMDA receptor-mediated intrinsic oscillations in embryonic amphibian spinal neurons, *Proc. R. Soc. Lond. (Biol.)*, 255, 139, 1994.

21. MacLean, J.N., Cowley, K.C., and Schmidt, B.J., NMDA receptor-mediated oscillatory activity in the neonatal rat spinal cord is serotonin dependent, *J. Neurophysiol.*, 79, 2804, 1998.

22. Jankowska, E., Hammar, I., Chojnicka, B., and Heden, C.H., Effects of monoamines on interneurons in four spinal reflex pathways from group I and/or group II muscle afferents, *Eur. J. Neurosci.*, 12, 701, 2000.

23. Jankowska, E., Hammar, I., Djouhri, L., Heden, C., Szabo, L.Z., and Yin, X.K., Modulation of responses of four types of feline ascending tract neurons by serotonin and noradrenaline, *Eur. J. Neurosci.*, 9, 1375, 1997.

24. Willis, W.D., Effects of peripherally and centrally administered serotonin on primate spinothalamic neurons, *Adv. Exp. Med. Biol.*, 133, 105, 1981.

25. Jordan, L.M., Kenshalo, D.R., Jr., Martin, R.F., Haber, L.H., and Willis, W.D., Depression of primate spinothalamic tract neurons by iontophoretic application of 5-hydroxytryptamine, *Pain*, 5, 135, 1978.

26. Jordan, L.M., Kenshalo, D.R., Jr., Martin, R.F., Haber, L.H., and Willis, W.D., Two populations of spinothalamic tract neurons with opposite responses to 5-hydroxytryptamine, *Brain Res.*, 164, 342, 1979.

27. Jacobs, B.L. and Fornal, C.A., 5-HT and motor control: A hypothesis, *Trends Neurosci.*, 16, 346, 1993.

28. Willis, W.D., Jr. and Coggeshall, R.E., *Sensory Mechanisms of the Spinal Cord*, Plenum Press, New York, 1991.

29. Wallis, D.I., 5-HT receptors involved in initiation or modulation of motor patterns: Opportunities for drug development, *Trends Pharmacol. Sci.*, 15, 288, 1994.

30. Peng, Y.B., Lin, Q., and Willis, W.D., The role of 5-HT3 receptors in periaqueductal gray-induced inhibition of nociceptive dorsal horn neurons in rats, *J. Pharmacol. Exp. Ther.*, 276, 116, 1996.

31. Zemlan, F.P., 5-HT(1A) Receptors mediate the effect of the bulbospinal serotonin system on spinal dorsal horn nociceptive neurons, *Pharmacology*, 48, 1, 1994.

32. Zhang, Z.-H., Yang, S.-W., Chen, J.-Y., Xie, Y.-F., Qiao, J.-T., and Dafny, N., Interaction of serotonin and norepinephrine in spinal antinociception, *Brain Res. Bull.*, 38, 167, 1995.

33. Elliott, P. and Wallis, D.I., Serotonin and L-norepinephrine as mediators of altered excitability in neonatal rat motoneurons studied *in vitro*, *Neuroscience*, 47, 533, 1992.

34. Calejesan, A.A., Ch'ang, M.H., and Zhuo, M., Spinal serotonergic receptors mediate facilitation of a nociceptive reflex by subcutaneous formalin injection into the hindpaw in rats, *Brain Res.*, 798, 46, 1998.

35. Wei, F., Dubner, R., and Ren, K., Nucleus reticularis gigantocellularis and nucleus raphe magnus in the brain stem exert opposite effects on behavioral hyperalgesia and spinal Fos protein expression after peripheral inflammation, *Pain*, 80, 127, 1999.

36. Hille, B., Modulation of ion-channel function by G-protein-coupled receptors, *Trends Neurosci.*, 17, 531, 1994.

37. Harris-Warrick, R.M. and Marder, E., Modulation of neural networks for behavior, *Annu. Rev. Neurosci.*, 14, 39, 1991.

38. Katz, P.S. and Frost, W.N., Intrinsic neuromodulation: Altering neuronal circuits from within, *Trends Neurosci.*, 19, 54, 1996.

39. Anwyl, R., Neurophysiological actions of 5-hydroxytryptamine in the vertebrate nervous system, *Prog. Neurobiol.*, 35, 451, 1990.

40. Aghajanian, G.K., Sprouse, J.S., Sheldon, P., and Rasmussen, K., Electrophysiology of the central serotonin system: receptor subtypes and transducer mechanisms, *Ann. NY Acad. Sci.*, 600, 93, 1990.

41. Roth, B.L., Lopez, E., Patel, S., and Kroeze, W.K., The multiplicity of serotonin receptors: Uselessly diverse molecules or an embarrassment of riches?, *The Neuroscientist*, 6, 252, 2000.

42. Dahlström, A. and Fuxe, K., Evidence for the existence of monoamine neurons in the central nervous system, *Acta. Physiol. Scand.*, Suppl. 64, 1, 1965.

43. Dahlström, A. and Fuxe, K., Localization of monoamines in the lower brain stem, *Experientia*, 20, 398, 1964.

44. Jones, B.E., Reticular formation: cytoarchitecture, transmitters, and projections, in Paxinos, G., Ed., *The Rat Nervous System,* Academic Press, San Diego, 1995, 155.

45. Steinbusch, H.W., Distribution of serotonin-immunoreactivity in the central nervous system of the rat-cell bodies and terminals, *Neuroscience*, 6, 557, 1981.

46. Marlier, L., Sandillon, F., Poulat, P., Rajaofetra, N., Geffard, M., and Privat, A., Serotonergic innervation of the dorsal horn of rat spinal cord: Light and electron microscopic immunocytochemical study, *J. Neurocytol.*, 20, 310, 1991.

47. Halliday, G., Harding, A., and Paxinos, G., Serotonin and tachykinin systems, in Paxinos, G., Ed., *The Rat Nervous System*, Academic Press, San Diego, 1995, 929.

48. Tork, I., Anatomy of the serotonergic system, *Ann. NY Acad. Sci.*, 600, 9, 1990.

49. Skagerberg, G. and Bjorklund, A., Topographic principles in the spinal projections of serotonergic and non-serotonergic brainstem neurons in the rat, *Neuroscience*, 15, 445, 1985.

50. Lauder, J.M., Ontogeny of the serotonergic system in the rat: serotonin as a developmental signal, *Ann. NY Acad. Sci.*, 600, 297, 1990.

51. Bregman, B.S., Development of serotonin immunoreactivity in the rat spinal cord and its plasticity after neonatal spinal cord lesions, *Dev. Brain Res.*, 34, 245, 1987.

52. Ziskind-Conhaim, L., Seebach, B.S., and Gao, B.-X., Changes in serotonin-induced potentials during spinal cord development, *J. Neurophysiol.*, 69, 1338, 1993.

53. Fitzgerald, M. and Koltzenburg, M., The functional development of descending inhibitory pathways in the dorsolateral funiculus of the newborn rat spinal cord, *Brain Res.*, 389, 270, 1986.

54. Miyata, Y., Nakano, S., and Yasuda, H., Postnatal transient expression of long-lasting descending inhibitory effect on spinal reflexes in the rat, *Neurosci. Res.*, 4, 268, 1987.

55. Wallis, D.I., Wu, J., and Wang, X., Descending inhibition in the neonate rat spinal cord is mediated by 5-hydroxytryptamine, *Neuropharmacology*, 32, 73, 1993.

56. Magnuson, D.S.K., Schramm, M.J., and MacLean, J.N., Long-duration, frequency-dependent motor responses evoked by ventrolateral funiculus stimulation in the neonatal rat spinal cord, *Neurosci. Lett.*, 192, 97, 1995.

57. Magnuson, D.S.K. and Trinder, T.C., Locomotor rhythm evoked by ventrolateral funiculus stimulation in the neonatal rat spinal cord *in vitro*, *J. Neurophys.*, 77, 200, 1997.

58. Brocard, F., Vinay, L., and Clarac, F., Gradual development of the ventral funiculus input to lumbar motoneurons in the neonatal rat, *Neuroscience*, 90, 1543, 1999.

59. Fitzgerald, M., The post-natal development of cutaneous afferent fiber input and receptive field organization in the rat dorsal horn, *J. Physiol. (Lond.)*, 364, 1, 1985.

60. Hokfelt, T., Broberger, C., Xu, Z.Q., Sergeyev, V., Ubink, R., and Diez, M., Neuropeptides — an overview, *Neuropharmacology*, 39, 1337, 2000.

61. Poulat, P., Marlier, L., Rajaofetra, N., and Privat, A., 5-Hydroxytryptamine, substance P and thyrotropin-releasing hormone synapses in the intermediolateral cell column of the rat thoracic spinal cord, *Neurosci. Lett.*, 136, 19, 1992.

62. Wu, W., Elde, R. and Wessendorf, M.W., Organization of the serotonergic innervation of spinal neurons in rats — III. Differential serotonergic innervation of somatic and parasympathetic preganglionic motoneurons as determined by patterns of co-existing peptides, *Neuroscience*, 55, 223, 1993.

63. Hokfelt, T., Arvidsson, U., Cullheim, S., Millhorn, D., Nicholas, A.P., Pieribone, V., Seroogy, K., and Ulfhake, B., Multiple messengers in descending serotonin neurons: localization and functional implications, *J. Chem. Neuroanat.*, 18, 75, 2000.

64. Schotland, J.L., Shupliakov, O., Grillner, S., and Brodin, L., Synaptic and nonsynaptic monoaminergic neuron systems in the lamprey spinal cord, *J. Comp. Neurol.*, 372, 229, 1996.

65. Zoli, M. and Agnati, L.F., Wiring and volume transmission in the central nervous system: The concept of closed and open synapses, *Prog. Neurobiol.*, 49, 363, 1996.

66. Hoyer, D., Clarke, D.E., Fozard, J.R., Hartig, P.R., Martin, G.R., Mylecharane, E.J., Saxena, P.R., and Humphrey, P.P.A., International union of pharmacology classification of receptors for 5-hydroxytryptamine (Serotonin), *Pharmacol. Rev.*, 46, 157, 1994.

67. Barnes, N.M. and Sharp, T., A review of central 5-HT receptors and their function, *Neuropharmacology*, 38, 1083, 1999.

68. Kennett, G.A., Serotonin receptors and their function, TOCRIS, 1998.

69. Ogilvie, J., Wigglesworth, M., Appleby, L., Kingston, T.O., and Clarke, R.W., On the role of 5-HT1B/1D receptors in modulating transmission in a spinal reflex pathway in the decerebrated rabbit, *Br. J. Pharmacol.*, 128, 781, 1999.

70. Huang, J.C. and Peroutka, S.J., Identification of 5-hydroxytryptamine binding site subtypes in rat spinal cord, *Brain Res.*, 436, 173, 1987.

71. Daval, G., Verge, D., Basbaum, A.I., Bourgoin, S., and Hamon, M., Autoradiographic evidence of serotonin 1 binding sites on primary afferent fibers in the dorsal horn of the rat spinal cord, *Neurosci. Lett.*, 83, 71, 1987.

72. Laporte, A.M., Fattaccini, C.M., Lombard, M.C., Chauveau, J., and Hamon, M., Effects of dorsal rhizotomy and selective lesion of serotonergic and noradrenergic systems on 5-HT1A, 5-HT1B, and 5-HT3 receptors in the rat spinal cord, *J. Neural Transm. Gen. Sect.*, 100, 207, 1995.

73. Marlier, L., Teilhac, J.-R., Cerruti, C., and Privat, A., Autoradiographic mapping of 5-HT_1, 5-HT_{1A}, 5-HT_{1B} and 5-HT_2 receptors in the rat spinal cord, *Brain Res.*, 550, 15, 1991.

74. Ridet, J.-L., Tamir, H., and Privat, A., Direct immunocytochemical localization of 5-hydroxytryptamine receptors in the adult rat spinal cord: A light and electron microscopic study using an anti-idiotypic antiserum, *J. Neurosci. Res.*, 38, 109, 1994.

75. Dickenson, A.H., Rivot, J.P., Chaouch, A., Besson, J.M., and Le Bars, D., Diffuse noxious inhibitory controls (DNIC) in the rat with or without pCPA pretreatment, *Brain Res.*, 216, 313, 1981.

76. Brown, L., Amedro, J., Williams, G., and Smith, D., A pharmacological analysis of the rat spinal cord serotonin (5-HT) autoreceptor, *Eur. J. Pharmacol.*, 145, 163, 1988.

77. Murphy, R.M. and Zemlan, F.P., Selective 5-HT1B agonists identify the 5-HT autoreceptor in lumbar spinal cord of rat, *Neuropharmacology*, 27, 37, 1988.

78. Castro, M.E., Pascual, J., Romon, T., del Arco, C., del Olmo, E., and Pazos, A., Differential distribution of [3H]sumatriptan binding sites (5-HT1B, 5-HT1D and 5-HT1F receptors) in human brain: focus on brainstem and spinal cord, *Neuropharmacology*, 36, 535, 1997.

79. Mills, A. and Martin, G.R., Autoradiographic mapping of [³H]sumatriptan binding in cat brain stem and spinal cord, *Eur. J. Pharmacol.*, 280, 175, 1995.

80. Lopez-Garcia, J.A., Serotonergic modulation of the responses to excitatory amino acids of rat dorsal horn neurons *in vitro*: implications for somatosensory transmission, *Eur. J. Neurosci.*, 10, 1341, 1998.

81. el Yassir, N. and Fleetwood-Walker, S.M., A 5-HT1-type receptor mediates the antinociceptive effect of nucleus raphe magnus stimulation in the rat, *Brain Res.*, 523, 92, 1990.

82. Noga, B.R., Bras, H., and Jankowska, E., Transmission from group II muscle afferents is depressed by stimulation of locus coeruleus/subcoeruleus, Kölliker-Fuse and raphe nuclei in the cat, *Exp. Brain Res.*, 88, 502, 1992.

83. Jankowska, E., Szabo Läckberg, Z., and Dyrehag, L.E., Effects of monoamines on transmission from group II muscle afferents in sacral segments in the cat, *Eur. J. Neurosci.*, 6, 1058, 1994.

84. Jankowska, E., Krutki, P., Szabo Läckberg, Z., and Hammar, I., Effects of serotonin on dorsal horn dorsal spinocerebellar tract neurons, *Neuroscience*, 67, 489, 1995.

85. Gharagozloo, A., Holohean, A.M., Hackman, J.C., and Davidoff, R.A., Serotonin and GABA-induced depolarizations of frog primary afferent fibers, *Brain Res.*, 532, 19, 1990.

86. Alhaider, A.A. and Wilcox, G.L., Differential roles of 5-hydroxytryptamine1A and 5-hydroxytryptamine 1B receptor subtypes in modulating spinal nociceptive transmission in mice, *J. Pharmacol. Exp. Ther.*, 265, 378, 1993.

87. el Yassir, N., Fleetwood-Walker, S.M., and Mitchell, R., Heterogeneous effects of serotonin in the dorsal horn of rat: the involvement of 5-HT1 receptor subtypes, *Brain Res.*, 456, 147, 1988.

88. Ali, Z., Wu, G., Kozlov, A., and Barasi, S., The actions of 5-HT1 agonists and antagonists on nociceptive processing in the rat spinal cord: results from behavioural and electrophysiological studies, *Brain Res.*, 661, 83, 1994.

89. Oyama, T., Ueda, M., Kuraishi, Y., Akaike, A., and Satoh, M., Dual effect of serotonin on formalin-induced nociception in the rat spinal cord, *Neurosci. Res.*, 25, 129, 1996.

90. Wu, S.Y., Wang, M.Y., and Dun, N.J., Serotonin via presynaptic 5-HT$_1$ receptors attenuates synaptic transmission to immature rat motoneurons *in vitro*, *Brain Res.*, 554, 111, 1991.

91. Wallis, D.I. and Wu, J., FAST and SLOW ipsilateral and contralateral spinal reflexes in the neonate rat are modulated by 5-HT, *Gen. Pharmacol.*, 23, 1035, 1992.

92. Clarke, R.W., Ogilvie, J., and Houghton, A.K., Enhancement and depression of spinal reflexes by 8-hydroxy-2-(di-n-propylamino)tetralin in the decerebrated and spinalized rabbit: involvement of 5-HT1A and non-5-HT1A receptors, *Br. J. Pharmacol.*, 122, 631, 1997.

93. Holohean, A.M., Hackman, J.C., and Davidoff, R.A., Changes in membrane potential of frog motoneurons induced by activation of serotonin receptor subtypes, *Neuroscience*, 34, 555, 1990.

94. Zhang, L., Effects of 5-hydroxytryptamine on cat spinal motoneurons, *Can. J. Physiol. Pharmacol.*, 69, 154, 1991.

95. Legendre, P., Guzman, A., Dupouy, B., and Vincent, J.D., Excitatory effect of serotonin on pacemaker neurons in spinal cord cell culture, *Neuroscience*, 28, 201, 1989.

96. Pranzatelli, M.R., Murthy, J.N., and Pluchino, R.S., Identification of spinal 5-HT1C binding sites in the rat: characterization of [3H]mesulergine binding, *J. Pharmacol. Exp. Ther.*, 261, 161, 1992.

97. Pazos, A., Cortes, R., and Palacios, J.M., Quantitative autoradiographic mapping of serotonin receptors in the rat brain. II. Serotonin-2 receptors, *Brain Res.*, 346, 231, 1985.

98. Maeshima, T., Ito, R., Hamada, S., Senzaki, K., Hamaguchi-Hamada, K., Shutoh, F., and Okado, N., The cellular localization of 5-HT2A receptors in the spinal cord and spinal ganglia of the adult rat, *Brain Res.*, 797, 118, 1998.

99. Cornea-Hebert, V., Riad, M., Wu, C., Singh, S.K., and Descarries, L., Cellular and subcellular distribution of the serotonin 5-HT2A receptor in the central nervous system of adult rat, *J. Comp. Neurol.*, 409, 187, 1999.

100. Helton, L.A., Thor, K.B., and Baez, M., 5-hydroxytryptamine$_{2A}$, 5-hydroxytryptamine$_{2B}$, and 5-hydroxytryptamine$_{2C}$ receptor mRNA expression in the spinal cord of rat, cat, monkey and human, *Neuroreport*, 5, 2617, 1994.

101. Molineaux, S.M., Jessell, T.M., Axel, R., and Julius, D., 5-HT1c receptor is a prominent serotonin receptor subtype in the central nervous system, *Proc. Natl. Acad. Sci. U.S.A.*, 86, 6793, 1989.

102. Pompeiano, M., Palacios, J.M., and Mengod, G., Distribution of the serotonin 5-HT2 receptor family mRNAs: comparison between 5-HT2A and 5-HT2C receptors, *Brain Res. Mol. Brain Res.*, 23, 163, 1994.

103. Butler, P.D., Pranzatelli, M.R., and Barkai, A.I., Regional central serotonin-2 receptor binding and phosphoinositide turnover in rats with 5,7-dihydroxytryptamine lesions, *Brain Res. Bull.*, 24, 125, 1990.

104. Pranzatelli, M.R., Neonatal 5,7-DHT lesions upregulate [3H]mesulergine-labelled spinal 5-HT1C binding sites in the rat, *Brain Res. Bull.*, 25, 151, 1990.

105. Crisp, T., Stafinsky, J.L., Spanos, L.J., Uram, M., Perni, V.C., and Donepudi, H.B., Analgesic effects of serotonin and receptor-selective serotonin agonists in the rat spinal cord, *Gen. Pharmacol.*, 22, 247, 1991.

106. Holohean, A.M., Hackman, J.C., Shope, S.B., and Davidoff, R.A., Activation of 5-HT$_{1C/2}$ receptors depresses polysynaptic reflexes and excitatory amino acid-induced motoneuron responses in frog spinal cord, *Brain Res.*, 579, 8, 1992.

107. Hori, Y., Endo, K., and Takahashi, T., Long-lasting synaptic facilitation induced by serotonin in superficial dorsal horn neurones of the rat spinal cord, *J. Physiol. (Lond.)*, 492, 867, 1996.

108. Tan, H. and Miletic, V., Diverse actions of 5-hydroxytryptamine on frog spinal dorsal horn neurons *in vitro*, *Neuroscience*, 49, 913, 1992.

109. Yamazaki, J., Fukuda, H., Nagao, T., and Ono, H., 5-HT$_2$/5-HT$_{1C}$ receptor-mediated facilitatory action on unit activity of ventral horn cells in rat spinal cord slices, *Eur. J. Pharmacol.*, 220, 237, 1992.

110. Fone, K.C., Johnson, J.V., Bennett, G.W., and Marsden, C.A., Involvement of 5-HT2 receptors in the behaviours produced by intrathecal administration of selected 5-HT agonists and the TRH analogue (CG 3509) to rats, *Br. J. Pharmacol.*, 96, 599, 1989.

111. Fone, K.C., Robinson, A.J., and Marsden, C.A., Characterization of the 5-HT receptor subtypes involved in the motor behaviours produced by intrathecal administration of 5-HT agonists in rats, *Br. J. Pharmacol.*, 103, 1547, 1991.

112. Watson, N.V. and Gorzalka, B.B., Concurrent wet dog shaking and inhibition of male rat copulation after ventromedial brainstem injection of the 5-HT2 agonist DOI, *Neurosci. Lett.*, 141, 25, 1992.

113. Eide, P.K. and Hole, K., Different role of 5-HT$_{1A}$ and 5-HT$_2$ receptors in spinal cord in the control of nociceptive responsiveness, *Neuropharmacology*, 30, 727, 1991.

114. Mjellem, N., Lund, A., and Hole, K., Different functions of spinal 5-HT$_{1A}$ and 5-HT$_2$ receptor subtypes in modulating behaviour induced by excitatory amino acid receptor agonists in mice, *Brain Res.*, 626, 78, 1993.

115. Nagano, N., Ono, H., and Fukuda, H., Functional significance of subtypes of 5-HT receptors in the rat spinal reflex pathway, *Gen. Pharmacol.*, 1, 789, 1988.

116. Yamazaki, J., Ono, H., and Nagao, T., Stimulatory and inhibitory effects of serotonergic hallucinogens on spinal mono- and polysynaptic reflex pathways in the rat, *Neuropharmacology*, 31, 635, 1992.

117. Clarke, R.W., Harris, J., and Houghton, A.K., Spinal 5-HT-receptors and tonic modulation of transmission through a withdrawal reflex pathway in the decerebrated rabbit, *Br. J. Pharmacol.*, 119, 1167, 1996.

118. Anderson, M.F., Mokler, D.J., and Winterson, B.J., Inhibition of chronic hindlimb flexion in rat: Evidence for mediation by 5-hydroxytryptamine, *Brain Res.*, 541, 216, 1991.

119. Jackson, D.A. and White, S.R., Receptor subtypes mediating facilitation by serotonin of excitability of spinal motoneurons, *Neuropharmacology*, 29, 787, 1990.

120. Nance, P.W., A comparison of clonidine, cyproheptadine and baclofen in spastic spinal cord injured patients, *J. Am. Paraplegia Soc.*, 17, 150, 1994.

121. Holohean, A.M., Hackman, J.C., and Davidoff, R.A., An *in vitro* study of the effects of serotonin on frog primary afferent terminals, *Neurosci. Lett.*, 113, 175, 1990.
122. Zhuo, M. and Gebhart, G.F., Spinal serotonin receptors mediate descending facilitation of a nociceptive reflex from the nuclei reticularis gigantocellularis and gigantocellularis pars alpha in the rat, *Brain Res.*, 550, 35, 1991.
123. Hamon, M., Gallissot, M.C., Menard, F., Gozlan, H., Bourgoin, S., and Verge, D., 5-HT3 receptor binding sites are on capsaicin-sensitive fibers in the rat spinal cord, *Eur. J. Pharmacol.*, 164, 315, 1989.
124. Gehlert, D.R., Gackenheimer, S.L., Wong, D.T., and Robertson, D.W., Localization of 5-HT3 receptors in the rat brain using [3H]LY278584, *Brain Res.*, 553, 149, 1991.
125. Laporte, A.M., Koscielniak, T., Ponchant, M., Verge, D., Hamon, M., and Gozlan, H., Quantitative autoradiographic mapping of 5-HT3 receptors in the rat CNS using [125I]iodo-zacopride and [3H]zacopride as radioligands, *Synapse*, 10, 271, 1992.
126. Kidd, E.J., Laporte, A.M., Langlois, X., Fattaccini, C.-M., Doyen, C., Lombard, M.C., Gozlan, H., and Hamon, M., 5-HT$_3$ receptors in the rat central nervous system are mainly located on nerve fibers and terminals, *Brain Res.*, 612, 289, 1993.
127. Laporte, A.M., Doyen, C., Nevo, I.T., Chauveau, J., Hauw, J.J., and Hamon, M., Autoradiographic mapping of serotonin 5-HT1A, 5-HT1D, 5-HT2A and 5-HT3 receptors in the aged human spinal cord, *J. Chem. Neuroanat.*, 11, 67, 1996.
128. Doucet, E., Miquel, M.C., Nosjean, A., Verge, D., Hamon, M., and Emerit, M.B., Immunolabeling of the rat central nervous system with antibodies partially selective of the short form of the 5-HT3 receptor, *Neuroscience*, 95, 881, 2000.
129. Tecott, L.H., Maricq, A.V., and Julius, D., Nervous system distribution of the serotonin 5-HT$_3$ receptor mRNA, *Proc. Natl. Acad. Sci. U.S.A.*, 90, 1430, 1993.
130. Kia, H.K., Miquel, M.-C., McKernan, R.M., Laporte, A.-M., Lombard, M.-C., Bourgoin, S., Hamon, M., and Vergé, D., Localization of 5-HT$_3$ receptors in the rat spinal cord: Immunohistochemistry and *in situ* hybridization, *Neuroreport*, 6, 257, 1995.
131. Tsuchiya, M., Yamazaki, H., and Hori, Y., Enkephalinergic neurons express 5-HT3 receptors in the spinal cord dorsal horn: single cell RT-PCR analysis, *Neuroreport*, 10, 2749, 1999.
132. Morales, R., Battenberg, E., and Bloom, F.E., Distribution of neurons expressing immunoreactivity for the 5HT$_3$ receptor subtype in the rat brain and spinal cord, *J. Comp. Neurol.*, 402, 385, 1998.
133. Rende, M., Morales, M., Brizi, E., Bruno, R., Bloom, F., and Sanna, P.P., Modulation of serotonin 5-HT3 receptor expression in injured adult rat spinal cord motoneurons, *Brain Res.*, 823, 234, 1999.
134. Alhaider, A.A., Lei, S.Z., and Wilcox, G.L., Spinal 5-HT$_3$ receptor-mediated antinociception: Possible release of GABA, *J. Neurosci.*, 11, 1881, 1991.
135. Bell, J.A. and Matsumiya, T., Inhibitory effects of dorsal horn and excitant effects of ventral horn intraspinal microinjections of norepinephrine and serotonin in the cat, *Life Sci.*, 29, 1507, 1981.
136. Giordano, J., Antinociceptive effects of intrathecally administered 2-methylserotonin in developing rats, *Brain Res. Dev. Brain Res.*, 98, 142, 1997.
137. Bardin, L., Lavarenne, J., and Eschalier, A., Serotonin receptor subtypes involved in the spinal antinociceptive effect of 5-HT in rats, *Pain*, 86, 11, 2000.
138. Glaum, S.R., Proudfit, H.K., and Anderson, E.G., Reversal of the antinociceptive effects of intrathecally administered serotonin in the rat by a selective 5-HT3 receptor antagonist, *Neurosci. Lett.*, 95, 313, 1988.
139. Glaum, S.R., Proudfit, H.K., and Anderson, E.G., 5-HT$_3$ receptors modulate spinal nociceptive reflexes, *Brain Res.*, 510, 12, 1990.

140. Holohean, A.M., Hackman, J.C., and Davidoff, R.A., Modulation of frog spinal cord interneuronal activity by activation of 5-HT$_3$ receptors, *Brain Res.*, 704, 184, 1995.
141. Gao, B.-X. and Ziskind-Conhaim, L., Development of chemosensitivity in serotonin-deficient spinal cords of rat embryos, *Dev. Biol.*, 158, 79, 1993.
142. Chesnoy-Marchais, D., Potentiation of chloride responses to glycine by three 5-HT$_3$ antagonists in rat spinal neurones, *Br. J. Pharmacol.*, 118, 2115, 1996.
143. Maksay, G., Bidirectional allosteric modulation of strychnine-sensitive glycine receptors by tropeines and 5-HT3 serotonin receptor ligands, *Neuropharmacology*, 37, 1633, 1998.
144. Larkman, P.M. and Kelly, J.S., Modulation of I$_H$ by 5-HT in neonatal rat motoneurones *in vitro*: Mediation through a phosphorylation independent action of cAMP, *Neuropharmacology*, 36, 721, 1997.
145. Wikström, M., Hill, R., Hellgren, J., and Grillner, S., The action of 5-HT on calcium-dependent potassium channels and on the spinal locomotor network in lamprey is mediated by 5-HT$_{1A}$-like receptors, *Brain Res.*, 678, 191, 1995.
146. Gerard, C., Martres, M.P., Lefevre, K., Miquel, M.C., Verge, D., Lanfumey, L., Doucet, E., Hamon, M., and el Mestikawy, S., Immuno-localization of serotonin 5-HT6 receptor-like material in the rat central nervous system, *Brain Res.*, 746, 207, 1997.
147. Gerard, C., el Mestikawy, S., Lebrand, C., Adrien, J., Ruat, M., Traiffort, E., Hamon, M., and Martres, M.P., Quantitative RT-PCR distribution of serotonin 5-HT6 receptor mRNA in the central nervous system of control or 5,7-dihydroxytryptamine-treated rats, *Synapse*, 23, 164, 1996.
148. Cina, C. and Hochman, S. Serotonin receptor phamacology of the locomotor CPG: Activation by a 5-HT7 receptor agonist in isolated rat spinal cord, *Soc. Neurosci. Abst.*, 28, 1998.
149. Hochman, S. and Garraway, S.M. Modulation of primary-afferent evoked responses in rat deep dorsal horn neurons with serotonin receptor ligands. *Soc. Neurosci. Abst.* 24, 392, 1998.
150. Connell, L.A. and Wallis, D.I., 5-hydroxytryptamine depolarizes neonatal rat motorneurones through a receptor unrelated to an identified binding site, *Neuropharmacology*, 28(6), 625, 1989.
151. Roberts, M.H., Davies, M., Girdlestone, D., and Foster, G.A., Effects of 5-hydroxytryptamine agonists and antagonists on the responses of rat spinal motoneurones to raphe obscurus stimulation, *Br. J. Pharmacol.*, 95, 437, 1988.
152. Zoli, M., Jansson, A., Sykova, E., Agnati, L.F., and Fuxe, K., Volume transmission in the CNS and its relevance for neuropsychopharmacology, *Trends Pharmacol. Sci.*, 20, 142, 1999.
153. Bowker, R.M., Westlund, K.N., Sullivan, M.C., Wilber, J.F., and Coulter, J.D., Descending serotonergic, peptidergic and cholinergic pathways from the raphe nuclei: a multiple transmitter complex, *Brain Res.*, 288, 33, 1983.
154. Wallis, D.I. and Wu, J., The pharmacology of descending responses evoked by thoracic stimulation in the neonatal rat spinal cord *in vitro*, *Naunyn Schmiedebergs Arch. Pharmacol.*, 347, 643, 1993.
155. Hadjiconstantinou, M., Panula, P., Lackovic, Z., and Neff, N.H., Spinal cord serotonin: a biochemical and immunohistochemical study following transection, *Brain Res.*, 322, 245, 1984.
156. Coderre, T.J., Katz, J., Vaccarino, A.L., and Melzack, R., Contribution of central neuroplasticity to pathological pain: review of clinical and experimental evidence [see comments], *Pain*, 52, 259, 1993.

157. Garraway, S.M., Pockett, S., and Hochman, S., Primary afferent-evoked synaptic plasticity in deep dorsal horn neurons from neonatal rat spinal cord *in vitro*, *Neurosci. Lett.*, 230, 61, 1997.
158. Liu, X.-G. and Sandkühler, J., Long-term potentiation of C-fiber-evoked potentials in the rat spinal dorsal horn is prevented by spinal *N*-methyl- D-aspartic acid receptor blockage, *Neurosci. Lett.*, 191, 43, 1995.
159. Sandkühler, J., Chen, J.G., Cheng, G., and Randic, M., Low-frequency stimulation of afferent Aδ-fibers induces long-term depression at primary afferent synapses with substantia gelatinosa neurons in the rat, *J. Neurosci.*, 17, 6483, 1997.
160. Liu, X.G., Morton, C.R., Azkue, J.J., Zimmermann, M., and Sandkühler, J., Long-term depression of C-fiber-evoked spinal field potentials by stimulation of primary afferent Aδ-fibers in the adult rat, *Eur. J. Neurosci.*, 10, 3069, 1998.
161. Svendsen, F., Tjølsen, A., and Hole, K., AMPA and NMDA receptor-dependent spinal LTP after nociceptive tetanic stimulation, *Neuroreport*, 9, 1185, 1998.
162. Durkovic, R.G. and Prokowich, L.J., D-2-Amino-5-phosphonovalerate, an NMDA receptor antagonist, blocks induction of associative long-term potentiation of the flexion reflex in spinal cat, *Neurosci. Lett.*, 257, 162, 1998.
163. Anderson, M.F. and Winterson, B.J., Properties of peripherally induced persistent hindlimb flexion in rat: Involvement of *N*-methyl-D-aspartate receptors and capsaicin-sensitive afferents, *Brain Res.*, 678, 140, 1995.
164. Chen, J., and Sandkühler, J., Induction of homosynaptic long-term depression at spinal synapses of sensory a delta-fibers requires activation of metabotropic glutamate receptors, *Neuroscience*, 98, 141, 2000.
165. Sandkühler, J. and Liu, X., Induction of long-term potentiation at spinal synapses by noxious stimulation or nerve injury, *Eur. J. Neurosci.*, 10, 2476, 1998.
166. Fenollosa, P., Pallares, J., Cervera, J., Pelegrin, F., Inigo, V., Giner, M., and Forner, V., Chronic pain in the spinal cord injured: statistical approach and pharmacological treatment, *Paraplegia*, 31, 722, 1993.
167. Levi, R., Hultling, C., Nash, M.S., and Serger, A., The Stockholm spinal cord injury study. 1. Medical problems in a regional SCI population, *Paraplegia*, 33, 308, 1995.
168. Mariano, A.J., Chronic pain and spinal cord injury, *Clin. J. Pain*, 8, 87, 1992.
169. Schouenborg, J., Holmberg, H., and Weng, H.-R., Functional organization of the nociceptive withdrawal reflexes. II. Changes of excitability and receptive fields after spinalization in the rat, *Exp. Brain Res.*, 90, 469, 1992.
170. Ashby, P., and McCrea, D.A., Neurophysiology of spinal spasticity, in Davidoff, R., Ed., *Handbook of the Spinal Cord*, Vol. 4 & 5, Marcel Dekker, New York, 1987, 119.
171. Sherrington, C.S., Flexion-reflex of the limb, crossed extension-reflex and reflex stepping and standing, *J. Physiol. (Lond.)*, 40, 28, 1910.
172. Holmqvist, B. and Lundberg, A., Differential supraspinal control of synaptic actions evoked by volleys in the flexion reflex afferents in alpha motoneurons, *Acta Physiol. Scand.*, 54, 1, 1961.
173. Woolf, C.J. and Wall, P.D., Relative effectiveness of C primary afferent fibers of different origins in evoking a prolonged facilitation of the flexor reflex in the rat, *J. Neurosci.*, 6, 1433, 1986.
174. Gozariu, M., Bragard, D., Willer, J.C., and Le-Bars, D., Temporal summation of C-fiber afferent inputs: competition between facilitatory and inhibitory effects on C-fiber reflex in the rat, *J. Neurophysiol.*, 78, 3165, 1997.
175. Basbaum, A.I. and Fields, H.L., Endogenous pain control systems: brainstem spinal pathways and endorphin circuitry, *Annu. Rev. Neurosci.*, 7, 309, 1984.

176. Fields, H.L. and Basbaum, A.I., Brainstem control of spinal pain-transmission neurons, *Annu. Rev. Physiol.*, 40, 217, 1978.

177. Hammond, D.L., Control systems for nociceptive afferent processing: The descending inhibitory pathways, in Yaksh, T., Ed., *Spinal Afferent Processing,* Plenum, New York, 1986, 363.

178. Gebhart, G.F., Modulatory effects of descending systems on spinal dorsal horn neurons, in Yaksh, T., Ed., *Spinal Afferent Processing,* Plenum, New York, 1986, 391.

179. Willis, W.D., Jr., Anatomy and physiology of descending control of nociceptive responses of dorsal horn neurons: comprehensive review, in *Progress in Brain Research,* Fields, H.L. and Besson, J.-M., Eds., Elsevier, Amsterdam, 1988, 1.

180. Villanueva, L., Bouhassira, D., and Le Bars, D., The medullary subnucleus reticularis dorsalis (SRD) as a key link in both the transmission and modulation of pain signals, *Pain*, 67, 231, 1996.

181. Martin, W.J., Gupta, N.K., Loo, C.M., Rohde, D.S., and Basbaum, A.I., Differential effects of neurotoxic destruction of descending noradrenergic pathways on acute and persistent nociceptive processing, *Pain*, 80, 57, 1999.

182. Zhuo, M. and Gebhart, G.F., Characterization of descending facilitation and inhibition of spinal nociceptive transmission from the nuclei reticularis gigantocellularis and gigantocellularis pars alpha in the rat, *J. Neurophysiol.*, 67, 1599, 1992.

183. Durkovic, R.G., Retention of a classically conditioned reflex response in spinal cat, *Behav. Neural Biol.*, 43, 12, 1985.

184. Woolf, C.J. and McMahon, S.B., Injury-induced plasticity of the flexor reflex in chronic decerebrate rats, *Neuroscience*, 16, 395, 1985.

185. Wall, P.D. and Woolf, C.J., Muscle but not cutaneous C-afferent input produces prolonged increases in the excitability of the flexion reflex in the rat, *J. Physiol.*, 356, 443, 1984.

186. Willcockson, W.S., Chung, J.M., Hori, Y., Lee, K.H., and Willis, W.D., Effects of iontophoretically released amino acids and amines on primate spinothalamic tract cells, *J. Neurosci.*, 4, 732, 1984.

187. Lozier, A.P. and Kendig, J.J., Long-term potentiation in an isolated peripheral nerve-spinal cord preparation, *J. Neurophysiol.*, 74, 1001, 1995.

188. Fisher, K. and Coderre, T.J., The contribution of metabotropic glutamate receptors (mGluRs) to formalin-induced nociception, *Pain*, 68, 255, 1996.

189. Ben-Ari, Y., Aniksztejn, L., and Bregestovski, P., Protein kinase C modulation of NMDA currents: An important link for LTP induction, *Trends Neurosci.*, 15, 333, 1992.

190. Chen, L. and Huang, L.-Y.M., Protein kinase C reduces Mg^{2+} block of NMDA-receptor channels as a mechanism of modulation, *Nature*, 356, 521, 1992.

191. Palecek, J., Paleckova, V., and Willis, W.D., The effect of phorbol esters on spinal cord amino acid concentrations and responsiveness of rats to mechanical and thermal stimuli, *Pain*, 80, 597, 1999.

192. Yashpal, K., Pitcher, G.M., Parent, A., Quirion, R., and Coderre, T.J., Noxious thermal and chemical stimulation induce increases in ^{3}H-phorbol 12,13-dibutyrate binding in spinal cord dorsal horn as well as persistent pain and hyperalgesia, which is reduced by inhibition of protein kinase C, *J. Neurosci.*, 15, 3263, 1995.

193. Mao, J.R., Price, D.D., Phillips, L.L., Lu, J.A., and Mayer, D.J., Increases in protein kinase C gamma immunoreactivity in the spinal cord dorsal horn of rats with painful mononeuropathy, *Neurosci. Lett.*, 198, 75, 1995.

194. Miller, J.F., Paul, K.D., Lee, R.H., Rymer, W.Z., and Heckman, C.J., Restoration of extensor excitability in the acute spinal cat by the 5-HT$_2$ agonist DOI, *J. Neurophysiol.*, 75, 620, 1996.

195. Woolf, C.J., Shortland, P., and Sivilotti, L.G., Sensitization of high mechanothreshold superficial dorsal horn and flexor motor neurones following chemosensitive primary afferent activation, *Pain*, 58, 141, 1994.

196. Machacek, D.W., Garraway, S.M., Shay, B., and Hochman, S., Serotonin induces a long-lasting reflex facilitation in isolated rat spinal cord. *Soc. Neurosci. Abst.* 29, 1918, 1999.

197. Jordan, L.M., Factors determining motoneuron rhythmicity during fictive locomotion, *Soc. Exp. Biol. Symp.*, 37, 423, 1983.

198. Jordan, L.M., Brainstem and spinal cord mechanisms for the initiation of locomotion, in Shimamura, S., Grillner, S., Edgerton, V.R., Eds., *Neurobiological Basis of Human Locomotion*, Japan Scientific Soc., Japan, 1991, 3.

199. Gossard, J.P. and Hultborn, H., The organization of the spinal rhythm generation in locomotion, in Wernig, A., Ed., *Plasticity of Motoneuronal Connections*, Elsevier, Amsterdam, 1991, 385.

200. Cazalets, J.R., Borde, M., and Clarac, F., Localization and organization of the central pattern generator for hindlimb locomotion in newborn rat, *J. Neurosci.*, 15, 4943, 1995.

201. Cazalets, J.R., Borde, M., and Clarac, F., The synaptic drive from the spinal locomotor network to motoneurons in the newborn rat, *J. Neurosci.*, 16, 298, 1996.

202. Kjaerulff, O. and Kiehn, O., Distribution of networks generating and coordinating locomotor activity in the neonatal rat spinal cord *in vitro*: A lesion study, *J. Neurosci.*, 16, 5777, 1996.

203. Hultborn, H., Conway, B.A., Gossard, J.P., Brownstone, R., Fedirchuk, B., Schomburg, E.D., Enríquez-Denton, M., and Perreault, M.C., How do we approach the locomotor network in the mammalian spinal cord?, *Ann. NY Acad. Sci.*, 860, 70, 1998.

204. Tresch, M.C. and Kiehn, O., Population reconstruction of the locomotor cycle from interneuron activity in the mammalian spinal cord, *J. Neurophysiol.*, 83, 1972, 2000.

205. Hochman, S., Jordan, L.M., and MacDonald, J.F., N-methyl-D-aspartate receptor-mediated voltage oscillations in neurons surrounding the central canal in slices of rat spinal cord, *J. Neurophysiol.*, 72, 565, 1994.

206. MacLean, J.N., Hochman, S., and Magnuson, D.S.K., Lamina VII neurons are rhythmically active during locomotor-like activity in the neonatal rat spinal cord, *Neurosci. Lett.*, 197, 9, 1995.

207. Kiehn, O., Johnson, B.R., and Raastad, M., Plateau properties in mammalian spinal interneurons during transmitter-induced locomotor activity, *Neuroscience*, 75, 263, 1996.

208. Tresch, M.C. and Kiehn, O., Motor coordination without action potentials in the mammalian spinal cord, *Natl. Neurosci.*, 3, 593, 2000.

209. Beato, M. and Nistri, A., Interaction between disinhibited bursting and fictive locomotor patterns in the rat isolated spinal cord, *J. Neurophysiol.*, 82, 2029, 1999.

210. Smith, J.C. and Feldman, J.L., *In vitro* brainstem-spinal cord preparations for study of motor systems for mammalian respiration and locomotion, *J. Neurosci. Meth.*, 21, 321, 1987.

211. Kudo, N. and Yamada, T., N-Methyl-D, L-aspartate-induced locomotor activity in a spinal cord-hindlimb muscles preparation of the newborn rat studied *in vitro*, *Neurosci. Lett.*, 75, 43, 1987.

212. Dai, X., Douglas, J.R., Nagy, J.I., Noga, B.R., and Jordan, L.M., Localization of spinal neurons activated during treadmill locomotion using the C-Fos immunohistochemical method, *Soc. Neurosci. Abst.*, 16, 889, 1990.

213. Viala, D., Buisseret-Delmas, C., and Portal, J.J., An attempt to localize the lumbar locomotor generator in the rabbit using 2-deoxy-[^{14}C]glucose autoradiography, *Neurosci. Lett.*, 86, 139, 1988.

214. Viala, D., Viala, G., and Jordan, M., Interneurones in the lumbar cord related to spontaneous locomotor activity in the rabbit. I. Rhythmically active interneurones, *Exp. Brain Res.*, 84, 177, 1991.

215. Noga, B.R., Fortier, P.A., Kriellaars, D.J., Dai, X., Detillieux, G.R., and Jordan, L.M., Field potential mapping of neurons in the lumbar spinal cord activated following stimulation of the mesencephalic locomotor region, *J. Neurosci.*, 15, 2203, 1995.

216. Kjærulff, O., Barajon, I., and Kiehn, O., Sulphorhodamine-labelled cells in the neonatal rat spinal cord following chemically induced locomotor activity *in vitro*, *J. Physiol. (Lond.)*, 478, 265, 1994.

217. Kremer, E. and Lev-Tov, A., Localization of the spinal network associated with generation of hindlimb locomotion in the neonatal rat and organization of its transverse coupling system, *J. Neurophys.*, 77, 1155, 1997.

218. Cina, C. and Hochman, S., Diffuse distribution of sulforhodamine-labeled neurons during serotonin-evoked locomotion in the neonatal rat thoracolumbar spinal cord, *J. Comp. Neurol.*, 423, 590, 2000.

219. Barbeau, H., Chau, C., and Rossignol, S., Noradrenergic agonists and locomotor training affect locomotor recovery after cord transection in adult cats, *Brain Res. Bull.*, 30, 387, 1993.

220. Sqalli-Houssaini, Y., Cazalets, J.-R., and Clarac, F., Oscillatory properties of the central pattern generator for locomotion in neonatal rats, *J. Neurophysiol.*, 70, 803, 1993.

221. Rossignol, S., Chau, C., Brustein, E., Giroux, N., Bouyer, L., Barbeau, H., and Reader, T.A., Pharmacological activation and modulation of the central pattern generator for locomotion in the cat, *Ann. NY Acad. Sci.*, 860, 346, 1998.

222. Zifa, E. and Fillion, G., 5-Hydroxytryptamine receptors, *Pharmacol. Rev.*, 44, 401, 1992.

223. van Wijngaarden, I., Tulp, M.T., and Soudijn, W., The concept of selectivity in 5-HT receptor research, *Eur. J. Pharmacol.*, 188, 301, 1990.

224. Feraboli-Lohnherr, D., Barthe, J.Y., and Orsal, D., Serotonin-induced activation of the network for locomotion in adult spinal rats, *J. Neurosci. Res.*, 55, 87, 1999.

225. Feraboli-Lohnherr, D., Orsal, D., Yakovleff, A., and Ribotta, M.G.Y., Privat, A., Recovery of locomotor activity in the adult chronic spinal rat after sublesional transplantation of embryonic nervous cells: Specific role of serotonergic neurons, *Exp. Brain Res.*, 113, 443, 1997.

226. Yakovleff, A., Cabelguen, J.M., Orsal, D., Ribotta, M.G.Y., Rajaofetra, N., Drian, M.J., Bussel, B., and Privat, A., Fictive motor activities in adult chronic spinal rats transplanted with embryonic brainstem neurons, *Exp. Brain Res.*, 106, 69, 1995.

227. Cowley, K.C. and Schmidt, B.J., A comparison of motor patterns induced by *N*-methyl-D-aspartate, acetylcholine and serotonin in the *in vitro* neonatal rat spinal cord, *Neurosci. Lett.*, 171, 147, 1994.

228. Hochman, S. and Schmidt, B.J., Whole cell recordings of lumbar motoneurons during locomotor like activity in the *in vitro* neonatal rat spinal cord, *J. Neurophys.*, 79, 743, 1998.

229. Wallis, D.I., Connell, L.A., and Kvaltinova, Z., Further studies on the action of 5-hydroxytryptamine on lumbar motoneurones in the rat isolated spinal cord, *Naunyn Schmiedebergs Arch. Pharmacol.*, 343, 344, 1991.

230. Beato, M. and Nistri, A., Serotonin-induced inhibition of locomotor rhythm of the rat isolated spinal cord is mediated by the 5-HT1 receptor class, *Proc. R. Soc. Lond. B Biol. Sci.*, 265, 2073, 1998.

231. Bracci, E., Beato, M., and Nistri, A., Extracellular K+ induces locomotor-like patterns in the rat spinal cord *in vitro*: comparison with NMDA or 5-HT induced activity, *J. Neurophys.*, 79, 2643, 1998.

232. Jovanovic, K., Petrov, T., Greer, J.J., and Stein, R.B., Serotonergic modulation of the mudpuppy (*Necturus maculatus*) locomotor pattern *in vitro*, *Exp. Brain Res.*, 111, 57, 1996.

233. Boess, F.G. and Martin, I.L., Molecular biology of 5-HT receptors, *Neuropharmacology*, 33, 275, 1994.

234. Clark, F.M. and Proudfit, H.K., The projection of noradrenergic neurons in the A7 catecholamine cell group to the spinal cord in the rat demonstrated by anterograde tracing combined with immunocytochemistry, *Brain Res.*, 547, 279, 1991.

235. Clark, F.M. and Proudfit, H.K., The projections of noradrenergic neurons in the A5 catecholamine cell group to the spinal cord in the rat: Anatomical evidence that A5 neurons modulate nociception, *Brain Res.*, 616, 200, 1993.

236. Holstege, J.C., Van Dijken, H., Buijs, R.M., Goedknegt, H., Gosens, T., and Bongers, C.M.H., Distribution of dopamine immunoreactivity in the rat, cat, and monkey spinal cord, *J. Comp. Neurol.*, 376, 631, 1996.

237. Rajaofetra, N., Ridet, J.-L., Poulat, P., Marlier, L., Sandillon, F., Geffard, M., and Privat, A., Immunocytochemical mapping of noradrenergic projections to the rat spinal cord with an antiserum against noradrenaline, *J. Neurocytol.*, 21, 481, 1992.

238. Fritschy, J.M. and Grzanna, R., Demonstration of two separate descending noradrenergic pathways to the rat spinal cord: evidence for an intragriseal trajectory of locus coeruleus axons in the superficial layers of the dorsal horn, *J. Comp Neurol.*, 291, 553, 1990.

239. Rajaofetra, N., Sandillon, F., Geffard, M., and Privat, A., Pre- and post-natal ontogeny of serotonergic projections to the rat spinal cord, *J. Neurosci. Res.*, 22, 305, 1989.

240. Weight, F.F. and Salmoiraghi, G.C., Responses of spinal cord interneurons to acetylcholine, norepinephrine and serotonin administered by microelectrophoresis, *J. Pharmacol. Exp. Ther.*, 153, 420, 1966.

241. Belcher, G., Ryall, R.W., and Schaffner, R., The differential effects of 5-hydroxytryptamine, noradrenaline and raphe stimulation on nociceptive and non-nociceptive dorsal horn interneurones in the cat, *Brain Res.*, 151, 307, 1978.

242. Headley, P.M., Duggan, A.W., and Griersmith, B.T., Selective reduction by noradrenaline and 5-hydroxytryptamine of nociceptive responses of cat dorsal horn neurones, *Brain Res.*, 145, 185, 1978.

243. Van Dijken, H., Dijk, J., Voorn, P., and Holstege, J.C., Localization of dopamine D_2 receptor in rat spinal cord identified with immunocytochemistry and *in situ* hybridization, *Eur. J. Neurosci.*, 8, 621, 1996.

244. Stone, L.S., Broberger, C., Vulchanova, L., Wilcox, G.L., Hokfelt, T., Riedl, M.S., and Elde, R., Differential distribution of alpha2A and alpha2C adrenergic receptor immunoreactivity in the rat spinal cord, *J. Neurosci.*, 18, 5928, 1998.

245. Bras, H., Cavallari, P., Jankowska, E., and McCrea, D., Comparison of effects of monoamines on transmission in spinal pathways from group I and II muscle afferents in the cat, *Exp. Brain Res.*, 76, 27, 1989.

246. Jankowska, E., Hammar, I., Chojnicka, B., and Heden, C.H., Effects of monoamines on interneurons in four spinal reflex pathways from group I and/or group II muscle afferents, *Eur. J. Neurosci.*, 12, 701, 2000.

247. Todd, A.J. and Millar, J., Receptive fields and responses to ionophoretically applied noradrenaline and 5-hydroxytryptamine of units recorded in laminae I-III of cat dorsal horn, *Brain Res.*, 288, 159, 1983.

248. Skoog, B. and Noga, B.R., Dopaminergic control of transmission from group II muscle afferents to spinal neurones in the cat and guinea-pig, *Exp. Brain Res.*, 105, 39, 1995.

249. Khasabov, S.G., Lopez-Garcia, J.A., and King, A.E., Serotonin-induced population primary afferent depolarisation *in vitro*: the effects of neonatal capsaicin treatment, *Brain Res.*, 789, 339, 1998.

250. Chitour, D., Dickenson, A.H., and Le Bars, D., Pharmacological evidence for the involvement of serotonergic mechanisms in diffuse noxious inhibitory controls (DNIC), *Brain Res.*, 236, 329, 1982.

251. Lakke, E.A., The projections to the spinal cord of the rat during development: a timetable of descent, *Adv. Anat. Embryol. Cell Biol.*, 135, 1, 1997.

252. Kuoppamaki, M., Syvalahti, E., and Hietala, J., Clozapine and N-desmethylclozapine are potent 5-HT1C receptor antagonists, *Eur. J. Pharmacol.*, 245, 179, 1993.

253. Contesse, V., Lenglet, S., Grumolato, L., Anouar, Y., Lihrmann, I., Lefebvre, H., Delarue, C., and Vaudry, H., Pharmacological and molecular characterization of 5-hydroxytryptamine(7) receptors in the rat adrenal gland, *Mol. Pharmacol.*, 56, 552, 1999.

4 Advances in Measuring Active Dendritic Currents in Spinal Motoneurons *in Vivo*

C. J. Heckman and Robert H. Lee

CONTENTS

Key words: voltage clamp, motoneuron, cat, persistent inward current, feedback gain, spinal cord

4.1 INTRODUCTION

The first 20 years of intracellular studies of neurons in mammalian species focused primarily on the spinal motoneuron in the lumbar cord of the cat. The reasons for this focus were technical: Spinal motoneurons are exceptionally large and the lumbar cord of the cat is relatively stable in terms of respiratory and blood pressure movements. Thus, stable recordings from these cells could be readily obtained via penetration with sharp microelectrodes.

The presumed location of penetration of the electrode is at or near the soma, as dendrites have a very narrow diameter. This is a significant limitation. In the spinal motoneuron, as in many types of neurons, the vast majority of synaptic input is on the dendritic tree. Considerable insights about dendritic processing of synaptic input were obtained using cable models of the dendritic tree,[1] but cable models required the assumption that the dendritic membranes did not possess voltage-sensitive channels, i.e., they were entirely passive.

89

The development of the slice preparation greatly expanded the types of neurons that could be studied intracellularly. Equally important, it became possible to record directly from the large diameter portions of the dendritic tree.[2] This is now done relatively routinely using the patch clamp technique.[3] Many studies have demonstrated that the dendrites of a wide variety of neurons contain strong voltage-sensitive channels.[4–6]

In vitro studies of spinal motoneuron lagged behind other neuron types because of the difficulty in getting these cells to survive *in vitro*. The major obstacle is the large size of motoneurons. The dendritic tree is especially large, and unlike Purkinje cells, does not usually have a particular orientation. Thus, slices thin enough to permit adequate diffusion of oxygen eliminate a huge proportion of the dendritic tree of motoneurons. However, at least three different types of *in vitro* preparations currently exist in which recordings of mature spinal motoneurons can be obtained. Hounsgaard and colleagues developed the turtle preparation,[7] whose resistance to anoxia allows for especially thick slices and thus, recordings from healthy adult motoneurons. This preparation has been essential in revealing the cellular mechanisms of motoneuron behaviors. Recently, slice preparations from functionally mature mice[8,9] and from an *in vitro* preparation of sacral spinal cord of the adult rat (David Bennett, personal communication) have also been successfully obtained. Direct recordings from the large diameter portion of dendritic branches have only been successfully obtained in cultured motoneurons,[10–12] but even in this preparation, recordings from the finer branches remain unobtainable. Unlike neocortical pyramidal cells, which have a large apical dendritic trunk, motoneuron dendrites undergo rapid branching and narrowing. In the adult mammalian motoneuron, the dendritic tree constitutes the vast majority of the surface area of the cell[13–16] and systematic understanding of active conductances in these regions cannot be achieved in reduced preparations such as cell cultures or slices obtained from neonatal animals. Techniques to quantify active conductances in fully intact motoneurons in adult preparations are the focus of this review.

Indirect evidence that the dendrites of adult motoneurons contained active currents was, in fact, obtained before the development of *in vitro* preparations. Redman and colleagues[17] showed that monosynaptic EPSPs from single Ia axons likely to originate on the distal dendritic tree were just as large as those originating in proximal sites. Moreover, they subsequently showed[18] that injection of K channel blockers into the cell increased EPSP amplitude.

The most important development for understanding the role of active dendritic conductances in motoneuron processing was obtained from recordings in the unanesthetized decerebrate preparation. The majority of motoneuron intracellular recordings had been obtained in deeply anesthetized preparations. The advantage of the decerebrate preparation over anesthetized preparations is that brainstem nuclei that are the source of potent neuromodulatory inputs to motoneurons are tonically active. The monoamines serotonin and norepinephrine have been shown to be particularly important in this regard.[19] Serotonin is released by axons descending from the caudal portion of the raphe nucleus, and norepinephrine is released by axons descending from the locus coeruleus.[20]

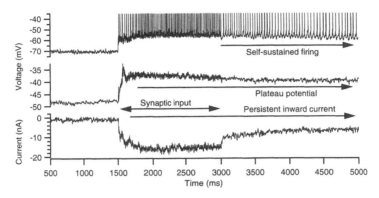

FIGURE 4.1 Activation of a persistent inward current (PIC) by a steady 1.5 s period of excitatory synaptic input from muscle spindle Ia afferents. The PIC (lowest trace) greatly amplifies the effective Ia synaptic current during the input and generates a sustained tail current after the input ends. This results in a sustained plateau potential (middle trace) recorded in a cell in which action potential were blocked with QX-314 (different cell than in the lower trace). In unclamped conditions with normal spike generation, the PIC generates strong firing during the input and self-sustained firing after the input ends (upper trace, same cell as lower trace). All three phenomena (PIC, plateau potential, and self-sustained firing) can be turned off by a brief period of hyperpolarization, giving two stable states for a given input level, or bistable behavior. Data are from intracellular recordings from triceps surae motoneurons in the decerebrate cat preparation. (Data from Lee, R.H. and Heckman, C.J., *J. Neurophysiol.,* 80, 572, 1998 and Lee, R.H. and Heckman, C.J., *J. Neurophysiol.,* 82, 2518, 1999. With permission.)

Hultborn and colleagues showed that the properties of motoneurons in the decerebrate are dramatically different from those in anesthetized preparations.[21] Excitatory inputs can generate prolonged plateau potentials that greatly increase the potency of the synaptic input while it is maintained. In addition, the plateau can generate prolonged self-sustained firing after the excitatory input ceases. These phenomena are illustrated in Fig. 4.1. Because a brief inhibitory input eliminates the self-sustained firing and returns the cell to the quiescent state, the motoneuron is said to be "bistable."[21] Hounsgaard, Kiehn, and colleagues then demonstrated that most of the plateau potential is generated by an L-type calcium current in turtle motoneurons.[22] Recent work has also established that an L-type calcium current plays a primary role in mouse motoneurons,[8] and it is generally assumed this same current is equally important in other vertebrate species.[23] It is important to realize that the plateau potential is generated by a persistent inward current (PIC), which is illustrated by the bottom trace in Fig. 4.1. The voltage clamp techniques to study this PIC and their importance for understanding dendritic processing are considered below.

One important effect of the plateau potential on motoneuron behavior strongly suggested that much of the plateau potential is generated in dendritic regions. A standard test of neuronal behavior is measuring its rhythmic firing properties in response to injected currents. When a motoneuron with a strong plateau potential is

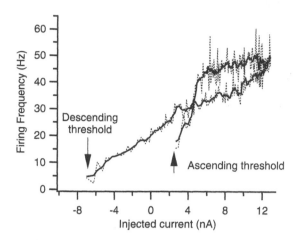

FIGURE 4.2 Hysteresis in the frequency-current (F-I) function in a motoneuron with a strong PIC. A triangular pattern of injected current (5 s duration on the ascending and descending portions) was applied to generate various levels of steady rhythmic firing. Note that firing ceases at a much more hyperpolarized current than at which it was initiated (see arrows). The inflection on the rising phase is thought to occur as the PIC becomes fully activated. Data are from intracellular recordings from triceps surae motoneurons in the decerebrate cat preparation. (Data from Lee, R.H. and Heckman, C.J., *J. Neurophysiol.*, 80, 572, 1988. With permission.)

subjected to an injected current with a triangular pattern, the resulting frequency-current (F-I) function reveals a strong hysteresis.[21,24,25] Termination of firing on the descending phase of the triangular input current occurs at a much lower current level than the initiation of firing on the ascending phase (Fig. 4.2). This hysteresis could be readily accounted for if the plateau potential is primarily generated in dendritic regions.[24,25] On the ascending phase, current injected at the soma would be relatively ineffective in activating a voltage-sensitive dendritic conductance due to current loss in the intervening membrane. For the same reason, once the plateau is activated in the dendrite, it becomes difficult to turn off by reducing current at the soma. Consequently, the current required to turn off the dendritic plateau is considerably hyperpolarized compared to the on current.

Direct evidence that plateau potentials do exist in the dendrites of turtle motoneurons was obtained by Hounsgaard and Kiehn.[26] Using the turtle slice preparation, they showed that extracellular fields that depolarized the dendrites but hyperpolarized the soma could produce plateau potentials in the presence of K+ channel blockers. The presence of plateau potentials in motoneuron dendrites suggests that synaptic input should be more effective in activating these plateaus than injected current, which is applied at the soma. Bennett and colleagues[24] have demonstrated this effectiveness in motoneurons in the cat. Simultaneous application of synaptic and injected current markedly lowered the onset of acceleration in firing rate due to plateau activation compared with injected current alone. In the following sections, we discuss how studying the effect of synaptic input during voltage clamp instead of current clamp provides direct evidence for the dendritic origin of the plateau in adult mammalian motoneurons.

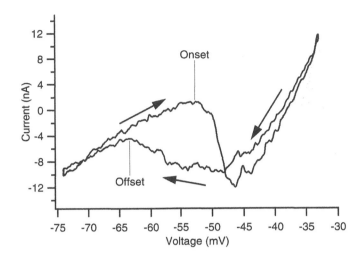

FIGURE 4.3 Hysteresis in the current-voltage relation (I-V) in a motoneuron with a strong PIC. A triangular voltage command (5 s on both ascending and descending portions) activated the PIC, which is evident as the onset of a negative slope region. On the descending limb, the offset of the PIC is considerably more hyperpolarized than its onset. Data are from intracellular recordings from triceps surae motoneurons in the decerebrate cat preparation. (Data from Lee, R.H. and Heckman, C.J., *J. Neurophysiol.*, 80, 583, 1998. With permission.)

4.2 VOLTAGE CLAMP IN MOTONEURONS *IN VIVO*

Voltage clamp studies in motoneurons were initiated by Araki and Terzuolo.[27] Systematic studies by Barrett and Crill,[28] Barrett et al.,[29] and Schwindt and Crill[30] quantified several of the important voltage-sensitive conductances in motoneurons. Schwindt and Crill[30,31] identified a persistent inward current that they believed was primarily carried by Ca^{2+}. In the presence of K^+ channel blockers, this current became quite large in their deeply anesthetized preparations, resulting in a region of negative slope in the steady-state motoneuron current-voltage (I-V) relationship. The instability imparted by the negative slope produced sustained plateau potentials and bistable behavior in unclamped conditions. As noted above, Hultborn and colleagues then showed that bistable behavior was present spontaneously in the decerebrate without K^+ channel blockers due to the presence of tonic activity in serotonergic and noradrenergic axons.

Measurements of the I-V function in the presence of the monoamines have now been achieved in spinal motoneuron in three preparations: adult turtle motoneurons *in vitro*,[32] adult cat motoneuron *in vivo*,[23] and juvenile mouse motoneurons *in vitro*.[8,9] The results proved to remarkably similar in all three preparations. PIC imparts a strong negative slope to the I-V function and, moreover, exhibits strong hysteresis in its activation and deactivation (see Fig. 4.3). This hysteresis is required for sustained plateau potentials and bistable behavior.[8,23] The I-V hysteresis accounts for the F-I hysteresis in unclamped conditions and, like the F-I hystersis, can be explained on the basis of dendritic plateau potentials lagging behind the soma in their activation and deactivation.

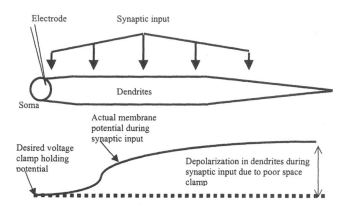

FIGURE 4.4 Poor space clamp in motoneuron dendrites during voltage clamp applied at the soma. This illustration is conjectural; the actual values of membrane potential in the dendrites are not known. However, it is likely that synaptic input could generate a substantial depolarization of the dendritic regions even as the clamp holds voltage at the soma constant. The extra current flow generated at the soma by the dendritic activation provided important information on the effect of voltage-sensitive dendritic conductances on synaptic integration. (Adapted from Lee, R.H. and Heckman, C.J., *J. Physiol. (Paris)*, 93, 97, 1999. With permission.)

4.3 VOLTAGE CLAMP MEASUREMENTS OF ACTIVE DENDRITIC CONDUCTANCES *IN VIVO*

The hysteresis discussed in the previous section raises a particularly important point: During voltage clamp applied at the electrode in the soma of the cell, the voltage control of dendritic regions may be very poor. This poor space clamp has long been recognized as a problem for voltage clamp of dendritic neurons.[33] The goal of our recent work has been to take advantage of this poor space clamp to obtain definitive evidence that much of the plateau potential is, in fact, located in dendritic regions. All of this work was achieved *in vivo*, in lumbar motoneurons in adult decerebrate cat preparations.

The cartoon in Fig. 4.4 illustrates the basic principles. The key element is to apply a steady synaptic input during voltage clamp. Because the clamp is applied at the soma while most of the synaptic input is applied to the dendritic tree, the synaptic input activates the PIC in the dendrites even though voltage at the soma stays constant. The resulting dendritic plateau potential is then measured as an increase in current at the electrode in the soma. It is important to realize that the voltage clamp does influence dendritic regions. Presumably, if the soma is clamped at a sufficiently hyperpolarized level, the corresponding hyperpolarization of the dendrites, though not as large as in the soma, will still be sufficient to prevent synaptic input from activating the PIC. These principles are illustrated in the following experimental results.

In our initial study to demonstrate a dendritic origin for PIC, we clamped the soma at various steady holding potentials and then applied a 1.5-s period of high-frequency

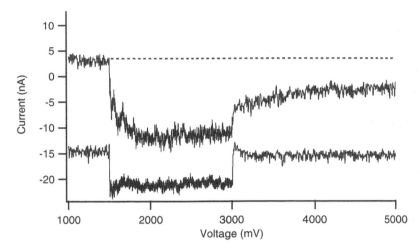

FIGURE 4.5 Differences in Ia effective synaptic current at two different hold potentials during voltage clamp, hyperpolarized (–85 mV) and depolarized (–50 mV). The hyperpolarization prevents activation of the PIC, which is clearly activated by the Ia input at the depolarized holding potential. Dashed line illustrates the difference between the steady current for the hold potential before the Ia input and the Ia effective synaptic current. Data are from intracellular recordings from triceps surae motoneurons in the decerebrate cat preparation. (Data from Lee, R.H. and Heckman, C.J., *J. Neurophysiol.*, 76, 2107, 1996. With permission.)

low-amplitude vibration to the Achilles tendon. This vibration produces steady high-frequency firing in muscle spindle Ia afferents, which monosynaptically excite motoneurons innervating the triceps surae muscles.[34] When a motoneuron is held at a hyperpolarized command level, the Ia input produces a steady inward current with a sharp onset and offset, as illustrated by the example in Fig. 4.5 (lower trace). The hyperpolarization applied at the soma is apparently sufficient to prevent the Ia input from activating the PIC in the poorly clamped but still somewhat hyperpolarized dendrites. In contrast, at depolarized holding potentials just above the level at which spikes are initiated in unclamped conditions, the Ia input activates PIC in dendritic regions (Fig. 4.5 upper trace). As a result, the total current generated by the Ia input at the soma of the cell, i.e., the Ia effective synaptic current,[35] is markedly amplified during the Ia input and persists long after the input ends. This long-lasting stable activation of PIC by the Ia input is what generates stable plateau potentials and bistable behavior (see Fig. 4.1).

To make sure that voltage-sensitive conductances at the soma did not contribute to either the amplification or the persistence of the Ia effective synaptic current, the membrane potential was held steady at the specified holding potential for several seconds before application of the Ia input. During this time period, all voltage-sensitive channels at the soma reached steady activation levels. If the voltage clamp works effectively to control voltage at the soma (see below for technical considerations for achieving high clamp feedback gains), application of the Ia input will not change the activation levels of the somatic voltage-sensitive conductances.

4.4 MINIMIZING ERRORS FOR VOLTAGE CLAMP ASSESSMENTS OF ACTIVE DENDRITIC CONDUCTANCES

A key assumption for the interpretation of Fig. 4.5 is that the Ia input is purely ionotropic. If this input acted via NMDA glutamate receptors or metabotropic glutamate (mGLU) receptors, at least some of the depolarization-dependent effects illustrated in Fig. 4.5 could be because these receptors boost Ia current at the soma or the dendrites. However, it is clear that Ia afferents do not act via NMDA receptors, as the Ia EPSP does not increase with depolarization.[36,37] The possibility that Ia afferents activate mGLU receptors has not been systematically studied but preliminary studies indicate that mGLU receptor antagonists have no significant actions on the reflex forces generated by Ia afferent (unpublished data, Miller and Heckman). Moreover, the sustained Ia EPSPs evoked by vibration exhibit no amplification with depolarization if the cord is acutely transected or if the preparation is deeply anesthetized. Both of these actions eliminate the effects of monoamines in motoneurons that are present in the decerebrate preparation with intact cord. Therefore, the assumption that the Ia input is ionotropic, probably acting via AMPA or kainate receptors, seems well supported.

There remains, however, an important technical concern with the interpretation that the amplification seen in Fig. 4.5 is due to PIC in the dendrites and not active somatic conductances. Voltage clamp gain is never infinite. This limitation is especially relevant for single electrode voltage clamp techniques, which involve high frequency switching between current and voltage.[38] Consequently, the Ia input generates a small degree of depolarization at the soma. Normally, this small error would not be a concern, but PIC imparts a negative slope to the I-V function (see Fig. 4.3). In theory, if the cell is sitting very close to the onset voltage for PIC, only the slightest of depolarizations could push the cell into the unstable negative slope region and fully activate PIC. Thus, it is possible that the large amplification of Ia current is due to this small somatic depolarization. To minimize this problem, we designed and implemented a simple external feedback loop for our Axon Instruments 2A amplifier to markedly enhance feedback gain.

The limit on feedback gain is that high frequency oscillations easily develop in the feedback loop. However, the Ia input produces a steady depolarization. Thus, it is possible to minimize this steady error in voltage during steady synaptic input by restricting high feedback gain to low frequencies.[39] To achieve this increased gain, we added an external feedback loop to our system using two of the AxoClamp's standard external connections: the output of the membrane potential (V_m) and the input for the voltage command (V_C). The basic circuit is illustrated in Fig. 4.6. The large rectangle (thick line) encloses the AxoClamp's internal feedback loop. The AxoClamp's external output of V_m is applied to a summing junction, where it is compared to the desired V_C. The resulting error signal (V_{Error}) is low-pass filtered (first order, –3 dB at 30 Hz) and amplified (with a gain, G_{Ext}, of 10). Next, this filtered, amplified version of the error signal is summed with another copy of the V_C. This sum is then applied to the input for V_C on the AxoClamp. A second comparison with V_m occurs at the summing junction within the AxoClamp and the

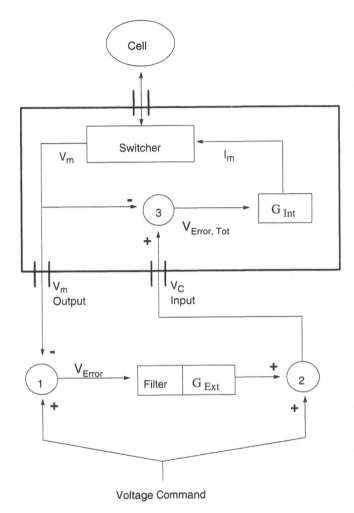

FIGURE 4.6 Basic circuitry for adding enhanced low frequency gain to the feedback provided by an Axoclamp 2A amplifier (Axon Instruments, Inc.). The abbreviations are defined in the text. The circuitry enclosed by the rectangle (thick lines) is internal to the amplifier. The numbered circles denote summing junctions.

resulting total error ($V_{Error, Tot}$) is then amplified by the internal gain (G_{Int}). Therefore, the total feedback gain for the low-frequency component of the error is $G_{Int}*(1+G_{Ext})$. Because G_{Ext} was set to 10, this means that the external circuit resulted in an 11-fold increase in feedback gain for low frequencies. At higher frequencies, the filter in the external loop means that there is no error signal for G_{Ext} to amplify and the feedback gain reduces to G_{Int}.

In our implementation of the external feedback loop, we had to take into account that the V_C input to the Axoclamp assumes an amplification factor of 50 (i.e., a 1.0 V input produces a 20 mV change in potential). In addition, the output of V_m from the Axoclamp is multiplied by a factor of 10. The first step was to boost this $10 \times$ V_m signal by another factor of 5 to reach the 50-fold amplification required to match the V_C input requirement on the AxoClamp. This was done by applying the signal to the positive input of an Axon Instruments model AI 2130 differential amplifier. Summing junction #1 in Fig. 4.6 was implemented with a standard differential amplifier for a Tectronics 5115 oscilloscope (model 5A22N). This amplifier was set to unity gain. The resulting output (i.e., $V_C - V_m$) was applied to a Princeton Applied Research amplifier (model 113) to provide the filtering and the additional 10-fold increase in gain for this error signal. Summing junction #2 in Fig. 4.6 was implemented by a second Tectronics model 5A22N, also set to unity gain. The dual positive sign for this summing junction was achieved by passing one of the signals through an inverter (provided by a Bak Digital Controller, Bak Instruments, Inc.). Alternatively, the inputs to the summing junction #1 could be reversed (V_m to positive and V_C to negative) and the filtered, amplified output applied to the negative input of summing junction #2. Note also that voltage commands typically have two components: the steady-state holding command and the desired change in voltage due to a step- or ramp-shaped function. The steps and ramps were supplied by the digital-to-analog (D-to-A) output from our computer data acquisition system (Cambridge Electronic Devices, Inc.). The computer files for the D-to-A output included the 50-fold amplification required by the AxoClamp's input for voltage commands. The hold and step/ramp components of the voltage command were combined before being added to the circuit shown in Fig. 4.6. This was done by applying the analog output of the computer to a third Tectronics 5A22N amplifier. The knob for controlling DC offset on this Tectronics amplifier was used to specify the holding command.

Before the external feedback loop was closed, the holding command knob on the front panel of the AxoClamp 2A amplifier was set to zero, leaving the cell at its resting membrane potential. V_m was monitored on an oscilloscope screen and the holding potential component of the voltage command to the external loop was adjusted to equal V_m. The external feedback loop was then closed. All subsequent adjustments in holding command were made via the DC offset control of the second Tectronics amplifier.

Typically, we are able to achieve gains of 10 to 30 nA/mV via the circuit built into the AxoClamp 2A amplifier. Motoneurons have input conductances of about 1 μS (typical range: 0.5 to 2.0 μS), so that a steady synaptic input generating a 10 mV change in membrane potential can be held to about a 0. 5 to 1 mV excursion during the clamp. As noted above, the circuit for enhanced low-frequency gain resulted in an 11-fold increase in gain, or about 100 to 300 nA/mV. Fig. 4.7 gives an example of the effectiveness of the additional circuit to enhance low-frequency feedback gain in eliminating small DC offsets in voltage. The Ia input lasted 1.5 s. In the unclamped state, this input depolarized the cell by more than 8 mV and caused it to discharge rhythmically (upper trace). The middle trace in Fig. 4.7 shows the membrane potential during voltage clamp of the same Ia input in the standard case, without the enhanced low-frequency gain. The clamp works fairly well, but there is still about a 1.0 mV peak change in potential followed by a 0.5 mV steady-state error. When the enhanced low-frequency gain is added to the feedback control circuit, this remaining offset is virtually eliminated (lowest trace in Fig. 4.7).

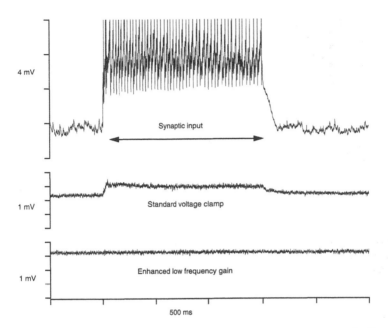

FIGURE 4.7 Effectiveness of the external circuit for enhanced low-frequency feedback gain in eliminating steady-state errors during voltage clamp. Intracellular recording from a medial gastrocnemius motoneuron in the decerebrate cat preparation. Upper trace: Changes in membrane potential produced by a 1.5-s period of Ia input. The resulting activation of the PIC was sufficient to drive the cell to discharge at about 20 spikes/s. Middle trace: Changes in membrane potential of the same input during discontinuous single electrode voltage clamp. Switching rate was 10 kHz and feedback gain was about 15 nA/mV. Note there is still a 0.5 to 1.0 mV excursion in membrane potential. Lowest trace: Changes in membrane potential during voltage clamp with the enhanced low frequency gain. The steady error is virtually eliminated. (Data from Lee, R.H. and Heckman, C.J., *J. Neurophysiol.,* 76, 2107, 1996. With permission.)

One possible error remains: The Ia input not only produces a steady input but also small oscillations at the tendon vibration frequency of 180 Hz. This frequency is only partly suppressed by the external feedback loop. However, PIC activates relatively slowly. We assumed, therefore, that the high frequency noise generated by the Ia input would not have a significant effect on PIC. This assumption has been tested by adding a 125 Hz sin wave (0.5 mV peak to peak amplitude) to the voltage ramps we use to generate I-V functions. We have found that this sin wave does not change the onset voltage for PIC nor does it affect its amplitude (Lee and Heckman, unpublished data).

Fig. 4.8 makes a further point (Lee and Heckman, unpublished data): A series of small voltage steps were applied just below and above the onset voltage for PIC. The small step that just exceeded PIC threshold produced a very slow activation of this current. Full amplitude was not reached for over 10 s. This shows that even if we did not routinely minimize low-frequency feedback gain with our external loop,

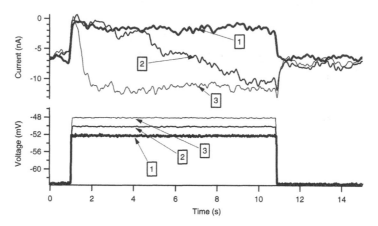

FIGURE 4.8 Small voltage steps near the threshold for activation of PIC. Voltage steps are illustrated in the lower panel. The resulting currents are in the upper panel. Note that the leak conductances have not been subtracted and that the steps are long lasting (10 s). The smallest voltage step (#1) was just subthreshold for activation of a PIC series of steps. A mere 2-mV increase in amplitude activates PIC (step #2), but the onset is extremely slow — over 10 s. Another 2-mV increment (step #3) is required to produce the normal onset dynamics for PIC in motoneurons. Data are from intracellular recordings from triceps surae motoneurons in the decerebrate cat preparation. (Unpublished data from Lee, R.H. and Heckman, C.J. With permission.)

the small depolarization produced by the Ia input could not generate the strong and relatively (0.5 s) rapid activation of PIC illustrated in Fig. 4.5. Certainly, the very small depolarization produced at the soma when low frequency feedback gain is enhanced 10-fold cannot account for the large amplification of Ia input.

Therefore, we conclude that both the amplification of Ia input and the generation of the sustained tail current are due to activation of PIC in dendritic regions. In the past few years, we have used this potent technique to systematically investigate the role of active dendritic conductances for synaptic integration in spinal motoneurons *in vivo*.

4.5 THE EFFECT OF THE PIC IN MOTONEURON DENDRITES ON SYNAPTIC INTEGRATION

Perhaps the most important point to emerge from our work thus far is that synaptic amplification occurs in every motoneuron we have recorded in the decerebrate preparation. In contrast, full bistability, which is manifest as long duration self-sustained firing, is seen in less than 10% of the motoneurons in the decerebrate. Adding an exogenous monoaminergic agonist to the decerebrate increases the frequency of bistable behavior but even in this case, only about 30% of the motoneurons are fully bistable. Thus, it is very likely that the amplification of synaptic input is the most physiologically important effect of PIC in the dendrites of motoneurons.

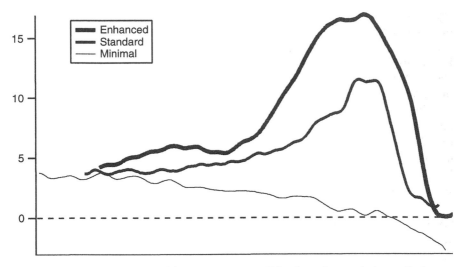

FIGURE 4.9 Effect of neuromodulatory state on amplification of synaptic input. Each trace shows Ia effective synaptic current as a function of voltage in a different cell. All data were recorded during voltage clamp. The minimal neuromodulatory state was defined by a pento-barbital-anesthetized preparation. The standard state was the decerebrate preparation and the enhanced state was the decerebrate plus exogenous administration of the noradrenergic alpha-1 agonist methoxamine. Data are from intracellular recordings from triceps surae motoneurons in the decerebrate cat preparation. (Data from Lee, R.H. and Heckman, C.J., *J. Neurosci.*, 20, 6734, 2000. With permission.)

Amplification has a tremendous impact on synaptic integration. The Ia input only generates about 2 to 3 nA of current in the pentobarbital anesthetized prepa-ration where the serotonergic and noradrenergic input to motoneurons is suppressed and the PIC in the dendrites is virtually undetectable. In the decerebrate, the tonic activity in the monoaminergic fibers generates a large dendritic PIC, so that the Ia effective synaptic current increases to over 12 nA.[41] When the noradrenergic alpha 1 agonist methoxamine is added to the decerebrate preparation, peak Ia effective synaptic current reaches 17 nA.[41] As a result, the firing rates generated by the Ia input in unclamped conditions are remarkably high: 30 Hz in the decerebrate and 50 Hz in the decerebrate plus methoxamine.[25,41] In type-S motor units, 30 Hz is sufficient to generate over 90% of the maximum force, while 50 Hz can exceed the rate required for maximum force.[35] In other words, the Ia input alone saturates the output of type S motoneurons. In constrast, in the pentobarbital-anesthetized preparation, the Ia input only increases motoneuron firing rates by about 5 Hz.[35] Therefore, PIC in the dendrites of S motoneurons completely transforms their integration of synaptic input. A small ionotropic synaptic input acts to control a highly excitable dendritic tree, with PIC in the dendritic tree providing the majority of current to drive rhythmic firing.

It is also clear from these results that the amplitude of PIC, and hence also the amplification of synaptic input, depend on the level of monoaminergic drive to the motoneurons. This dependency is illustrated in Fig. 4.9. Each trace in this figure shows the relationship between Ia effective synaptic current and membrane potential for one cell. In the cell recorded in the pentobarbital-anesthetized preparation, Ia input sharply declines with depolarization. In the decerebrate and decerebrate plus methoxamine preparations, marked amplification is present. Note also that amplification is followed by a step decline in Ia-effective synaptic current. In all three cells, Ia-effective synaptic current becomes negative above −35 mV. Because this is far short of the reversal potential of 0 mV for the Ia synapse,[37] it is likely due to activation of voltage-sensitive outward currents in the motoneuron's dendrites.[18,26]

The consequences of this saturation of synaptic current at depolarized levels for normal generation of rhythmic firing are unclear. In human motor unit firing patterns, low threshold units do exhibit a sharp decline in slope of the relationship between unit firing rate and total muscle force after an initial period of steep rate modulation.[35] However, a recent study of input summation in the decerebrate cat preparation showed that two separate input systems, both of which underwent depolarization-dependent amplification, nonetheless summed linearly with respect to their effects on firing rate.[42] Considerable further work needs to be done before synaptic integration in motoneurons with a dendritic PIC can be fully understood. Two particularly important points for synaptic integration are the existence of systematic differences in PIC among motoneurons and the effect of synaptic inhibition on the activation of the dendritic PIC.

On average, PIC is activated at more hyperpolarized levels (around −50 mV) and is more persistent (often being stable for long time periods) in low-input conductance motoneurons.[23] In the high-input conductance motoneurons, PIC is activated around −40 mV and typically decays within a few seconds. This decay accounts for the lack of bistable behavior in high-input conductance cells.[25] Peak amplitude of PIC in high-input conductance motoneurons is, if anything, slightly larger than in low-input conductance cells. As a result, amplification of synaptic input in high-input conductance motoneurons is very strong but occurs at a more depolarized level than in low-input conductance motoneurons.[41] Because low-input conductance motoneuron tend to innervate slow (S) muscle units and high-input conductance motoneurons tend to innervate fast (F) muscle units, the differences in PIC are likely to be functionally important. The stronger persistence of PIC in S motoneurons makes sense with the high fatigue resistance of their muscle units and the usage of these units in postural tasks. The relatively large but brief dendritic PIC in F units may assist in recruiting them for high force tasks. These considerations further emphasize the importance of Henneman's size principle,[35,43] which postulates orderly recruitment of units from low input conductance to high input conductance, in understanding the functional organization of the motoneuron pool.

What happens when inhibitory synaptic input is applied to the motoneuron? Systematic studies of inhibition have yet to be completed in our lab, but the preliminary work indicates that inhibitory input is also profoundly affected by the PIC in the dendrites (Lee and Heckman, unpublished data). In Fig. 4.10, the lower trace shows the inhibitory effective synaptic current generated by continuous stimulation of the common peroneal nerve at a strength of about 3 times its threshold. This inhibition, therefore, includes reciprocal inhibition from Ia afferent in muscles antagonistic to the triceps surae and also inhibition from higher threshold afferents in the group II class. The upper trace shows the Ia effective synaptic current in the same

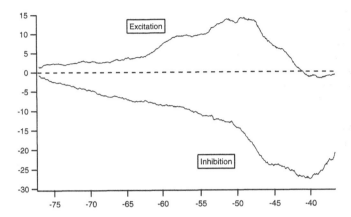

FIGURE 4.10 Dendritic amplification of synaptic inhibition compared to that of excitation. The lower trace shows inhibitory effective synaptic current as a function of voltage, while the upper trace shows the excitatory Ia effective synaptic current in the same cell. The inhibition was generated by continuous electrical stimulation of the common peroneal nerve at 5 times its threshold at 100 Hz. Data are from intracellular recordings from triceps surae motoneurons in the decerebrate cat preparation. (Unpublished data from Lee, R.H. and Heckman, C.J. With permission.)

motoneuron. It is clear that the inhibition peaks in its efficacy just as the Ia input starts to decline. These results suggest a complex integration of excitatory and inhibitory synaptic inputs in motoneurons with a strong PIC in their dendrites. Considerable further study of these issues is required, but even at this early stage it is evident that descending motor commands can, by adjusting the level of activity in the descending monoaminergic inputs, dramatically alter the integration of synaptic inputs in motoneuron dendrites. It has been suggested[32,41] that this control may provide motor commands with the capacity to adjust motoneuron processing to suit the demands of different motor tasks. As yet, it is not clear what sort of synaptic processing might be the optimal fit for a given motor task, but it is remarkable how greatly our view of synaptic processing in motoneurons has changed in just the past few years.

ACKNOWLEDGMENT

This work was supported by the National Institutes of Health (NINDS grant NS34382).

REFERENCES

1. Rall, W., Core conductor theory and cable properties of neurons, *Handbook of Physiology, The Nervous System, Cellular Biology of Neurons*, American Physiological Society, Bethesda, MD, 1977, 39.

2. Llinas, R. and Sugimori, M., Electrophyisological properties of *in vitro* Purkinje cell dendrites in mammalian cerbellar slices, *J. Physiol.* 305, 197, 1980.

3. Stuart, G.J., Dodt, H.U., and Sakmann, B., Patch-clamp recordings from the soma and dendrites of neurons in brain slices using infrared video microscopy, *Pflügers Arch.,* 423, 511, 1993.

4. Johnston, D., Magee, J.C., Colbert, C.M., and Cristie, B.R., Active properties of neuronal dendrites, *Annu. Rev. Neurosci.* 19, 165, 1996.

5. Yuste, R. and Tank, D.W., Dendritic integration in mammalian neurons, a century after Cajal, *Neuron,* 16, 701, 1996.

6. Stuart, G., Spruston, N., Sakmann, B., and Hausser, M., Action potential initiation and backpropagation in neurons of the mammalian CNS, *Trends Neurosci.,* 20, 125, 1997.

7. Hounsgaard, J., Hultborn, H., Jespersen, B., and Kiehn, O., Intrinsic membrane properties causing a bistable behaviour of alpha-motoneurones, *Exp. Brain Res.,* 55, 391, 1984.

8. Carlin, K.P., Jones, K.E., Jiang, Z., Jordan, L.M., and Brownstone, R.M., Dendritic L-type calcium currents in mouse spinal motoneurons: implications for bistability, *Eur. J. Neurosci.,* 12, 1635, 2000.

9. Carlin, K.P., Jiang, Z., and Brownstone, R.M., Characterization of calcium currents in functionally mature mouse spinal motoneurons, *Eur. J. Neurosci.,* 12, 1624, 2000.

10. Larkum, M.E., Rioult, M.G., and Luscher, H.R., Propagation of action potentials in the dendrites of neurons from rat spinal cord slice cultures, *J. Neurophysiol.,* 75, 154, 1996.

11. Larkum, M.E., Launey, T., Dityatev, A., and Luscher, H.R., Integration of excitatory postsynaptic potentials in dendrites of motoneurons of rat spinal cord slice cultures, *J. Neurophysiol.,* 80, 924, 1998.

12. Luscher, H.R. and Larkum, M.E., Modeling action potential initiation and backpropagation in dendrites of cultured rat motoneurons, *J. Neurophysiol.,* 80, 715, 1998.

13. Clements, J.D. and Redman, S.J., Cable properties of cat spinal motoneurones measured by combining voltage clamp, current clamp and intracellular staining, *J. Physiol. (Lond.)* 409, 63, 1989.

14. Burke, R.E., Dum, R.P., Fleshman, J.W., Glenn, L.L., Lev, T.A., O'Donovan, M.J., and Pinter, M.J., A HRP study of the relation between cell size and motor unit type in cat ankle extensor motoneurons, *J. Comp. Neurol.,* 209, 17, 1982.

15. Kernell, D. and Zwaagstra, B., Input conductance, axonal conduction velocity and cell size among hindlimb motoneurones of the cat, *Brain Res.,* 204, 311, 1981.

16. Chen, X.Y. and Wolpaw, J.R., Triceps surae motoneuron morphology in the rat: a quantitative light microscopic study, *J. Comp. Neurol.,* 343, 143, 1994.

17. Redman, S., A quantitative approach to the integrative function of dendrites, *Int. Rev. Physiol.: Neurophysiol.,* 10, 1, 1976.

18. Clements, J.D., Nelson, P.G., and Redman, S.J., Intracellular tetraethylammonium ions enhance group Ia excitatory post-synaptic potentials evoked in cat motoneurones, *J. Physiol. (Lond.),* 377, 267, 1986.

19. Baldissera, F., Hultborn, H., and Illert, M., Integration in spinal neuronal systems, in *Handbook of Physiology, The Nervous System, Motor Control,* American Physiological Society, Bethesda, MD, 1981, 509.

20. Björklund, A. and Skagerberg, G., Descending monoaminergic projections to the spinal cord, *Brain Stem Control of Spinal Mechanisms,* Elsevier, Amsterdam, 1982, 55.

21. Hounsgaard, J., Hultborn, H., Jespersen, B., and Kiehn, O., Bistability of alpha-motoneurones in the decerebrate cat and in the acute spinal cat after intravenous 5-hydroxytryptophan, *J. Physiol.,* 405, 345, 1988.

22. Hounsgaard, J. and Kiehn, O., Serotonin-induced bistability of turtle motoneurones caused by a nifedipine-sensitive calcium plateau potential, *J. Physiol. (Lond.)* 414, 265, 1989.

23. Lee, R.H. and Heckman, C.J., Bistability in spinal motoneurons *in vivo*: systematic variations in persistent inward currents, *J. Neurophysiol.*, 80, 583, 1998.

24. Bennett, D.J., Hultborn, H., Fedirchuk, B., and Gorassini, M., Synaptic activation of plateaus in hindlimb motoneurons of decerebrate cats, *J. Neurophysiol.*, 80, 2023, 1998.

25. Lee, R.H. and Heckman, C.J., Bistability in spinal motoneurons *in vivo*: systematic variations in rhythmic firing patterns, *J. Neurophysiol.*, 80, 572, 1998.

26. Hounsgaard, J. and Kiehn, O., Calcium spikes and calcium plateaus evoked by differential polarization in dendrites of turtle motoneurones *in vitro.*, *J. Physiol. (Lond.)*, 468, 245, 1993.

27. Araki, T. and Terzuolo, C.A., Membrane currents in spinal motoneurons associated with the action potential and synaptic activity, *J. Neurophysiol.*, 25, 772, 1962.

28. Barrett, J.N. and Crill, W.E., Voltage clamp of cat motoneurone somata: properties of the fast inward current, *J. Physiol. (Lond.)*, 304, 231, 1980.

29. Barrett, E.F., Barrett, J.N., and Crill, W.E., Voltage-sensitive outward currents in cat motoneurones, *J. Physiol. (Lond.)*, 304, 251, 1980.

30. Schwindt, P.C. and Crill, W.E., Properties of a persistent inward current in normal and TEA-injected motoneurons, *J. Neurophysiol.*, 43, 1700, 1980.

31. Schwindt, P.C. and Crill, W.E., Effects of barium on cat spinal motoneurons studied by voltage clamp, *J. Neurophysiol.*, 44, 827, 1980.

32. Svirskis, G. and Hounsgaard, J., Transmitter regulation of plateau properties in turtle motoneurons, *J. Neurophysiol.*, 79, 45, 1998.

33. Rall, W. and Segev, I., Space clamp problems when voltage clamping branched neurons with intracellular microelectrodes, *Voltage and Patch Clamping with Microelectrodes,* American Physiological Society, Bethesda, MD, 1985, 191.

34. Matthews, P.B.C., Mammalian muscle receptors and their central actions, *Monogr. Physiolog. Soc.* 23, 1, 1972.

35. Binder, M.D., Heckman, C.J., and Powers, R.K., The physiological control of motoneuron activity, in *Handbook of Physiology. Exercise: Regulation and Integration of Multiple Systems,* Oxford University Press, New York, 1996, 1.

36. Brownstone, R.M., Gossard, J.-P., and Hultborn, H., Voltage-dependency of the motoneuronal locomotor drive potentials during fictive locomotion in the decerebrate cat, *J. Physiol. (Lond.)*, 438, 216P, 1991.

37. Coombs, J.S., Eccles, J.C., and Fatt, P., The specific ionic conductances and the ionic movements across the motoneuronal membrane that produce the inhibitory postsynaptic potential, *J. Physiol. (Lond.)*, 130, 326, 1955.

38. Finkel, A.S. and Redman, S.J., Optimal voltage clamping with single microelectrode, *Voltage and Patch Clamping with Microelectrodes,* American Physiological Society, Bethesda, MD, 1985, 95.

39. Misgeld, U., Muller, W., and Polder, H.R., Potentiation and suppression by eserine of muscarinic synaptic transmission in the guinea-pig hippocampal slice, *J. Physiol. (Lond.)*, 409, 191, 1989.

40. Gustafsson, B. and Pinter, M.J., Relations among passive electrical properties of lumbar alpha-motoneurones of the cat, *J. Physiol. (Lond.)*, 356, 401, 1984.

41. Lee, R.H. and Heckman, C.J., Adjustable amplification of synaptic input in the dendrites of spinal motoneurons *in vivo*, *J. Neurosci.* 20, 6734, 2000.

42. Prather, J.F., Powers, R.K., and Cope, T.C., Relation between effective synaptic current and firing rate modulation in medial gastrocnemius motoneurons studied in the decerebrate cat, *Soc. Neurosci. Abstr.* 24, 911, 1998.

43. Henneman, E. and Mendell, L.M., Functional organization of motoneuron pool and its inputs, in *Handbook of Physiology, The Nervous System, Motor Control,* American Physiological Society, Bethesda, MD, 1981, 423.

44. Lee, R.H. and Heckman, C.J., Paradoxical effect of QX-314 on persistent inward currents and bistable behavior in spinal motoneurons *in vivo, J. Neurophysiol.,* 82, 2518, 1999.

45. Lee, R.H. and Heckman, C.J., Influence of voltage-sensitive dendritic conductances on bistable firing and effective synaptic current in cat spinal motoneurons *in vivo, J. Neurophysiol.* 76, 2107, 1996.

5 Investigating the Synaptic Control of Human Motoneurons: New Techniques, Analyses, and Insights from Animal Models

Randall K. Powers and Kemal S. Türker

CONTENTS

0-8493-0006-1/01/$0.00+$1.50

5.1   INTRODUCTION

The contraction of a group of muscle fibers is directly dependent upon the activity of the motoneuron connected to those fibers, and there is a one-to-one relation between the occurrence of action potentials in the motoneuron axon and those in its innervated muscle fibers. For this reason, the effects of activity in afferents, interneurons, and descending fibers on motor behavior are dependent upon their ability to modulate the discharge of motoneurons. The unique importance of the motoneuron in motor control was recognized by Sherrington,[1] who introduced the concept of the motoneuron as the final common path between activity in the central nervous system and movement. The one-to-one relation between the occurrence of action potentials in a motoneuron and in the muscle fibers they innervate makes it possible to record the discharge behaviour of single motoneurons using intramuscular electrodes. Consequently, motoneurons are the only CNS neurons whose individual discharge behaviour can be recorded in human subjects during the execution of normal movements.

The ability to record the activity of human motor units has made it possible to draw inferences regarding the organization of synaptic inputs to human motoneurons during various motor tasks, in both healthy subjects and in subjects suffering from a variety of nervous system disorders. These inferences are often based on the effects of stimulating peripheral or descending afferents on motoneuron discharge probability. It is generally accepted that excitatory synaptic inputs lead to an increase in discharge probability, whereas inhibitory synaptic inputs lead to a decrease in discharge probability. However, the exact relation between the time course of a synaptic potential and its effects on motoneuron discharge probability is still a matter of some controversy. Nonetheless, there have been a number of methodological and theoretical advances in the last 20 years that have led to an improved understanding of the synaptic control of human motoneurons. In the following review, we focus on four different advances related to measuring and interpreting synaptic effects on the discharge of human motoneurons: (1) improvements in isolating the activity of single motor units; (2) new techniques for stimulating different afferent inputs; (3) new methods of analyzing afferent effects on motor unit discharge; and (4) recent insights from animal models.

5.2   MOTOR UNIT ISOLATION

Although it is possible to record the activity of single motor units from the muscle surface, the contribution of any motor unit to the surface electromyogram (SEMG) depends upon its size and its distance from the surface electrodes. Therefore, whereas action potentials from large motor units situated close to the electrodes appear as large spikes on the SEMG, action potentials from small motor units situated in the deep portions of the muscle can be in the noise level.

Insertion of needle or wire electrodes into muscle is commonly used to record the activity of a more limited sample of motor units. The number of motor unit action potentials (MUAPs) recorded using intramuscular electrodes depends upon the extent of the uninsulated (active) area.[2] As the size of the active area of recording is increased, so do the number of units recorded. Recording from a large number of motor units is a useful technique to get the overall picture of a muscle's activity patterns. Furthermore, quantification of multi-unit recording is easier and more reliable than the SEMG records (see 5.3). It is also possible to record the activity of one or a few MUAPs using wire or needle electrodes with a smaller active recording area.[2] From the few-unit record, it is possible to isolate one of the MUAPs and study its response to a given stimulus.

Selection of a single MUAP from a few-unit record is not straightforward but requires experience and special electronic circuits or computer programs. The most common criterion used to discriminate the units is their peak amplitude. This is achieved with simple level crossing circuitry. However, the units often may have similar amplitudes but differ in the time taken to reach to the maximal amplitude (frequency component of the MUAP). It is possible in some cases to produce an amplitude difference between such units using bandpass filtering. In other cases, some peculiarities of the MUAP shapes can be used to distinguish different units. Time-amplitude window circuits can be used for selecting such units. This technique uses a combination of the slope of the leading edge and the amplitude of the unit and may require two experienced persons (four hands!) working very closely together.

The most powerful approaches for discriminating single motor units use some sort of computer-based pattern recognition or template-matching algorithm to characterize the entire MUAP waveform. This has been described by a number of laboratories,[3-7] and commercial waveform discriminators are now widely available. These various motor unit recognition programs often use the regular nature of motor unit discharge together with interaction of the computer operator to minimize missed or incorrectly classified MUAPs. One of the first approaches to sorting multiple motor units utilized several different recording channels to improve discrimination,[3] since two motor units that exhibited similar shapes on a single channel often were easily differentiated on one of the other channels. This approach has recently been used to allow single unit discrimination based on an array of surface EMG electrodes.[8]

Motor unit recognition is generally performed offline but in some cases[5] can be used online based on a short epoch of previously collected data. In the latter case, the operator first sets a threshold voltage for incoming unit signals. This threshold needs to be above the noise level but below the peak of the MUAP of interest. Whenever the input signal crosses this threshold, the system is triggered; i.e., it will now consider a millisecond or so of data on each side of the threshold crossing as a potential spike. The template/s is established before the experimental run begins by running a few seconds of data containing MUAPs of interest. The operator chooses one (or a few) MUAP waveforms and stores them in the computer's memory as the templates.

During the experimental run, the system is triggered each time the incoming signal exceeds the threshold. A millisecond of the incoming signal on each side of the trigger is then compared with the previously established templates. If any of the templates match the incoming MUAP shape, the computer accepts that point as the discharge of the unit. The discharge times of the motor unit can be saved and used in variety of the analysis programs to estimate the synaptic potential that is developed on a motoneuron by the stimulus (see 5.4).

5.3 STIMULATION TECHNIQUES

Stimulating one afferent fiber type without affecting others has been a great challenge for a number of years. Without invasive techniques, completely selective activation of a single type of afferent fiber is generally not possible. However, given sufficient attention to stimulus parameters, it is often possible to apply stimuli that predominantly activate one class of afferent fibers.

5.3.1 ELECTRICAL STIMULATION

Electrical stimuli can be applied with ease to the skin to study the synaptic connection of the skin afferents to motoneurons. Usually, the sensory perception threshold (T) of the subject is used to standardize the stimulus intensity. Intensities of 1 to 3T are used to stimulate low-threshold afferents that convey information about touch sensation.[9,10] When the stimulus intensity is increased, however, as well as stimulating the low-threshold afferent fibers, the stimulus current begins to activate the higher threshold afferents that convey information about squeeze, pinprick, and pain to the central nervous system. Even though some methods can be developed to study the stimulation of one type of afferents by working during the application of pressure or local anaesthetics to the region, such experiments are technically challenging and the results are difficult to interpret.[11]

Electrical stimuli can also be applied near mixed or muscle nerves in order to directly activate afferent axons. This technique is most commonly used to activate primary muscle spindle (Ia) afferents, since these afferents have relatively low electrical thresholds and make monosynaptic excitatory connections onto motoneurons innervating the same and synergist muscles.[12] Reproducible activation of a given population of Ia afferents requires careful placement of the stimulating electrodes and relatively brief (0.5 ms) stimulus pulses.[12] To ensure that a constant proportion of Ia afferents is activated, the stimulus intensity is generally increased to a level that will directly activate a small proportion of motoneuron axons, producing an M-wave. A constant amplitude M-wave is then taken as evidence that the effective stimulus strength is constant.[12] Stimuli that are suprathreshold for producing an M-wave will also activate Golgi tendon organ (Ib) afferent fibers in muscle nerves and low-threshold cutaneous afferents in mixed nerves, complicating the interpretation of the reflex effects of electrical nerve stimulation.[13]

5.3.2 MECHANICAL STIMULATION

Mechanical stimulation is more difficult to standardize than electrical stimulation since its application requires fine control of the duration, the intensity, the shape,

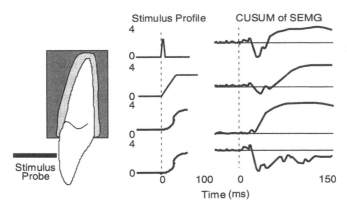

FIGURE 5.1 The effect of the stimulus profile on the masseteric reflex in one subject. The left column illustrates the force profiles and the right column is the CUSUM of the ipsilateral masseter muscle SEMG. The effective force applied to the tooth is indicated in Newtons. Stimuli were delivered at time zero. In all cases, the number of stimuli used was 150; the push force was about 2.5 N; all had contraction levels of about 10% MVC. Note that the probability of eliciting an excitatory reflex increases with the increase in the smoothness of the force delivery. Also note that when the preload is not applied (bottom trace in left column), even when using the smoothest force profile, the speed of the force delivery increases (not shown, cf. 14) inducing an inhibitory reflex response.

and the exact location of the stimulus. Furthermore, the profile of the stimulus shape, including the rate of rise of the stimulus, is difficult to standardize since it changes with the physical relationship between the stimulating probe and the stimulated area. If this relationship is not fixed, the stimulus profile and the rate of rise of the stimulus will also change. It is, therefore, best to physically connect the probe to the area to be stimulated either by gluing, or by applying some preload to take up the slack and the space between the probe and the area to be stimulated. The existence of a preload minimizes the fast component of the force and, hence, is more likely to deliver the exact stimulus profile that is specified by the wave generating system (see Fig. 5.1).

The exact profile of the delivered force is likely to determine the relative activation of different types of mechanoreceptors, which in some cases have opposite reflex effects. An example is given below where an upper incisor tooth of an individual was stimulated using a probe attached to a vibrator. Various mechanical force profiles were delivered to the tooth. Some of the profiles had sharp edges (top two profiles in the left column of Fig. 5.1) that preferentially activate periodontal mechanoreceptors that are particularly sensitive to abrupt changes in force, and which induce inhibition in jaw closing muscles. However, when the stimulus profile is smoothed (third waveform from top in the left column in Fig. 5.1), the applied force preferentially activates receptors with excitatory actions on jaw closing muscles. The same force profile, however, induces an inhibitory reflex response when no preload is applied to take up the slack between the stimulating probe and the tooth. This is due to the fact that the probe now moves rapidly to take up the slack and the abrupt change in applied force (not shown here; see Figure 3 in Reference 14) causes an inhibitory reflex.

Mechanical stimuli applied to the tendons of muscles generally produce short- and long-latency reflex responses.[15] Both the components of the response are thought to result from the activation of primary muscle spindle (Ia) afferents. The short latency response is thought to result from a monosynaptic relay through the spinal cord, whereas the long latency reflex is believed to be mediated by a transcortical pathway. As in the case of activation of periodontal mechanoreceptors, the delivery of the stimulus needs to be standardized using the above-mentioned precautions of probe attachment and continuous assessment of the effective profile of the stimulus to ensure reproducible reflex responses.

5.3.3 CORTICAL STIMULATION

In 1980, it was discovered that the human brain could be stimulated through the intact scalp using a specially designed electrical stimulator (high-voltage, low-output impedance stimulator[16]). Very large transient voltages (around 500 V) are required to reduce the interelectrode resistance to very low values so that stimulation of the cortex can be achieved. Although electrical stimulation of the cortex, and especially the motor cortex, is a reliable and repeatable method, it has not become a common method due to the pain it generates. A new and virtually painless method of stimulating the brain, based on magnetic fields, was later introduced (transcranial magnetic brain stimulator[17]). Magnetic brain stimulation is now becoming a common form of assessing human motor pathways. It is believed that electrical brain stimulation directly activates corticospinal fibers deep in the brain, whereas magnetic brain stimulation trans-synaptically activates corticospinal neurons.[18] A single electrical or magnetic stimulus to the human scalp causes repetitive high frequency discharge of the corticospinal neurons which induce rapid excitatory postsynaptic potentials and discharge in motoneurons.[19]

Standardization of the stimulus intensity involves delivering a fixed percentage of the maximum output of the device or a threshold intensity to elicit a recognizable motor-evoked potential on the surface of the muscle of interest. The position of the electrodes (for the electrical stimulation) and the coil (for the magnetic stimulation) also need to be fixed to deliver repeatable stimulation.

5.3.4 MICRONEUROGRAPHY

None of the stimulation methods covered in the previous sections can initiate activity in a single nerve fiber. Stimulation of a single human nerve fiber in the periphery has become possible since the early 1980s when intraneural microstimulation was first described.[20] This method allows the study of the synaptic connections of a single identified nerve fiber to other neurons, as well as of the ability of human subjects to perceive the activation of single afferents. The microstimulation method has already been used by a number of investigators to describe the perceptual responses to selective stimulation of fibers supplying the skin, joints, and muscles. These studies showed that cutaneous (except the slowly adapting type IIs) and joint receptors had the strongest synaptic security and induced specific perceptual sensation in most of the experiments.[21] Similar findings on the connection of identified single fibers to motoneurons have been described. Although discharges of single muscle spindle afferents have not been found to generate any responses in the surface EMG activity of the muscle,[22] discharges of single cutaneous afferents have been shown to induce significant changes in surface EMG activity.[23]

5.4 ANALYZING AFFERENT EFFECTS ON MOTOR UNIT DISCHARGE

The effects of a synaptic input on motor unit discharge can be assessed either by recording the activity of a population of motor units via surface or intramuscular electrodes, or by isolating the discharge of single motor units using intramuscular electrodes. Multi-unit recordings are relatively easy to obtain, but can be difficult to interpret, due to the possibility of heterogeneous responses of different motor units and the probability that motor unit discharge is affected by both the stimulus and the recent discharge history of the motoneurons. Although the effects of discharge history also complicate the interpretation of stimulus-evoked effects on the discharge of single motor units, new methods of analysis have been developed to separate stimulus-related from discharge history-related effects on motor unit discharge probability.

5.4.1 SURFACE ELECTROMYOGRAM (SEMG)

Surface EMG recordings are simple to obtain but difficult to interpret. Depending on the size of the muscle and the spatial relationship of the muscle to the recording electrodes on the skin surface, the recordings may be affected by activity in neighbouring muscles (cross talk). The recordings are also prone to electrical noise and mechanical artifact, both of which can be reduced by using low-impedance ground electrodes.[24] Quantification of surface EMG is equally problematic since the amplitude and frequency content of the recording not only represent the number and frequency of active motor units but also the amplitude and shapes of the MUAPs, which may change during the course of a contraction.

Despite these drawbacks, it is still possible to get a rough measure of the sign and strength of reflex connections to a muscle using various quantification measures of surface EMG activity. The most common technique is full-wave rectification and averaging of the SEMG around the time of stimulation. It has been claimed that this approach can illustrate the strength of the synaptic potential. Several methods of quantifying the rectified averaged SEMG record have been proposed, including the area,[25] the sum of the absolute surfaces outside of a confidence interval,[26] and the percentage modulation of the mean SEMG level.[27,28]

The interpretation of longer-latency effects on SEMG activity is complicated by two potential errors arising from the regularity of motoneuron discharge: those due to the synchronization of motoneurons spikes by the arrival of a postsynaptic potential, and those due to the low probability of discharge immediately following a spike.

Motoneurons tend to discharge at fairly regular intervals; at all but the lowest firing frequencies, there is a Gaussian distribution of interspike intervals with a fairly low (0.1 to 0.2) coefficient of variation.[29–31] As a result, the autocorrelogram exhibits several peaks and troughs at intervals corresponding to the mean interspike interval.[31] Similar features can be induced in the averaged SEMG record due to phase advancing or delaying the occurrence of action potentials (spikes) in bulk. An excitatory postsynaptic potential (EPSP) causes a phase advancement of the occurrence of the spikes. The phase-advanced spikes are generally followed by several peaks and troughs at intervals determined by the discharge rates of the affected units.[32–34] In an analogous fashion, the synchronous activation of the phase delayed spikes by an inhibitory postsynaptic potential (IPSP) induces peaks and troughs in the averaged SEMG record.[35] Therefore, an increase in the SEMG level, following an inhibitory event, may not always indicate an excitatory synaptic connection but may be caused by the synchronous recurrence of underlying spikes.[35,36]

The decrease in the probability of spike occurrence following a spike can lead to a short-latency decrease in the averaged SEMG record immediately following an excitatory reflex.[14] During this time of relative silence, many of the motoneurons cannot fire since the EPSP caused them to fire only a few milliseconds earlier. For the above reasons, only the initial SEMG response is likely to reflect the synaptic potentials induced in the responding motoneurons. The peaks and troughs that follow the initial response in the averaged SEMG records can be caused by the first event and may not have any synaptic basis.

It may be possible to identify synaptically induced secondary features in the averaged SEMG by subtracting out the mean pre-stimulus baseline level and integrating the remainder (cumulative sum or CUSUM).[37] For example, the spikes that are phase delayed by an inhibitory input should be followed by a recurrence at the mean pre-stimulus interspike interval, bringing the CUSUM trace back to the zero line (mean pre-stimulus level; see Fig. 5.2). Any further increase in the CUSUM trace above the zero line that is larger than the largest prestimulus deflection (error box; Fig. 5.3) and before the minimum reaction time to the stimulus may reflect a long-latency excitatory synaptic connection between the stimulated afferents and the motoneurons that innervate the muscle.[14,38]

It has been claimed that the rectification process may induce an excitation-like peak preceding an inhibitory reflex response.[39] This is because that strong inhibition abruptly stops the discharge of the whole motoneuron pool, so that the last event before the inhibition of the SEMG activity is the repolarization of the last group of active motor units. Since this happens at a fixed latency from the stimulus, it generates a substantial peak in the rectified SEMG record and can be confused with genuine excitatory reflex responses.[39] This problem is especially evident in short-latency reflex pathways (trigeminal reflexes) where temporal dispersion of action potentials is minimal. It is, therefore, suggested that unless an excitatory reflex response is apparent in the unrectified records, peaks that precede inhibitory periods should not be labeled as excitatory reflex responses.[39] Poliakov and Miles[40] proposed that the integral of the average of the unrectified EMG provides a better representation of the underlying motor unit activity in trigeminal reflexes. However, for this analysis to work properly, the surface representation of the motor unit action potentials should be biphasic

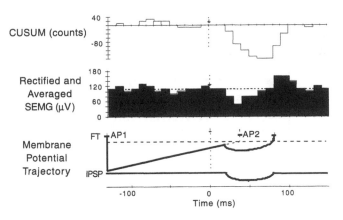

FIGURE 5.2 Simulated representations of the SEMG and its CUSUM. Bin width for these graphs is 10 ms and the stimulus is delivered at time zero (down arrow and dotted line). The average pre-stimulus bin value (K) was 110 µV in the SEMG (middle trace). SEMG displays an inhibitory response lasting for 5 bins followed by an excitatory response lasting for 3 bins. CUSUM (top trace) is calculated by subtracting the value in each bin in the SEMG record from K and adding the difference to the value of the next bin. The first bin value in CUSUM (S_1) is obtained by subtracting its value from K [$S_1 = (110 - 110) = 0$]; the second bin value in CUSUM [$S_2 = S_1 + (120 - 110) = 10$], etc. After the stimulus, the CUSUM values decrease for five consecutive bins since the bin values in the SEMG are consistently lower than K, therefore, the inhibitory period. This period is followed by a period of increased CUSUM activity since the SEMG values during that period are consistently above K. An investigation using the SEMG alone would have resulted in a claim that the stimulus had caused an inhibition, followed by an excitation. However, we argue that since the CUSUM did not exceed the zero level during the excitatory phase, the extra activity in the SEMG was not an excitation but simply delayed spikes recurring synchronously (lower trace). The normal rise toward the firing threshold (FT) of the membrane potential by voluntarily driven inputs was delayed by the addition of the inhibitory postsynaptic potential (IPSP) induced by the stimulus. AP = action potential.

and symmetrical. Furthermore, the excitatory responses should be evident in individual unrectified responses[39] before labeling any peaks as excitation.

5.4.2 INTRAMUSCULAR MULTI-UNIT EMG

The use of intramuscular electromyography (IM-EMG) for the assessment of synaptic potentials is preferred if the muscle of interest is small, situated deep in the limb, or when the synaptic input to the motoneurons that innervate defined parts (compartments) of a muscle is to be studied. The major advantage of IM-EMG is that it is specific to the area of recording and is not as subject to artifacts (such as cross talk, stimulus, and movement artifacts) as the SEMG. However, intramuscular recording is also subject to the same synchronization- and count-related artifacts as the SEMG. Similar steps as those described for the SEMG, such as rectification, averaging, and CUSUM calculation can be used for quantification of the reflex responses from IM-EMGs (see Figs. 5.2 and 5.3).

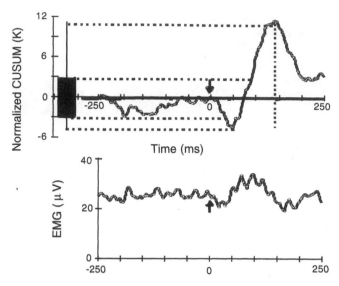

FIGURE 5.3 Methodology from representing the reflex response in the surface EMG. Arrows indicate the timing of the stimulus (time zero). From the pre-stimulus period of the CUSUM records, maximal positive and negative deflections were obtained. The larger of the two values was used to make a symmetrical box for the CUSUM record (filled box to the left of the CUSUM). The box, therefore, illustrated the largest deflection to either side of the zero line during the pre-stimulus period (error box). Any post-stimulus deflection that was larger than the error box and occurred within 140 ms (vertical line indicating reaction time) after the stimulus was considered a reflex response. (Adapted from Türker, K.S., Yang, J., and Brodin, P., *Arch. Oral Biol.*, 42, 121, 1997. With permission.).

5.4.3 SINGLE MOTOR UNIT DISCHARGE

In addition to the problems noted above, the interpretation of multi-unit recordings from either surface or intramuscular electrodes is complicated by the fact that the differences in the background discharge rates and the conduction velocities of different motoneurons will lead to a dispersion of the synaptic effects on the recorded activity. Recording the activity of single motor units provides the most direct estimate of the underlying synaptic potential, since motor unit activity directly represents the output of individual motoneurons. However, despite over 20 years of research on the topic, there is still no consensus on the quantitative relation between the time course and magnitude of a synaptic potential and its effects on motoneuron discharge probability.[41–45]

The most common response measure is the peristimulus time histogram (PSTH[46,47]), which is constructed from the firing of one motor unit over many stimulus applications to assess the effect of that stimulus on firing probability. As in the case of the average stimulus-evoked SEMG, secondary features appear in the PSTH that may reflect the autocorrelation function of the motoneuron, rather than direct stimulus effects.[33,48,49] For example, electrical activation of primary muscle spindle afferents shortens the interspike intervals of tonically discharging motoneurons.[50] However, because of the large number of counts that occur in a very short time period at the reflex latency, the firing of the motor unit is now synchronized to the stimulus. This synchronized firing may induce a series of peaks in the PSTH that gradually diminish.[34] Therefore, it has been proposed that besides neuronal excitation as the usual reason for peak, a PSTH peak can also be due to another PSTH peak occurring previously.[33]

A strong inhibitory stimulus can also induce a synchronizing effect on the firing of motor units by lengthening the interspike interval,[50] causing the action potentials to occur at a certain time after the stimulus. The timing of occurrence of the action potentials after the inhibitory postsynaptic potential (IPSP) is fixed in relation to the stimulus and thus induces several peaks and troughs in the PSTH. Like excitatory reflexes, these peaks and troughs in the PSTH may not represent a series of excitatory and inhibitory synaptic potentials since they could have been caused by the synchronous firing pattern of the unit that is set by the inhibitory stimulus.[35]

5.4.4 ALTERNATIVE METHODS OF ESTIMATING SYNAPTIC EFFECTS ON SINGLE MOTOR UNITS

A number of different methods have been proposed to separate direct stimulus effects from effects due to the discharge history of the motoneuron. Three types of alternatives to the standard PSTH have been proposed. The first two alternatives are to quantify stimulus-evoked effects in terms of stimulus-locked changes in interspike interval[33,51–53] or instantaneous firing rate.[34,54] Figure 5.4 compares these methods with the standard PSTH analysis of the effects of an excitatory input on motoneuron discharge probability. The data were derived from the responses of a tonically discharging rat hypoglossal motoneuron to repeated application of a current transient that mimicked the synaptic current associated with activation of a large number of excitatory afferents.[55] The filled bars in Fig. 5.4A are the PSTH, representing the number of action potentials occurring within a given 1-ms time bin before and after the onset of the excitatory current transient. The solid trace is the CUSUM, calculated by subtracting the mean bin count at negative time lags from the PSTH, and integrating the remainder.[37] (This trace has been normalized by dividing by the number of stimuli.) The dotted trace represents the simulated excitatory postsynaptic potential (EPSP) produced in response to the current transient. The CUSUM trace closely follows the time course of the EPSP for about 50 ms, consistent with the suggestion that the spike-triggering efficacy of a large EPSP is proportional to the EPSP derivative.[56] However, later peaks appear in the CUSUM at lags longer than the EPSP duration, reflecting the regular recurrence of spikes synchronized by the rising phase of the EPSP.

Fig. 5.4B illustrates a peristimulus frequencygram (PSF),[34] compiled by plotting the instantaneous frequency (the reciprocal of the interspike interval) as a function of the time between the stimulus onset and the last spike in the interspike interval. The PSF indicates the total duration and profile of the EPSP, and does not contain secondary peaks occurring after the end of the EPSP. For example, although relatively few action potentials occur on the falling phase of the EPSP, the instantaneous firing rate is greater than the background rate over nearly the entire duration of the EPSP. As illustrated in the Fig. 5.4C, a similar picture may be obtained by plotting

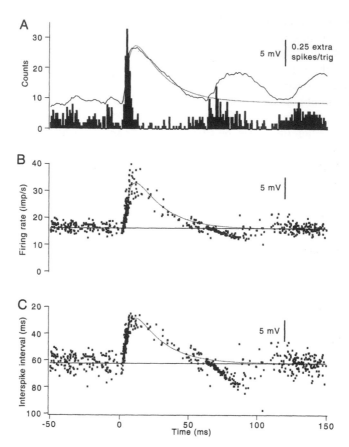

FIGURE 5.4 Three alternative representations of the effects of an EPSP on motoneuron discharge. The dotted trace in each panel shows the time course of a simulated excitatory postsynaptic potential (EPSP) produced by an injected current transient. (The voltage scale is indicated by the calibration bar in each trace.) (A) Peristimulus time histogram (PSTH, solid bars) and its associated CUSUM (solid trace). (B) The scatter plot shows a peristimulus frequencygram (PSF) obtained by plotting the instantaneous frequency of each interval as a function of time between the onset of the EPSP and the last spike in the interval. (C) The scatter plot shows the length of each interval as a function of time from the EPSP to the last spike. (Note that the ordinate has been reversed so that shorter interspike intervals are at the top of the plot.)

the interspike interval instead of its reciprocal. (The ordinate has been reversed so that shorter interspike intervals are displayed as upward deflections.)

An alternative method of separating direct stimulus effects from those related to motoneuron discharge history is to correct the PSTH counts based on the number of spike counts expected in the absence of a stimulus.[57,58] Fig. 5.5 illustrates the application of this type of correction to the PSTH presented in Fig. 5.4A. The thick trace in Fig. 5.5A represents the cumulative spike density following a stimulus, and is calculated in the same fashion as the CUSUM in Fig. 5.4A, except that the pre-stimulus baseline counts have not been subtracted out prior to the integration. The

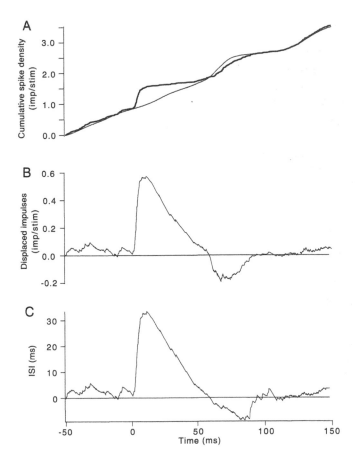

FIGURE 5.5 Correcting the PSTH and CUSUM for the effects of the motoneuron's autocorrelogram. (A) Cumulative spike density as a function of time since EPSP onset (thick) trace and cumulative spike density expected in the absence of a stimulus (thin trace). These functions were calculated from the same data as that used for the plots in Fig. 5.4. (B) Displaced impulses function, calculated as the difference between the two curves in (A). (C) Interspike interval change function, calculated from the horizontal distance between the two curves in (A).[33]

thin trace represents the expected cumulative spike density in the absence of a stimulus, and is calculated by adding a list of control interspike intervals obtained in the absence of stimulation to the times of spike occurrence relative to stimulus onset.[57] Fig. 5.5B illustrates the difference between the observed cumulative spike density and that expected in the absence of a stimulus effect. This function represents the impulses that have been displaced by the stimulus, and is analogous to the normalized CUSUM illustrated in Fig. 5.4A, except that the contribution of the motoneuron's autocorrelogram has been eliminated. Fig. 5.5C illustrates the function obtained by plotting the horizontal difference between the two curves in Fig. 5.5A, which represents the change in interspike interval produced by the stimulus.

Although all three alternative methods described above appear to avoid some of the errors associated with the interpretation of the PSTH, there is still the issue of the exact quantitative relation between a given response measure and the underlying synaptic potential. A direct estimate of this relation is only possible in an animal model in which it is possible to measure both the synaptic potential and its effect on motoneuron discharge probability. Early comparisons of PSTH features with the time course and amplitudes of postsynaptic potentials (PSPs) have generally relied on pooling data from different cells.[43,45,56] We will describe this work first, followed by a description of more recent work using injected current waveforms to mimic the currents associated with evoked synaptic potentials and background synaptic noise. This latter approach has allowed systematic examination of a number of factors affecting the relation between PSPs and their effects on motoneuron discharge, including (1) the magnitude and sign of the PSP, (2) the background discharge rate of the motoneuron, and (3) the magnitude and frequency content of the background synaptic noise.

5.5 INSIGHTS FROM WORK ON ANIMAL MODELS

5.5.1 RELATION OF SYNAPTIC POTENTIAL TIME COURSE TO EFFECTS ON FIRING PROBABILITY

Most analyses of the effects of PSPs on firing probability have used the PSTH as the response measure, and have concentrated on the initial effect of the PSP on neuronal firing probability. Three different linear models of the relation between PSP and PSTH features have been proposed. The PSTH has been approximated as a scaled version of the PSP,[48] the PSP derivative[44,56] or a linear combination of the two.[41] The degree to which the PSTH peak resembles the PSP, its derivative, or a combination of the two depends upon the experimental conditions in general and upon the ratio of the amplitude of the PSP to that of the background noise in particular.[43,45,56] Although most PSTHs can be fit with a scaled version of the PSP and its derivative,[43] the values of the scaling constants differ vary widely among different motoneurons.[43] In addition, the effects of inhibitory inputs (IPSPs) on motoneuron firing probability do not appear to be well fit by any of the linear models.[56]

5.5.2 PREDICTIONS FROM THRESHOLD-CROSSING MODELS

An alternative approach to estimating synaptic potentials from stimulus-evoked changes in motoneuron discharge is to use a threshold-crossing model of motoneuron discharge.[53,59,60] These models are based primarily on recordings of the repetitive discharge of cat lumbar motoneurons elicited by steps of injected current. Under these conditions, the interspike voltage trajectories are fairly stereotyped, consisting of an initial postspike hyperpolarization followed by a linear rise to threshold.[61,62] In models based on this stereotyped trajectory, spikes are advanced by an EPSP whenever its rising phase exceeds the gap between membrane potential and threshold. The advantage of such models is that quantitative relations between EPSP and PSTH parameters can be predicted from simple geometrical considerations based on the angle between the membrane potential and the threshold over the latter portion of the interspike interval.[56,60,63,64] However, significant errors in estimates based on these models may arise from the omission of important biophysical features of real motoneurons, such as interspike variations in conductance, interspike variations in the voltage threshold for spike initiation, and deviations of the interspike membrane potential trajectory from a straight line.[55,65,66] More realistic approximations to motoneuron behaviour can be obtained by incorporating additional known biophysical features of motoneurons.[65,67] However, there is still considerable uncertainty concerning the biophysical properties of different types of motoneurons, as well as increasing evidence that these properties are under neuromodulatory control.[68] For these reasons, it may still be premature to use more complicated biophysical motoneuron models to estimate synaptic potentials from their effects on motoneuron discharge.

5.5.3 USING INJECTED CURRENT TRANSIENTS TO MIMIC SYNAPTIC POTENTIALS

The use of injected currents to mimic the current delivered from the synapses to the soma allows precise experimental control of a number of variables known to influence motoneuron discharge. The rationale for this approach is that the site of spike initiation in motoneurons (as in most neurons) is in a segment of the axon adjacent to the soma.[69] For this reason, currents injected into the soma through a microelectrode should have the same effect as an equivalent amount of current delivered from dendritic synapses. This appears to be the case for the effects of steady synaptic currents on motoneuron discharge,[70–73] and has also been demonstrated for the effects of synaptic transients on discharge probability in neocortical neurons.[74]

Variations in injected current can also be used to mimic different levels of background synaptic noise and to vary the background discharge rate of the motoneuron. In addition, the ability to inject synaptic currents of different amplitude and time course in the same motoneuron allows rigorous comparisons of the ability of different response measures to indicate the entire time course of a synaptic potential. The following sections will examine the effects of the sign, amplitude, and time course of simulated synaptic potentials on motoneuron discharge, followed by a brief consideration of the effects of the background discharge rate of the motoneuron and the level of background noise.

5.5.3.1 Effects of Simulated Excitatory Synaptic Inputs on Motoneuron Discharge

Figure 5.6 illustrates four different measures of the effects of an excitatory current transient on the discharge of a rat hypoglossal motoneuron, using the same data as presented in Fig. 5.4 and 5.5. A tonic background discharge rate of about 16 imp/s was elicited by a suprathreshold 35-s step of injected current. A random noise waveform with a Gaussian amplitude distribution was superimposed upon the current step in order to produce a range of interspike intervals comparable to that seen during voluntary activation of human motor units. Finally, a train of identical current transients was superimposed to mimic periodic activation of an afferent input. The time course of the current transient is indicated by the dashed traces in Fig. 5.6, and

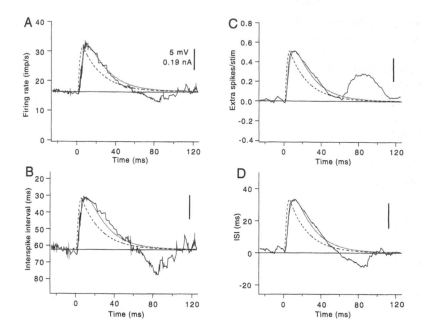

FIGURE 5.6 Comparison of the ability of different measures of changes in motoneuron discharge to reflect the time course of the EPSP (dotted trace in each panel) and the underlying injected current transient (dashed trace in each panel). (A) Smoothed version of the peristimulus frequencygram (PSF) shown in Fig. 5.4B. (B) Smoothed version of the interspike interval superposition plot shown in Fig. 5.4C. (C) CUSUM illustrated in Fig. 5.4A. (D) Interspike interval change function from Fig. 5.5C. Note that all the functions follow the initial portion of the EPSP fairly well, but deviate at later times.

the dotted lines indicate the EPSP that would result if the current transient was applied at the resting potential. The solid traces in Fig. 5.6A and B were derived from the plots of instantaneous frequency and interspike interval of Fig. 5.4B and C by sorting the individual values by the time relative to the onset of the transient and then computing a running average of ten consecutive values. Both the averaged frequency and interspike interval traces follow the initial time course of the EPSP quite closely, but the averaged frequency traces follow the falling phase of the EPSP until about 40 ms after the stimulus onset, whereas the interspike interval trace begins to diverge at about 25 ms.

Figures 5.6C and D compare the EPSP time course to the PSTH CUSUM (C) and the change in interspike interval function (IICF)[57] calculated from the corrected PSTH CUSUM values (D). As discussed above, the CUSUM shows a second period of excitation related to the regular recurrence of action potentials synchronized by the EPSP. This feature is absent from the IICF, which follows the rising phase and much of the falling phase of the EPSP. The PSTH and the various alternative measures can be used to provide a quantitative estimate of the initial portion of an excitatory synaptic input. For example, we have recently shown that for relatively large EPSPs, there is a linear relation between EPSP amplitude and the peak value of the running average of the discharge frequency record, as well as between EPSP amplitude and the area of the PSTH peak.[55] In addition, the response measures other than the PSTH also allow some estimation of the later time course of the EPSP; however, the various alternative response measures shown in Fig. 5.6A, B, and D all show a decrease in firing rate starting about 60 ms after the onset of the stimulus.

The delayed decrease in firing rate is commonly seen following large excitatory stimuli,[55] and is likely to be due to summation of the conductance underlying the post-spike afterhyperpolarization (AHP).[75,76] In a variety of motoneurons, the potassium conductance underlying the AHP is activated by calcium entry during the spike.[68] The calcium concentration in the vicinity of the channels apparently does not decay to resting levels for 50 to 200 ms following a spike. As a result, during repetitive discharge, calcium may accumulate over several interspike intervals, so that the conductance following a given spike is summed on top of the residual conductance left from the previous discharge. For intervals shortened by EPSPs, this residual conductance is likely to be higher than that remaining at the end of unaffected intervals, so that the peak AHP conductance is increased in the subsequent interval, and that interval is longer than normal. Similarly, intervals following IPSP-lengthened intervals are shortened,[55] which may reflect a decrease in the amount of AHP conductance left at the end of the affected interval.

The effects of AHP summation thus limit the quantitative analysis of long-lasting or complex synaptic potentials, since secondary effects evoked by the early portion of the synaptic potential are likely to add to the primary effects of the later portion of the PSP. These secondary effects are particularly prominent with large initial stimulus-evoked changes in the interspike interval. For example, when two large EPSPs are applied in quick succession, the increase in firing rate produced by the second EPSP is clearly less than that of the first, reflecting the decrease in excitability associated with AHP summation caused by the initial shortened interval.[77]

5.5.3.2 Effects of Simulated Inhibitory Synaptic Inputs on Motoneuron Discharge

Quantitative analysis of the inhibitory synaptic effects is complicated by the fact that large inhibitory inputs may completely suppress spike activity over much of their initial time course, precluding an estimate of peak hyperpolarization. Figure 5.7 illustrates the effects of repeated application of an inhibitory current transient on the different response measures. Spikes are delayed until about 30 ms after the onset of the IPSP. As a result, the continuous traces representing the running average of firing rate (A) and interspike interval (B) exhibit a straight line connecting the data points prior to and 30 ms after IPSP onset, and the CUSUM (C) and IICF (D) exhibit a diagonal line over this time period. All of the response measures provide some estimate of the repolarizing phase of the IPSP, and we have shown that the both the peak decrease in frequency and the decrease in firing probability are linearly related to IPSP amplitude.[55] As was the case for EPSPs, the initial change in interspike interval (lengthening in the case of IPSPs) induces secondary effects on firing rate and interspike interval, seen at about 80 to 100 ms after the IPSP onset as an increase in firing rate.

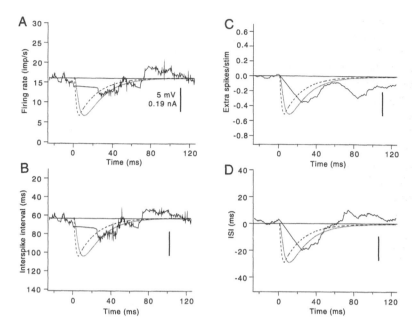

FIGURE 5.7 Comparison of the ability of different measures of changes in motoneuron discharge to reflect the time course of the IPSP (dotted trace in each panel) and the underlying injected current transient (dashed trace in each panel). (A) Smoothed PSF. (B) Smoothed interspike interval superposition plot. (C) CUSUM. (D) Interspike interval change function. Note that due to the absence of any spikes, none of the functions can represent the initial portion of the IPSP, but they do give some indication of the decrease in firing rate on the repolarizing phase of the IPSP.

5.5.3.3 Effects of Background Motoneuron Discharge Rate

The ability of the different response measures to represent the time course of the underlying synaptic potential is dependent upon the background discharge rate of the motoneuron, particularly in the case of IPSPs. Figure 5.8 illustrates the running averages of the PSFs elicited by applying the same EPSP (left column) or IPSP (right column) at different background discharge rates, ranging from about 10 imp/s (top row) to about 18 imp/s (bottom row). The rising phase of the EPSP is well represented in the PSFs regardless of the background discharge rate, but the falling phase is not well represented at the lowest background rates because very few spikes occur at this time. The falling phase is better represented at the higher discharge rates, except for the secondary decrease in firing rate reflecting AHP summation. In the case of IPSPs, there is no indication of the initial hyperpolarizing phase at any of the background discharge rates, due to the absence of spikes at this time. As the background discharge rate is increased, an increasing proportion of the IPSP is represented in the PSF.[36]

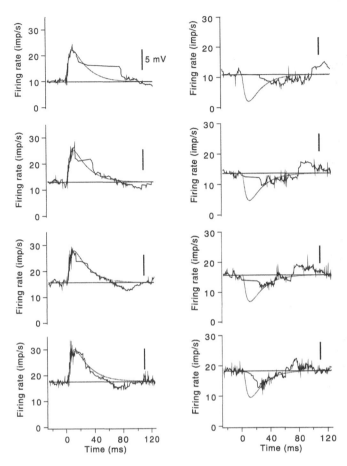

FIGURE 5.8 Effects of background firing rate on PSP-evoked changes in motoneuron firing rate. The solid traces in each panel are smoothed perstimulus frequencygrams (PSFs) evoked by simulated EPSPs (left) and IPSPs (right). At the lowest background firing rates (top), stimulus-evoked changes in firing rate provide only a rough indication of the time course of the underlying PSPs. As background firing rate increases (top to bottom), more of the time course of the EPSP and IPSP are represented by the changes in motoneuron discharge rate.

5.5.3.4 Effects of Background Noise

Threshold-crossing motoneuron models suggest that the addition of background synaptic noise should produce threshold-crossings over a larger proportion of an evoked synaptic potential, leading to an increase in the duration of the PSTH peak[78,79] (see also, H. Bostock's model[80]). Comparisons of the effects of stretch-evoked PSPs in motoneurons with different levels of background synaptic noise provided some experimental support for this idea.[43] More recently, the use of injected current to mimic small EPSPs and different levels of background synaptic noise demonstrated that the most marked effect of increasing the noise level was to reduce the size of the PSTH peak, with little or no change in its duration,[81] resulting in a decrease in peak area. The reduction in spike-triggering efficacy was related to the amplitude and frequency content of the noise, and could be as much as 50% for the highest levels of broadband noise.[81] These results suggest that estimates of the relative strength of different synaptic inputs based on changes in motoneuron firing probability could vary considerably with task or contraction level.

5.5.4 WHITE-NOISE ANALYSIS OF SPIKE ENCODING IN MOTONEURONS

Since the AHP summation, motoneuron firing rate, the sign of the synaptic potential, and the background noise level can all influence the effect of a synaptic potential on motoneuron firing probability, there is a clear need for the development of a more general model of spike encoding in motoneurons. An efficient method of deriving a general transform describing the effects of any current transient on motoneuron discharge is through the application of the white-noise method of system identification.[82,83] This approach is particularly useful for the analysis of nonlinear systems. Using it, the response of a system to any input is characterized by a series of Wiener kernels, h_0, $h_1(\tau)$, $h_2(\tau_1,\tau_2)$, etc., of increasing order. In the case of a discrete output (i.e., the train of motoneuron discharges at times t_1, t_2, ... t_N), the kernels are easily estimated by calculating the first- and second-, and higher-order cross-correlations between the motoneuron spikes and the values of the input signal preceding them.[83-85]

The zero-order kernel, h_0, is a constant equivalent to the mean firing rate. The first-order kernel, $h_1(\tau)$, is estimated from the first-order cross-correlation between the input and the output. For a system with a discrete output, $h_1(\tau)$ becomes the spike-triggered average of the input signal, reversed in time and multiplied by the coefficient h_0/P, where P is the power of the white-noise input. The second-order kernel, $h_2(\tau_1,\tau_2)$, is estimated from the second-order cross-correlation, and reflects the interaction between the two portions of the input signal in the past. A non-zero, second-order kernel is indicative of nonlinear behavior of the system.

Figure 5.9A shows the first-order kernel calculated from the response of a rat hypoglossal motoneuron to a white noise-injected current waveform superimposed upon a suprathreshold step of injected current.[86] The first-order kernel represents the linear component of the average change in firing rate produced by a brief pulse of current with an area of 1 nA-ms. For both cat and rat motoneurons, this waveform has a characteristic shape, consisting of an increase in firing probability followed by a more prolonged decrease. Figure 5.9B is a contour diagram of the second-order kernel calculated in the same motoneuron. The prominent features of this kernel are a peak with a maximal value at the point $\tau_1 = \tau_2 = 1.5$ ms and two symmetric depressions at lags of about 10 to 15 ms along the lines $\tau_1 = 1.5$ ms and $\tau_2 = 1.5$ ms. The second-order kernel describes the deviation of the output from that predicted by the first-order (linear) model in response to two separate inputs. The nature of this nonlinearity is indicated in Fig. 5.9C and D; 5.9C shows the change in firing probability produced by a single pulse of current (thin line), one expected in a linear

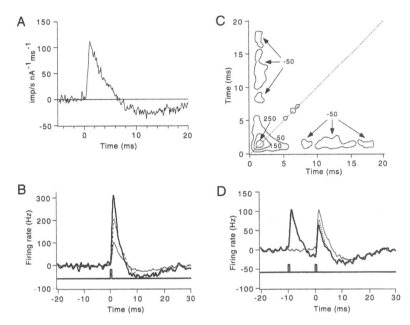

FIGURE 5.9 General representation of the input-output transform of a rat hypoglossal moto-neuron based on white-noise analysis. (A) and (B) show the first (A) and second-order (B) Wiener kernels. (C) Predicted response to a single brief input (top thin trace), along with predicted linear (dashed line) and nonlinear (thick line) responses to two brief input pulses applied simultaneously. (D) Predicted linear and nonlinear responses to two input pulses applied at different times. (Modified from Poliakov, A.V., Powers, R.K., and Binder, M.D., *J. Physiol. (Lond.)*, 504, 401, 1997. With permission.)

system if a second pulse of current is superimposed at the same time (dotted line), and one predicted based on the correction provided by the second-order kernel (bold line). The second-order model shows a greater-than-linear increase in firing probability with increasing input amplitude. Figure 5.9D shows the predicted effects of applying two pulses at different times based on the first- (dotted line) and second-order models (bold line). In this case, the second-order model shows that the preceding input reduces the response to a second pulse below that expected for a linear system.

The response to any current waveform can be calculated by convolving that waveform with the first- and second-order kernels.[86] Figure 5.10A shows simulated PSPs (lower dotted traces) and the PSTHs associated with them (upper jagged traces) in a cat spinal motoneuron. The thin lines superimposed upon the PSTHs represent the best first-order approximations of the response to the simulated synaptic inputs. The superimposed thick lines represent the best second-order approximations. In this and other cases, the first-order model underestimates the amplitude of the response to an excitatory input. For an inhibitory input, the first-order model over-estimated the minimal values of PSTH troughs, often predicting negative values, which, of course, the real PSTHs could not attain. The second-order predictions were asymmetric and provided a better match to the PSTHs for both excitatory and

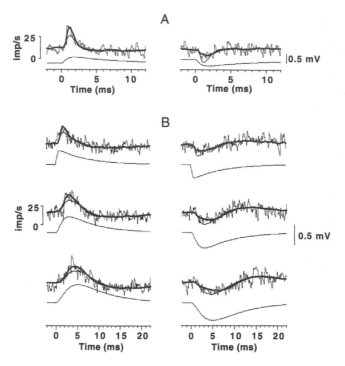

FIGURE 5.10 Calculated and predicted changes in discharge rate produced by simulated EPSPs and IPSPs in a cat spinal motoneuron (A) and rat hypoglossal motoneuron (B). The lower trace in each panel shows the simulated PSP. The jagged traces represents the change in discharge rate calculated from the PSTHs. The smooth thin lines show the predicted responses based only on the first-order Wiener kernel, whereas the thick lines show the predictions based on the first- and second-order Wiener kernels. (Modified from Poliakov, A.V., Powers, R.K., and Binder, M.D., *J. Physiol.* (*Lond.*), 504, 401, 1997. With permission.)

inhibitory inputs. Figure 5.10B shows the PSTHs obtained in a rat hypoglossal motoneuron along with the first-order (thin lines) and second-order (thick lines) predictions for three different excitatory inputs (Fig. 5.10B, left column), and symmetric inhibitory inputs (right column). The second-order predictions provided a good match to all of the illustrated PSTHs, whereas the first-order fits tended to underestimate the PSTH peaks produced by depolarizing inputs and overestimate the amplitudes of the PSTH troughs produced by hyperpolarizing inputs.

These results indicate that even the first-order Wiener model provides a good prediction of the PSTH features produced by a fairly wide range of current transients. Considering that a single set of model parameters is used to predict a range of responses, this represents a considerable improvement of previously proposed linear models. However, this set of predictions only holds for a given background firing rate and background noise level, since both factors were found to affect the calculated kernels.[86] It may be possible to derive an even more general description of spike encoding by calculating a kernel that reflects the previous discharge history of the neuron.[87]

5.6 SUMMARY

Although synaptic potentials cannot be directly measured in human motoneurons, there have been a number of recent technological and theoretical developments that have improved our ability to estimate the time course of a synaptic potential based on its effects on motoneuron firing probability and frequency. Improved techniques for stimulating different inputs and isolating the discharge of single motor units have allowed the examination of an increasing number of different inputs to human motoneurons. There is greater appreciation of potential artifacts associated with quantitative measurements of stimulus-evoked changes in motoneuron discharge. Finally, the use of animal models and the ability to mimic synaptic currents with injected currents has made it possible to test a number of different quantitative theories regarding the relation between the characteristics of synaptic potentials and their effects on the timing and rate of motoneuron spikes.

REFERENCES

1. Sherrington, C.S., The correlation of reflexes and the principle of the common path, *Br. Ass. Rep.*, 74, 728, 1904.
2. Basmajian, J.V. and De Luca, C.J., *Muscles Alive: Their Functions Revealed by Electromyography*, Williams & Wilkins, Baltimore, MD, 1985.
3. Mambrito, B. and De Luca, C.J., A technique for the detection, decomposition and analysis of the EMG signal, *Electroencephalogr. Clin. Neurophysiol.*, 58, 175, 1984.
4. Loudon, G.H., Jones, N.B., and Sehmi, A.S., New signal processing techniques for the decomposition of EMG signals, *Med. Biol. Eng. Comput.*, 30, 591, 1992.
5. Türker, K.S., Miles, T.S., Smith, N., and Nordstrom, M.A., On-line discrimination of unit potentials on the basis of their waveforms: a new approach implemented on a personal computer, in *Electromyography of Jaw Reflexes in Man,* D. van Steenberghe and A. De Laat, Eds., Leuven University Press, Belgium, 1989, 445.
6. Stashuk, D. and Qu, Y., Adaptive motor unit action potential clustering using shape and temporal information, *Med. Biol. Eng. Comput.*, 34, 41, 1996.
7. Fang, J., Agarwal, G.C., and Shahani, B.T., Decomposition of multiunit electromyographic signals, *IEEE Trans. Biomed. Eng.*, 46, 685, 1999.
8. Kleine, B.U., Blok, J.H., Oostenveld, R., Praamstra, P., and Stegeman, D.F., Magnetic stimulation-induced modulations of motor unit firings extracted from multi-channel surface EMG, *Muscle Nerve*, 23, 1005, 2000.
9. Türker, K.S. and Miles, T.S., The effect of stimulus intensity and gape on electrically-evoked jaw reflexes in man, *Arch. Oral Biol.*, 30, 621, 1985.
10. Türker, K.S., A method for standardization of silent period measurements in human masseter muscle, *J. Oral Rehabil.*, 15, 91, 1988.
11. Godaux, E. and Desmedt, J.E., Human masseter muscle: H- and tendon reflexes. Their paradoxical potentiation by muscle vibration, *Arch. Neurol.*, 32, 229, 1975.
12. Capaday, C., Neurophysiological methods for studies of the motor system in freely moving human subjects, *J. Neurosci. Meth.*, 74, 201, 1997.
13. Burke, D., Critical examination of the case for or against fusimotor involvement in disorders of muscle tone, *Adv. Neurol.*, 39, 133, 1983.
14. Türker, K.S., Yang, J., and Brodin, P., Conditions for excitatory or inhibitory masseteric reflexes elicited by tooth pressure in man, *Arch. Oral Biol.*, 42, 121, 1997.

15. Matthews, P.B.C., The human stretch reflex and the motor cortex, *TINS*, 14, 87, 1991.

16. Merton, P.A. and Morton, H.B., Stimulation of the cerebral cortex in the intact human subject, *Nature*, 285, 227, 1980.

17. Barker, A.T., Jalinous, R., and Freeston, I.L., Non-invasive magnetic stimulation of the human motor cortex, *Lancet*, i, 1106, 1985.

18. Rothwell, J.C., Burke, D., Hicks, R., Stephen, J., Woodforth, I., and Crawford, M., Transcranial electrical stimulation of the motor cortex in man: further evidence for the site of activation, *J. Physiol. (Lond.)*, 481, 243, 1994.

19. Mills, K.R., Boniface, S.J., and Schubert, M., The firing probability of single motor units following transcranial magnetic stimulation in healthy subjects and patients with neurological disease, *EEG Clin. Neurophysiol.*, Suppl. 43, 100, 1991.

20. Ochoa, J.L. and Torebjörk, H.E., Sensations evoked by intraneural microstimulation of single mechanoreceptor units innervating the human hand, *J. Physiol. (Lond.)*, 342, 633, 1983.

21. Gandevia, S.C. and Burke, D., Does the nervous system depend on kinesthetic information to control natural limb movements?, in *Movement Control*, P. Cordo and S. Harnad, Eds., Cambridge Univ. Press, Cambridge, 1994, 12.

22. Gandevia, S.C., Burke, D., and McKeon, B., Coupling between human muscle spindle endings and motor units assessed using spike-triggered averaging, *Neurosci. Lett.*, 71, 181, 1986.

23. McNulty, P.A., Türker, K.S., and Macefield, V.G., Evidence for strong synaptic coupling between single tactile afferents and motoneurones supplying the human hand, *J. Physiol. (Lond.)*, 518, 883, 1999.

24. Türker, K.S., Electromyography: some methodological problems and issues, *Phys. Ther.*, 73, 698, 1993.

25. Goldberg, L.J., Masseter muscle excitation induced by stimulation of periodontal and gingival receptors in man, *Brain Res.*, 32, 369, 1971.

26. van der Glas, H.W., Weytjens, J.L., De Laat, A., van Steenberghe, D., and Pardaens, J.L., The influence of clenching level on the post-stimulus EMG complex, including silent periods, of the masseter muscles in man, *Arch. Oral Biol.*, 29, 51, 1984.

27. Evans, A.L., Harrison, L.M., and Stephens, J.A., Task-dependent changes in cutaneous reflexes recorded from various muscles controlling finger movement in man, *J. Physiol. (Lond.)*, 418, 1, 1989.

28. Cadden, S.W. and Newton, J.P., The effects of inhibitory controls triggered by heterotopic noxious stimuli on a jaw reflex evoked by perioral stimuli in man, *Arch. Oral Biol.*, 39, 473, 1994.

29. Person, R.S. and Kudina, L.P., Discharge frequency and discharge pattern of human motor units during voluntary contraction of muscle, *Electroencephalogr. Clin. Neurophysiol.*, 32, 471, 1972.

30. Kranz, H. and Baumgartner, G., Human alpha motoneurone discharge, a statistical analysis, *Brain Res.*, 67, 324, 1974.

31. Clamann, H.P., Statistical analysis of motor unit firing patterns in a human skeletal muscle, *Biophys. J.*, 9, 1233, 1969.

32. Miles, T.S., Le, T.H., and Türker, K.S., Biphasic inhibitory responses and their IPSPs evoked by tibial nerve stimulation in human soleus motor neurones, *Exp. Brain Res.*, 77, 637, 1989.

33. Awiszus, F., Feistner, H., and Schafer, S.S., On a method to detect long-latency excitation and inhibitions of single hand muscle motoneurons in man, *Exp. Brain Res.*, 86, 440, 1991.

34. Türker, K.S. and Cheng, H.B., Motor-unit firing frequency can be used for the estimation of synaptic potentials in human motoneurones, *J. Neurosci. Meth.*, 53, 225, 1994.

35. Miles, T.S. and Türker, K.S., Decomposition of the human electromyogramme in an inhibitory reflex, *Exp. Brain Res.*, 65, 337, 1987.

36. Miles, T.S. and Türker, K.S., Does reflex inhibition of motor units follow the "size principle"?, *Exp. Brain Res.*, 62, 443, 1986.

37. Ellaway, P.H., Cumulative sum technique and its application to the analysis of peristimulus time histograms, *Electroencephalogr. Clin. Neurophysiol.*, 45, 302, 1978.

38. Brodin, P., Türker, K.S., and Miles, T.S., Mechanoreceptors around the tooth evoke inhibitory and excitatory reflexes in the human masseter muscle, *J. Physiol. (Lond.)*, 464, 711, 1993.

39. Widmer, C.G. and Lund, J.P., Evidence that peaks in EMG averages can sometimes be caused by inhibition of motoneurons, *J. Neurophysiol.*, 62, 212, 1989.

40. Poliakov, A.V. and Miles, T.S., Quantitative analysis of reflex responses in the averaged surface electromyogram, *J. Neurosci. Meth.*, 43, 195, 1992.

41. Kirkwood, P.A. and Sears, T.A., The synaptic connexions to intercostal motoneurones as revealed by the average common excitation potential, *J. Physiol. (Lond.)*, 275, 103, 1978.

42. Kirkwood, P.A., On the use and interpretation of cross-correlations measurements in the mammalian central nervous system, *J. Neurosci. Meth.*, 1, 107, 1979.

43. Gustafsson, B. and McCrea, D., Influence of stretch-evoked synaptic potentials on firing probability of cat spinal motoneurones, *J. Physiol. (Lond.)*, 347, 431, 1984.

44. Knox, C.K., Cross-correlation functions for a neuronal model, *Biophys. J.*, 14, 567, 1974.

45. Cope, T.C., Fetz, E.E., and Matsumura, M., Cross-correlation assessment of synaptic strength of single Ia fiber connections with triceps surae motoneurones in cats, *J. Physiol. (Lond.)*, 390, 161, 1987.

46. Gerstein, G.L. and Kiang, N.Y.-S., An approach to the quantitative analysis of electrophysiological data from single neurons, *Biophys. J.*, 1, 15, 1960.

47. Perkel, D.H., Gerstein, G.L., and Moore, G.P., Neuronal spike trains and stochastic point processes. I. The single spike train, *Biophys. J.*, 7, 391, 1967.

48. Moore, G.P., Segundo, J.P., Perkel, D.H., and Levitan, H., Statistical signs of synaptic interaction in neurons, *Biophys. J.*, 10, 876, 1970.

49. Türker, K.S., Yang, J., and Scutter, S.D., Tendon tap induces a single long-lasting excitatory reflex in the motoneurons of human soleus muscle, *Exp. Brain Res.*, 115, 169, 1997.

50. Kudina, L.P., Reflex effects of muscle afferents on antagonist studied on single firing motor units in man, *Electroencephalogr. Clin. Neurophysiol.*, 50, 214, 1980.

51. Awiszus, F., Continuous functions determined by spike trains of a neuron subject to stimulation, *Biol. Cybern.*, 58, 321, 1988.

52. Awiszus, F., On the description of neuronal output properties using spike train data, *Biol. Cybern*, 60, 323, 1989.

53. Poliakov, A.V., Miles, T.S., and Nordstrom, M.A., A new approach to the estimation of post-synaptic potentials in human motoneurones, *J. Neurosci. Meth.*, 53, 143, 1994.

54. Bessou, P., Laporte, Y., and Pages, B., A method of analysing the responses of spindle primary endings to fusimotor stimulation, *J. Physiol. (Lond.)*, 196, 37, 1968.

55. Türker, K.S. and Powers, R.K., Effects of large excitatory and inhibitory inputs on motoneuron discharge rate and probability, *J. Neurophysiol.*, 82, 829, 1999.

56. Fetz, E.E. and Gustafsson, B., Relation between shapes of post-synaptic potentials and changes in firing probability of cat motoneurones, *J. Physiol. (Lond.)*, 341, 387, 1983.

57. Awiszus, F., Quantification and statistical verification of neuronal stimulus responses from noisy spike train data, *Biol. Cybern.*, 68, 267, 1993.

58. Osborn, C.E. and Poppele, R.E., A method for determining the primary effect of a stimulus in tonically firing neurons using spike train analysis, *J. Neurosci. Meth.*, 24, 125, 1988.

59. Ashby, P. and Zilm, D., Relationship between EPSP shape and cross-correlation profile explored by computer simulation for studies on human motoneurons, *Exp. Brain Res.*, 47, 33, 1982.

60. Miles, T.S., Türker, K.S., and Le, T.H., Ia reflexes and EPSPs in human soleus motor neurones, *Exp. Brain Res.*, 77, 628, 1989.

61. Calvin, W.H. and Stevens, C.F., Synaptic noise and other sources of randomness in motoneuron interspike intervals, *J. Neurophysiol.*, 31, 574, 1968.

62. Schwindt, P.C. and Calvin, W.H., Membrane-potential trajectories between spikes underlying motoneuron rhythmic firing, *J. Neurophysiol.*, 35, 311, 1972.

63. Miles, T.S., Estimating post-synaptic potentials in tonically discharging human motoneurons, *J. Neurosci. Meth.*, 74, 167, 1997.

64. Nordstrom, M.A., Fuglevand, A.J., and Enoka, R.M., Estimating the strength of common input to human motoneurons from the cross-correlogram, *J. Physiol. (Lond.)*, 453, 547, 1992.

65. Powers, R.K.D.B. and Binder, M.D., Experimental evaluation of input-output models of motoneuron discharge, *J. Neurophysiol.*, 75, 367, 1996.

66. Powers, R.K. and Binder, M.D., Models of spike encoding and their use in the interpretation of motor unit recordings in man, *Prog. Brain Res.*, 123, 83, 1999.

67. Jones, K.E. and Bawa, P., Computer simulation of the responses of human motoneurons to composite 1A EPSPS: Effects of background firing rate, *J. Neurophysiol.*, 77, 405, 1997.

68. Binder, M.D., Heckman, C.J., and Powers, R.K., The physiological control of motoneuron activity, in *Handbook of Physiology, Exercise: Regulation and Integration of Multiple Systems,* L.B. Rowell and J.T. Shepherd, Eds., Oxford University Press, New York, 1996, 3.

69. Coombs, J.S., Curtis, D.R., and Eccles, J.C., The generation of impulses in motoneurones, *J. Physiol. (Lond.)*, 139, 232, 1957.

70. Powers, R.K., Robinson, F.R., Konodi, M.A., and Binder, M.D., Effective synaptic current can be estimated from measurements of neuronal discharge, *J. Neurophysiol.*, 68, 964, 1992.

71. Powers, R.K. and Binder, M.D., Effective synaptic current and motoneuron firing rate modulation, *J. Neurophysiol.*, 74, 793, 1995.

72. Schwindt, P.C. and Calvin, W.H., Equivalence of synaptic and injected current in determining the membrane potential trajectory during motoneuron rhythmic firing, *Brain Res.*, 59, 389, 1973.

73. Schwindt, P.C. and Calvin, W.H., Nature of conductances underlying rhythmic firing in cat spinal motoneurons, *J. Neurophysiol.*, 36, 955, 1973.

74. Reyes, A.D. and Fetz, E.E., Effects of transient depolarizing potentials on the firing rate of cat neocortical neurons, *J. Neurophysiol.*, 69, 1673, 1993.

75. Baldissera, F., Gustafsson, B., and Parmiggiani, F., Saturating summation of the afterhyperpolarization conductance in spinal motoneurones: a mechanism for 'secondary range' repetitive firing, *Brain Res.*, 146, 69, 1978.

76. Baldissera, F. and Gustafsson, B., Firing behaviour of a neuron model based on the afterhyperpolarization conductance time-course. First interval firing, *Acta Physiol. Scand.*, 91, 528, 1974.

77. Türker, K.S. and Powers, R.K., Estimation of synaptic potentials using discharge times and frequencies of motoneurons, *Soc. Neurosci. Abstr.*, 25, 123, 1999.

78. Polyakov, A.V., Synaptic noise and the cross-correlation between motoneuron discharges and stimuli, *Neuroreport*, 2, 489, 1991.

79. Midroni, G. and Ashby, P., How synaptic noise may affect cross-correlations, *J. Neurosci. Meth.*, 27, 1, 1989.

80. Kirkwood, P.A. and Sears, T.A., Cross-correlation analyses of motoneuron inputs in a coordinated motor act, in *Neuronal Cooperativity*, J. Kruger, Ed., Springer-Verlag, Heidelberg, 1991, 225.

81. Poliakov, A.V., Powers, R.K., Sawczuk, A., and Binder, M.D., Effects of background noise on the response of rat and cat motoneurones to excitatory current transients, *J. Physiol. (Lond.)*, 495, 143, 1996.

82. Sakai, H.M., White-noise in neurophysiology, *Physiol. Rev.*, 72, 491, 1992.

83. Marmarelis, P.Z. and Marmarelis, V.Z., *Analysis of Physiological Systems. The White Noise Approach*, Plenum Press, New York, 1978.

84. Bryant, H.L. and Segundo, J.P., Spike initiation by transmembrane current: a white-noise analysis, *J. Physiol. (Lond.)*, 260, 279, 1976.

85. Lee, Y.W. and Schetzen, M., Measurement of the Wiener kernels of a non-linear system by cross-correlation., *Int. J. Control*, 2, 237, 1965.

86. Poliakov, A.V., Powers, R.K., and Binder, M.D., Functional identification of the input-output transforms of motoneurones in the rat and cat, *J. Physiol. (Lond.)*, 504, 401, 1997.

87. Joeken, S., Schwegler, H., and Richter, C.-P., Modeling stochastic spike train responses of neurons: an extended Wiener series analysis of pigeon auditory nerve fibers, *Biol. Cybern.*, 76, 153, 1997.

6 The Use of Correlational Methods to Investigate the Organization of Spinal Networks for Pattern Generation

Thomas M. Hamm, Martha L. McCurdy,
Tamara V. Trank, and Vladimir V. Turkin

CONTENTS

6.1 INTRODUCTION

Correlation has been used to determine the organization and connections of neurons that are otherwise inaccessible or difficult to record. It is, therefore, useful for determining the organization of complex neural circuits and networks in the vertebrate nervous system. In this chapter we focus on the application of correlational techniques, primarily in the frequency domain, to the investigation of spinal circuits involved in the generation of rhythmic motor patterns, such as locomotion and scratching. Studies on the use of correlation to investigate neural systems and studies of central pattern generation are extensive, so citations to these fields are necessarily quite selective. Our intent is to establish a basic framework for the application of correlation to study neural systems, discuss the implementation of correlational techniques in the frequency domain, and briefly consider the use of composite recordings in correlation. Finally, we present examples of these applications from our studies on fictive locomotion and scratching.

6.2 THE TIME DOMAIN: CORRELATION AS AN INDICATOR OF NEURONAL CONNECTIONS

A variety of studies have explored the use of correlation to examine neuron organization, including direct connections between neurons, common synaptic input to neurons from branched presynaptic axons, or synchronized presynaptic inputs to neurons. Most studies have used correlations in the time domain; many reviews are available on these methods and their application.[1-2]

6.2.1 BASIC CONCEPTS AND TERMINOLOGY

Correlation functions describe the dependence of one variable on a second variable at earlier and later times. The variables are the same in the case of the auto-correlation function:

$$R_{xx}(\tau) = (1/T)\int x(t)x(t-\tau)dt, \qquad (6.1)$$

which indicates how the value of a signal, $x(t)$, depends statistically on its values displaced by the interval τ. This information is related to the frequency content of the signal, or its bandwidth, and its tendency to include periodicities. The cross-correlation function expresses the dependence between two signals, $x(t)$ and $y(t)$:

$$R_{yx}(\tau) = (1/T)\int y(t)x(t-\tau)dt. \qquad (6.2)$$

Using a finite period of integration, T, in practical applications provides estimates of these functions whose reliability increases with longer integration intervals, provided the statistical properties of the signals remain constant. If $x(t)$ and $y(t)$ are causally related, the cross-correlation function contains information on the process that relates them, in addition to information contained in the auto-correlation function of each signal.

Application of these equations to studies of neural function requires their adaptation for use with spike trains in place of continuous processes. By representing spike trains by values of 1 at times of spike occurrence and 0 at other times, the products in eqs. 6.1 and 6.2 are only non-zero when spikes occur in both trains at an interval of τ. The integral eqs. 6.1 and 6.2 are then replaced by simple summations of the numbers of spikes in the two trains separated by interval τ to $\tau + \Delta\tau$, yielding the familiar auto- and cross-correlation histograms. Dividing histogram counts by the number of reference spikes (those of train $x(t)$) and the bin width $\Delta\tau$ yields probability density functions in units of frequency. Alternatives include the cross-interval density histogram, which shows the time of occurrence only of spikes in train $y(t)$ that immediately precede or follow each spike in the reference train $x(t)$.

6.2.2 CROSS-CORRELATION AS AN INDICATOR
OF NEURONAL CONNECTIONS

Dependencies between spike trains can be produced by fundamental physiological processes, such as monosynaptic or oligosynaptic projections between neurons or common synaptic inputs from branched, presynaptic axons. Recognition of this fact led several investigators to consider applying correlational methods to determine the probable connections between neurons. Perkel et al.[3] discussed the uses of cross-correlation histograms and interval histograms to determine whether two spike trains were statistically dependent and to form guidelines for interpreting these histograms if dependence was demonstrated. On the basis of simulation, they suggested that (1) common synaptic input to neurons from branched presynaptic neurons is more difficult to detect than monosynaptic or oligosynaptic projections between neurons; (2) oligosynaptic connections are more difficult to detect than monosynaptic projections; and (3) several configurations can lead to the same form of correlation. A subsequent study described characteristic features of cross-correlation histograms produced by several simple neuronal circuits, based on simulations and recordings in *Aplysia*.[4] This study concluded that "fairly precise statements about the waveform, amplitude and polarity of the intracellular synaptic potential which couples the correlated cells" can be made using cross-correlation histograms based on spike trains. Furthermore, the existence of other neurons present in the network, like a common source of input, can be inferred from these histograms, even though the activity of these neurons is not observed directly. Cross-correlation and cross-interval histograms can be supplemented with other methods[5] to determine the configuration of neural circuits.

One limitation of this work was that rather large PSPs were used, while most synaptic inputs, in the absence of composite stimulation, are quite small.[6] Nevertheless, the net effect of many small PSPs can have a clear and measurable effect on neuron discharge. Calvin and Stevens[7] showed that background synaptic noise is sufficient to produce the variability observed in motoneuron discharge by causing threshold crossings sooner or later than the mean interspike interval. Sears and Stag[8] hypothesized that EPSPs produced by many presynaptic fibers shared by motoneurons would increase their probability of discharge during the rising phase of the EPSPs. Cross-correlation histograms between the discharge of pairs or small groups of intercostal motoneurons contained short-term synchronization, central peaks with widths of ±3 msec, consistent with this hypothesis. This work was further supported by the demonstration of an EPSP-like depolarization, the average common excitatory (ACE) potential, revealed by averaging the intracellular potentials in one motoneuron while using the spike discharge of another as a trigger.[9] A theory relating the waveform of the EPSP to an increased probability of discharge (see 6.2.3) successfully accounted for both the shape of the ACE potential and short-term synchronization.

6.2.3 IDENTIFYING THE ORGANIZATION OF SYNAPTIC INPUTS TO MOTONEURONS BASED ON CROSS-CORRELATION HISTOGRAMS

Identifying probable neuronal circuits based on correlation functions is discussed in several of the publications cited above. We confine our remarks to the issue of identifying the organization of synaptic inputs to motoneuron pools using correlations. Several correlating mechanisms can be distinguished in cross-correlation histograms between motoneurons. For example, Kirkwood et al.[10] show that cross-correlation histograms between respiratory motoneurons can exhibit short-term synchronization associated with common input, broad peaks which appear to be produced by correlated interneuron inputs, and correlation peaks associated with high-frequency oscillations originating in medullary neurons (see 6.3.2).

As Kirkwood and Sears[9] suggested originally, the form of the cross-correlation histogram for two motoneurons whose discharge is correlated by common input can be predicted from the convolution of their primary correlation kernels (PCK), in the terminology of Knox,[11] which describe the increased probability of neuron discharge produced by the PSP. Kirkwood and Sears found that a PCK expressed by a linear combination of the EPSP and its derivative was sufficient to account for the shape of both the cross-correlation peak and the ACE potential. Application of this theory to human motor unit recordings[12] suggests that synchrony in the discharge of human motor units occurs as a result of common inputs, probably from branched corticospinal fibers.[13] The dependence of this short-term synchronization on various physiological factors has been investigated in several studies.[14-16]

Clearly, the relationship between EPSP characteristics and the change in the probability of discharge is critical in the interpretation of cross-correlation histograms. The increased probability of discharge produced by an EPSP has been described as most directly related to the profile of the EPSP,[4] the derivative of the EPSP,[11] or a combination of the EPSP profile and its derivative.[9] Several studies have examined the relationship between the EPSP (or IPSP) received by a motoneuron and its effect on discharge probability.[17-19] These studies show that this relationship depends on PSP size in relation to the level of synaptic noise.[20] Moreover, the increased discharge probability produced by an EPSP is determined by its amplitude[19] or the amplitude of the EPSP and the derivative of its rising phase.[18] Demonstration that even the EPSPs produced by single afferents can increase the probability of motoneuron discharge[19] indicates that cross-correlation may be sensitive enough to detect dependencies between spike trains produced by neuronal circuits with a variety of connection patterns.

A central problem in this area is distinguishing the correlation peak produced by common, branched input fibers from other forms of correlating input, such as input fibers with correlated activity (presynaptic synchronization). Making this distinction can be difficult, as discussed by Kirkwood and Sears.[21] A central correlation peak produced by presynaptic synchronization should be wider than if produced by common input. But how much wider should it be? If the presynaptic neurons are synchronized by common input and project monosynaptically to motoneurons, then the peak should by widened by an additional convolution with the PCK of the presynaptic neurons. Any dispersion in the arrival time of action potentials in the set of synchronized presynaptic neurons would widen the peak as well. However, this increase in peak width may be rather slight, particularly if presynaptic synchronization occurs in neurons close to the motoneuron pools, as might be expected for interneuronal inputs. Kirkwood and Sears[21] suggest that correlation peaks with half-widths of 2.1 msec or less can be assumed to indicate the presence of common input, as opposed to presynaptic synchronization or some combination of the two. This decision must be based on the particular conditions of the system under study. A recent, careful application of this approach is given in Vaughn and Kirkwood.[22] We consider this issue with respect to interpreting correlations between motor pool activities during fictive locomotion in 6.5.2.2.

The precision with which the characteristics of PSPs and the organization of presynaptic inputs can be identified has not been fully resolved. As indicated above, the relationship between the profile of the PSP and the probability of motoneuron discharge is subject to PSP size relative to background synaptic noise. Since good estimates of this noise are unavailable in many, if not most, applications this variability introduces some uncertainty into the process of determining the organization of synaptic inputs to motoneurons from correlations in their outputs. An additional problem is determining the strength of the synaptic input from the correlation peak. This problem has received recent attention from Powers, Binder, and colleagues.[20,23,24] The level of background synaptic noise in the motoneuron affects both the size and area of the cross-correlation peak. Application of white-noise analysis reveals second-order nonlinear contributions to the change in motoneuron discharge probability resulting from injected current pulses, suggesting that the amplitudes of correlating synaptic inputs are related to the probability of discharge in a nonlinear manner. The dependence of several measures of cross-correlation peak amplitude on discharge rate is another problem.[25] Thus, the problem of accurately determining the strength of synaptic input to motoneurons from cross-correlation peaks is one of some difficulty.

6.3 THE FREQUENCY DOMAIN: COHERENCE AS AN INDICATOR OF NEURONAL CONNECTIONS

The use of correlation as an indicator of neuronal connections can be extended to the frequency domain via the coherence function. This function is a standard component in the application of spectral analysis techniques that has been used by many investigators to examine the correlation between signals in the frequency domain, as well as the linearity of the system that relates the signals.[26,27] Rosenberg and colleagues have explored the use of coherence specifically in the study of neural systems over the last several years and published several useful articles on this topic.[28,29]

6.3.1 Basic Terminology and Concepts

The coherence function, $\gamma^2(f)$, is a measure of statistical dependence between the components of two signals at each frequency in their spectra. A signal $x(t)$ is represented in the frequency domain by its Fourier transform:

$$X(f) = \int x(t)\exp(-j2\pi ft)dt, \tag{6.3}$$

where $X(f)$ is a complex-valued function of frequency, f, and the integral is evaluated over a finite length of sample record. The real-valued power spectral density function, or power spectrum, of $x(t)$ is then given by the product of $X(f)$ and its complex conjugate, $X^*(f)$:

$$\Phi_{xx}(f) = X(f)X^*(f). \tag{6.4}$$

The cross-spectral density function, or cross-spectrum, between two signals, $X(f)$ and $Y(f)$ is then given by

$$\Phi_{YX}(f) = Y(f)X*(f). \tag{6.5}$$

The power spectrum of a signal expresses the incremental power (modulus squared) of the signal for each frequency interval over the bandwidth of the signal; for a signal with mean of zero, the integral of the power spectrum over frequency equals the variance of the signal. The cross-spectrum is complex, and indicates the product and phase relation between the two signals. In practice, these functions are determined over multiple segments of sample data, with the finite segment length determining the resolution of the power spectra, i.e., the size of the frequency intervals. They are statistical variables, subject to noise in the signals and the statistical properties of the signals themselves. Thus, their accuracy as representations of the signals increases with the number of segments used in their determination. If the two signals $x(t)$ and $y(t)$ are unrelated (i.e., not correlated), then the values of the cross-spectrum, $\Phi_{YX}(f)$ will approach zero as the number of segments increases. The practical computation of spectral functions is presented and discussed in a variety of texts.[26,30]

From these signals, the coherence is determined by

$$\gamma_{YX}^2(f) = \Phi_{YX}(f)\Phi_{YX}^*(f)/\Phi_{YY}(f)\Phi_{XX}(f). \tag{6.6}$$

Note the similarity in form between this expression and the square of the correlation coefficient, or coefficient of determination. The value of the coherence function ranges from 0, indicating that no correlation exists between $X(f)$ and $Y(f)$ at frequency f, to 1, which occurs when $X(f)$ and $Y(f)$ are perfectly correlated. Confidence limits for coherence functions can be determined.[29]

6.3.2 PREVIOUS STUDIES USING COHERENCE

Many investigators have used coherence functions in the analysis of neural systems, and only a few examples are cited here to illustrate the experimental questions that can be addressed with this tool. These studies reflect the broad uses for coherence functions, which have been used to examine motor unit synchrony during tremor,[31] synchronization between muscle afferents,[32] and controls for cross-talk between EMGs.[33] Other investigators have used coherence functions to assess common drive in sympathetic activity in different limbs under various conditions,[34] or synchrony in the discharge of thalamic neurons.[35]

Of most relevance to the central issue of this article, coherence functions have been used to assess drive from central neurons involved in the generation and control of a centrally generated pattern, respiration. High frequency oscillations (HFOs), which are synchronized in the range of 50 to100 Hz, have been observed in the discharge[36] and membrane potentials[37] of medullary respiratory neurons. The significance of HFOs is unclear, since they do not appear necessary for the operation of the respiratory CPG.[38] Nevertheless, HFOs are evident in correlations between medullary inspiratory neurons and inspiratory nerve activity,[39] and between the discharge of individual phrenic and recurrent laryngeal motoneurons and the neurograms of these nerves.[39,40] The prevalence of HFOs among central and motor respiratory neurons suggests these rhythms originate in a common source closely associated with the respiratory pattern generator, and some investigators have used HFOs to indicate central respiratory drive and to obtain information about the functional connectivity between different groups of respiratory neurons.[41] Significant peaks at HFO frequencies occur in coherence functions between EMGs of respiratory muscles during respiration; these peaks are absent or reduced during other forms of motor activity involving these muscles.[42,43] These studies demonstrate that frequencies of activity generated in central neurons associated with the generation of respiration can be detected in motoneuron and muscle nerve activities, and that the expression of these rhythms is specific to normal respiration. It is worth noting that coherent activity has been observed in left and right masseter muscles during chewing, at somewhat lower frequencies than observed for HFOs, and that these peaks in the coherence functions were reduced during other forms of motor tasks using these muscles. This coherent activity was interpreted as sign of central drive from the CPG for mastication.[43] Similarly, we have observed coherent activity between motor pools during fictive locomotion and scratching at frequencies similar to those observed for modulated interneuron discharge during production of these rhythmic patterns (see 6.5.3.2.2.).

Several studies have also used coherence functions to examine the central drive to motoneurons during maintained and patterned voluntary contractions. Farmer et al.[44] found coherence peaks between motor units in two frequency ranges, from 1 to 12 Hz and from 16 to 32 Hz, suggesting that the latter peak represented periodic activity in presynaptic inputs to the motoneurons. Comparisons of coherence functions recorded from control subjects with those from stroke patients and patients with peripheral deafferentation indicated that this source was central neurons. This suggestion has been supported by studies demonstrating significant peaks over this frequency range in the coherence function between EMG and cortical activity, as indicated by magnetoencephalogram and electroencephalogram recordings.[45–47] Coherence functions have also been used to study correlations in the modulations of motor unit discharge or EMG during slow voluntary and precision movements.[47–49]

6.3.3 WHAT INFORMATION DOES THE COHERENCE FUNCTION PROVIDE?

The coherence function and other frequency-domain functions contain the same information as the corresponding time-domain functions, as is evident from the fact that the Fourier transform and its inverse transform can be used to generate one set of functions from the other. However, each set of functions emphasizes features of the data that are complementary to those emphasized by functions in the other domain,[28] so that using both types of functions is a useful approach to interpreting correlations between neuron activities (see 6.5.3.1.1).[50,51] While the central peak of the cross-correlation emphasizes the time course of interaction between pre- and

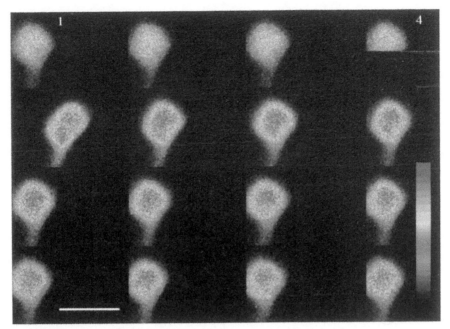

COLOR FIGURE 1 Response of a CiD cell during an escape. Images of a CiD cell are shown at 400-msec intervals. An escape was elicited in frame 4. The cell moved out of the frame during the escape, but upon its return in frame 5 it had increased in intensity and gradually returned toward baseline in the following frames. The complete recovery is not shown. The color bar at the right shows the intensity scale with red the brightest and blue the darkest. The intensity increased by 41%. Scale bar = 10 μm.

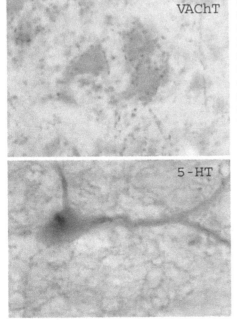

VAChT

5-HT

COLOR FIGURE 2 Contrasting patterns of synaptic input to motoneuron somata. The upper image (rat spinal cord) illustrates cholinergic input labeled by antibodies against the vesicular acetylcholine transporter, VAChT. Many of the large boutons on the soma are likely to be C-terminals. The lower image shows serotoninergic innervation of a cat motoneuron. Note that the 5-HT boutons are rather small, and that there are rather few in proximity to the cell body. However, 5-HT boutons are abundant in the surrounding neuropil, with numerous appositions on the motoneuron dendrites. Calibration: 7 mm equals 25 μm.

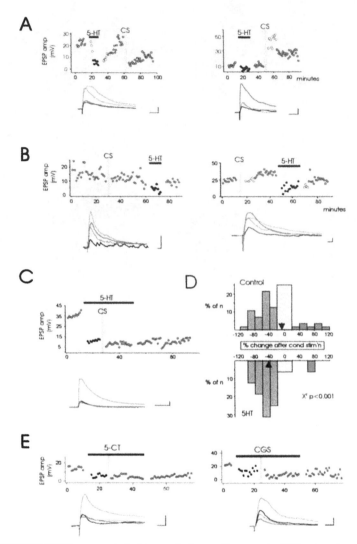

COLOR FIGURE 3 5-HT increases the incidence of primary afferent-evoked LTD. (A), (B) and (C) compare the actions of 5-HT (horizontal black bar) to conditioning stimulation of primary afferents (vertical gray bar). The ability of 5-HT to depress primary afferent input is independent of conditioning stimulation-evoked LTD or LTP whether applied before (A) or after (B) the conditioning stimulus. However, when applied during conditioning stimulation of primary afferents, (C) 5-HT almost always supports the expression of LTD (D). These actions are best reproduced by selective activation of 5-HT$_1$ receptor agonists (E). In (A), (B), (C) and (E), mean EPSP waveforms for the color-coded epochs in the histograms above them are presented overlapped and color-coded for comparison. Scale bars are 5 mV, 100 ms.

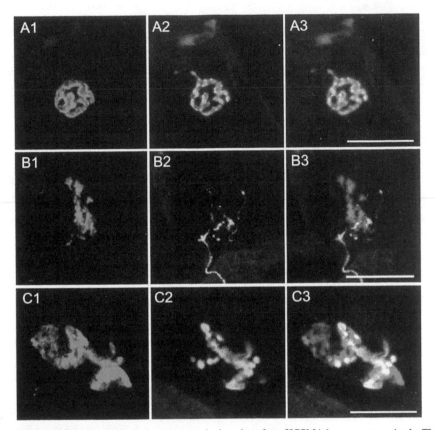

COLOR FIGURE 4 Immunostained neuromuscular junctions from HCSMA homozygous animals. The first column (A1–C1, red) shows junctions labeled for postsynaptic ACh receptors with rhodamine-labeled bungarotoxin. The second column (A2–C2, green) shows combined labeling for presynaptic motor nerve terminals (mAB for synaptophysin) and axon immunostaining (mAB for phosphorylated neurofilament protein). The third column (A3–C3) shows overlaid images from columns 1 and 2 illustrating alignment between pre- and postsynaptic labeling. (See Reference 27 for further details.) (A1–A3) Images obtained from the MG muscle of a homozygote in which failing motor units were found. The excellent alignment of pre- and postsynaptic labeling illustrated in (A3) is typical of NMJs observed in normal animals. Thus, despite the presence of motor unit failure in these muscles, junctions had normal appearances. (B) and (C). These images were obtained from more proximal muscles in HCSMA homozygotes in which frank denervation was present. (B1–B3) Images obtained from the pectineus muscle. In this case, poor alignment between pre- and postsynaptic labeling and decreased presynaptic labeling indicates the presence of nerve terminal degeneration. (C1–C3) Images obtained from the superficial gluteus muscle showing intermediate loss of presynaptic labeling. Scale bars: 25 μm (A, B); 10 μm (C).

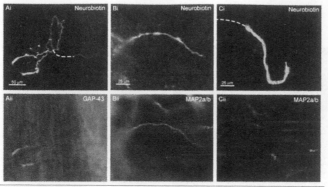

COLOR FIGURE 5

Distribution of MAP2a/b and GAP-43 in distal processes and dendrites of intact and axotomized neck motoneurons. The motoneurons were intracellularly stained with neurobiotin and visualized with the fluorochrome, Alexa 488. MAP2a/b and GAP-43 were detected using well-characterized, phosphorylation-state independent primary antibodies coupled to secondary antibodies tagged with Cy3. The top and bottom panels in (A), (B), and (C) show corresponding fields of view. (A) GAP-43 immunoreactivity in two unusually thick distal processes from an axotomized neck motoneuron. GAP-43 immunoreactivity was confined to the terminal 50 μm of each process. These processes originated from the isolated dendritic segment to the right of the twisting distal arborization. The missing link between these branches (indicated by the dashed line) was found on an adjacent section. (B) MAP2a/b immunoreactivity in the distal dendrite of a neck motoneuron with an intact axon. Note that MAP2a/b extends to the terminal of this dendrite. This dendrite was located in the white matter. As a consequence, the number of dendrites within the field of view was small. Similar fields of view in the gray matter contained a dense collection of MAP2a/b stained processes due to the much larger number of dendrites in the gray matter. (C) Absence of immunoreactivity for MAP2a/b in a thick distal process from an axotomized neck motoneuron. This process, like the distal dendrite in B, was located in the white matter. Hence, the absence of MAP2a/b in the neurobiotin-stained process can be easily detected due to the relative (compared to the gray matter) paucity of dendrites from other neurons. The proximal segment that gave rise to this process was found on an adjacent section. Its trajectory is indicated by the dashed line.

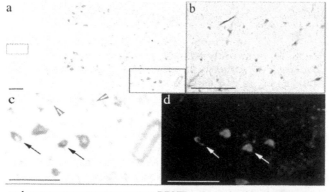

COLOR FIGURE 6

Neurotrophin expression in spinal cord astrocytes and interneurons. As an example of spinal cord cell types expressing neurotrophins, immunohistochemistry for BDNF was performed on a rat lumbar spinal cord tissue section (a, b, and c). BDNF-immunopositive astrocytes in the white matter are illustrated at higher magnification. Both white and gray matter astrocytes express BDNF as determined by double-labeling with an antibody directed against the astrocyte-specific glial fibrillary acidic protein (GFAP)(not shown). (c) A higher magnification view of the black box in (a) demonstrates BDNF-positive glial cells (red arrowheads, small cells) and larger cells with neuronal morphology (black arrows). The larger cells are Renshaw cell interneurons as indicated in the same section double-labeled with an antibody directed against calbindin. (d) White arrows indicate the same cells as black arrows in (c). Calbindin is preferentially expressed by Renshaw cells in the spinal cord. Scale bars = 50 μm.

postsynaptic activity, the coherence function emphasizes the frequencies at which the correlations between two signals occur.

The frequencies at which these correlations occur depend upon the frequency content of synaptic inputs and the transfer functions of neurons on which they act. The Fourier transform of a spike train[52] indicates its mean (or carrier) rate as well as any frequencies that modulate that rate. In the extreme (and unrealistic) case of a perfectly regular spike train, the power spectrum will show a peak at that rate and its harmonics (that is, at integer multiples of the basic rate). For the more typical case of a fairly regular spike train with some variability in the interspike interval, the power spectrum shows a peak for the mean frequency with additional contributions depending on the source of variability in the interspike interval. For example, if the variability in interspike interval is produced by cyclical modulation of the mean rate, then the power spectrum will show a peak at the frequency of modulation, a peak covering the range of frequencies over which the spike train was modulated, and harmonics of this peak. The power spectrum of a purely random spike train with a Poisson distribution will be broad band and flat. A significant feature of a spike train's power spectrum is its representation of the frequencies produced by modulation. These frequencies, in turn, provide information about the modulating processes.

The transformation of synaptic input to the discharge of a motoneuron is determined by the convolution of the input with the physiological processes that successively produce the synaptic currents, potentials, and action potentials. In the frequency domain, the product of the Fourier transforms of the signal and process describes each step. Considering the brief duration of the conductance change produced at many synapses,[53,54] the frequency content of the synaptic inputs to a motoneuron is largely preserved in postsynaptic conductances. Higher frequencies in the consequent synaptic potentials are attenuated primarily by the well-known low-pass filtering of the passive membrane,[55,56] particularly for distal synapses in which the prolongation of rise-time and half-width of potentials is greater. The overall effect of this filtering on the coherence function of the discharge of two model motoneurons subject to broadband common synaptic input has been shown by Farmer et al.[44]

To a first approximation, the spectrum of the synaptic noise in the neuron should be a summation of the spectra produced by the individual synaptic inputs. Interactions between synaptic conductances,[57,58] or activation of intrinsic conductances[59] may produce some departures from linear summation, but a linear summation of synaptic inputs provides a sufficient description of motoneuron functions under many conditions.[59]

The generation of action potentials by synaptic inputs determines the final stage in the transfer function of the motoneuron. The first-order Wiener kernel determined by Poljakov et al.,[23] which describes the relation between injected current transients and the probability of discharge, provides an estimate of the impulse response of the motoneuron. The magnitude of this kernel's Fourier transform, providing an estimate of the transfer function, decreases moderately with increasing frequency; the resulting attenuation is less than produced by passive membrane properties. Cross-spectra between injected current and motoneuron spike discharge in another recent study show little change with increasing frequency.[60] The caveat here is the potential distortions to the transfer function produced by nonlinearities, as represented by the second-order Wiener kernel. The contribution of this element occurs mainly with current transients of large amplitude; the first-order, linear model sufficiently describes motoneuron behavior for a wide range of current transients.[23] Consequently, the primary factor determining the transfer function of the motoneuron would appear to be its passive electrotonic properties, although this conclusion must be provisional pending a more direct examination of responses in the frequency domain. The possibility of substantial changes with activation of neuromodulatory pathways or voltage-dependent currents during rhythmic activities must also be considered.[61]

Based on the preceding considerations, the frequency content of synaptic inputs to motoneurons should be largely preserved in motoneuron spike trains, although with attenuation of higher frequencies. Consequently, significant peaks in the coherence function of two motoneuron spike trains, or of the activities of motoneuron pools, should indicate the discharge rates of synchronizing presynaptic inputs to the motoneurons or the frequencies at which these rates are modulated. Several lines of evidence support this expectation. One is the presence of HFOs in the activity of respiratory motoneurons or respiratory nerves, as described above. In this case, the correlated discharges of medullary neurons associated with the generation of the respiratory pattern are also found within the motoneuron pools at these frequencies.

Simple, but reasonable models of neuronal circuits also support this argument. For example, simulations of a pair of neurons with a common input or pairs of common inputs show that the discharge of the two neurons is coherent at the mean frequencies of the common inputs and at the frequencies at which these mean rates are modulated.[62] A recent paper by Halliday[63] explores the coherence produced in two dendritic motoneuron models driven by large sets of synaptic inputs, parts of which are shared by the two neurons. For Poisson input trains, the coherence function is significant through most of the spectrum, decreasing with frequency as determined by the low-pass characteristics of the motoneurons' passive, electrotonic properties. However, uncorrelated common inputs must form a large percentage of inputs before significant correlations between motoneurons are seen; common input of 80% is needed to demonstrate coherence over the full range of frequencies in the input. Coherence is stronger and more readily detectable when the inputs are discharging periodically with relatively small interspike variability (coefficient of variation of 0.1). The coherence functions under these conditions show peaks at the discharge rate of the synaptic inputs and, with decreasing amplitude, at the harmonics of the mean input rate. If the inputs are weakly correlated, then the strength of coherence is increased and can readily be detected with common inputs of 5 or 10%. The stronger effect of correlated common inputs indicates that presynaptic synchronization should be seriously considered as a correlating mechanism when strong peaks in the coherence function are detected. Both studies[62,63] also show that the mean discharge rates of the output neurons, determined by the overall strength of synaptic drive and intrinsic motoneuron properties, do not produce peaks in the coherence function. We also find that coherence functions between motor pool activities during fictive locomotion display significant peaks at frequencies mostly distinct from rates of motoneuron discharge (see 6.5.3.1.1.).

These studies show that peaks in the coherence function indicate the power spectra of correlating synaptic inputs to the motoneurons. These frequency components indicate the rates of discharge *or* the frequencies at which they are modulated. This distinction is important. Variations in activity levels during motor tasks are likely associated with modulated input frequencies to many motoneuron pools. DeLuca and colleagues[64] have shown correlations at low frequency in the discharge frequencies of motor units in a variety of tasks. The "common drive" indicated by such correlations at low frequency may be related to moment-to-moment fluctuations in activity and such well-established features of spinal organization as the size principle.[65] This common drive is ultimately related to the neuronal organization of the inputs to the motoneuron pools, of course, but we suspect it provides a less direct measure of inputs shared by motoneurons than correlations at higher frequencies, which appear to indicate the rates of discharge of the inputs. More work on this problem would be useful in the interpretation of the coherence functions observed during motor activities.

6.3.4 PARTIAL COHERENCE FUNCTIONS

In many cases, an investigator wishes to determine whether two signals are correlated by the influence of a third signal, or if the two signals would be correlated without the influence of the third. In this instance, a partial cross-spectral density, $\Phi_{YX/Z}(f)$, and partial coherence function, $\gamma^2_{XY/Z}(f)$, can be computed. These functions give the product of $X(f)$ and $Y(f)$ and the correlation between them, respectively, after the effect of $Z(f)$ is removed. The partial cross-spectral density is given by

$$\Phi_{YX/Z} = \Phi_{YX} - \Phi_{YZ}\,\Phi_{ZX}/\Phi_{ZZ}. \qquad (6.7)$$

Similar to eq. 6.6, the partial coherence function is given by:

$$\gamma^2_{XY/Z} = \Phi_{YX/Z}\,\Phi^*_{YX/Z}\Big/\Big[\Phi_{YY}\big(1-\gamma^2_{YZ}\big)\Phi_{XX}\big(1-\gamma^2_{ZX}\big)\Big]. \qquad (6.8)$$

These equations are based on the assumption that $X(f)$, $Y(f)$ and $Z(f)$ are related linearly, so that the effect of $Z(f)$ on the other two signals can be removed by subtraction. Confidence limits can be determined for partial coherence functions as they are for coherence functions.[29]

The partial coherence function provides a useful tool for interpreting the correlations between several recorded signals, since it enables the investigator to dissect out the contributions of individual signals to the correlations. This ability is useful in the analysis of neural circuits, determining the factors responsible for correlated effects in physiological studies, and controlling for the effects of a known correlation source. As described by Halliday et al.,[29] Fourier techniques can also be used to determine partial cross-correlation functions, providing a time-domain representation in which the effect of the correlating factor, or predictor, has been removed. Partial cross-correlation histograms permit the investigator to analyze the characteristics of central peaks or other features in the histograms without the complicating effects produced by a third source of correlation.

Rosenberg et al.[62] present several examples of the coherence, partial coherence, and cross-correlation functions between the discharge of neurons in simple circuits, illustrating the types of interactions that each circuit produces. Similarly, in studies of neural function that use stimulation to study the effects of one set of neurons on another (e.g., reflex studies) or induce a pattern of activity like fictive locomotion, partial coherence functions can be used to distinguish the effects of the stimulus from other correlating effects (see 6.5.3.1.1.). The utility of partial coherence functions is demonstrated by studies of complex physiological processes like tremor, in which the interacting effects of central drive to motoneurons, mechanical loading, and reflex actions complicate data interpretation.[66] Using partial coherence spectra, Halliday et al.[67] demonstrated that correlations in motor unit activity in two frequency bands, one of which has been attributed to supraspinal influences, contribute to physiological tremor.

6.3.5 LIMITATIONS OF COHERENCE AND PARTIAL COHERENCE FUNCTIONS

The coherence function readily shows the frequencies at which the activities of two neurons are correlated. However, the relations between the form of the coherence function and different forms of neuronal circuits have not been explored as thoroughly as the relations between cross-correlations and circuit organization, despite some recent contributions.[62] Thus, the use of cross-correlation techniques remains a valuable complement to coherence functions, particularly in such issues as distinguishing common input from presynaptic synchronization.

When the partial coherence function is used to distinguish the contributions of different correlating factors, the assumption of linearity in its computation must be recognized. If this assumption is invalid, then the partial coherence function may overstate the correlation between the two signals $X(f)$ and $Y(f)$ that is independent of correlations produced by the third signal, $Z(f)$, or otherwise mislead the investigator about the relation between the three signals.[62] Thus, tests of linearity of the system should be made to ensure this condition is met, or alternative controls should be considered, as discussed in 6.5.3.1.1.

6.4 DETECTING CORRELATIONS, COHERENCE IN COMPOSITE SIGNALS

Composite signals like EMGs and neurograms are often employed to assess motor and sensory activity because these signals are readily accessible. Although several laboratories in recent years have utilized techniques for making simultaneous multiple recordings from central neurons,[68–70] few examples of this type of recording are available for spinal systems, although some progress has been made in this area.[71] Due to this limitation and the ease with which EMGs and neurograms can be recorded in a variety of experimental situations, we discuss in this section the use of these recordings to detect correlations in populations of motoneurons.

6.4.1 The Use of Neurograms and EMGs for Composite Recordings

Rectified neurograms and EMGs are useful in detecting synchronization in populations of motor units or sensory neurons, as demonstrated in several previous investigations. Milner-Brown et al.[72] used spike-triggered averages of rectified EMG to detect motor unit synchrony. A single motor unit action potential was used as a trigger to average muscle force and rectified EMG. The former provided the twitch waveform of the reference motor unit; the latter provided a test for synchronization between the trigger and other units, indicated by a peak in the average broader than expected for the trigger unit alone. A similar approach has been used for detecting synchrony among muscle afferents.[73] An average can be compared to the profile expected if no synchronization exists using relatively simple calculations.[72,73] Confidence limits can also be calculated.[74]

Rectified signals have also been used to determine the projections from single neurons to motoneuron pools. Synaptic input from a central neuron to motoneurons may be evident in the correlations between the single unit's activity and the rectified EMG in the form of post-spike facilitations. Inhibitory projections and mixed projections can also be detected in such averages. Several laboratories have used this approach profitably.[75-77] Evaluation of this technique shows that the areas of post-spike facilitations in rectified EMGs are good estimators of synaptic input to a motoneuron pool.[78]

6.4.2 The Effects of Rectification on Composite Recordings

The use of rectified signals is based on the assumption that full wave rectification provides information about the timing of action potentials composing the signal of interest. The unrectified signal is dominated by the high-frequency components of the individual action potentials that constitute the neurogram or EMG, and the low-frequency components that are often of the greatest functional interest are less well represented. On the other hand, the variance of the signal is determined by the number of active units and their discharge rates. The expected value of a rectified composite signal is directly related to signal variance,[72] so the rectified signal estimates population activity and its moment-to-moment modulation. However, given the stochastic nature of composite signals, this estimate contains much low-frequency noise.[79] Moreover, the amplitude of the rectified signal depends in a nonlinear way on signal amplitude.[72,74] Consequently, despite the ease with which it can be employed, rectified signals have limitations in representing population activity.

The ability to detect synchrony in rectified neurograms was explored by Roscoe et al.[80] Synchrony of a unit is readily detectable if its signal is of sufficient size (approximately 1 to 1.5 times the standard deviation of the background neurogram activity). A unit's contribution to the peak in the rectified neurogram average increases approximately linearly above this point, but it is difficult to detect for smaller signals. Consequently, correlated activity of smaller motor or sensory units may not be detected in rectified averages of EMGs or neurograms, depending on the overall level of activity in the nerve. This issue is considered more fully by Roscoe et al.[80] Despite these limitations, this study demonstrated that synchrony among muscle afferents was demonstrated as readily using rectified neurograms as with conventional cross-correlation histograms. Moreover, rectified neurograms are equally sensitive to changes in synchrony produced by different numbers of synchronized units and by different strengths of synchronization.

Other evidence shows that rectified signals may provide reasonably accurate measures of neuronal activity. For example, Hoffer et al.[81] suggested that rectified EMGs reflected the synaptic drive to motoneuron pools during locomotion at frequencies at 30 Hz and below. This suggestion was based on their ability to inject currents proportional to the envelope of EMG into motoneurons and obtain discharge patterns very similar to those recorded during locomotion. Recently, Halliday et al.[29] compared coherence and correlation functions among tremor, motor unit activities and rectified EMGs. They found that the associations with the rectified EMG were quite similar to those with the motor unit spike trains, indicating that the rectified EMG reflects mainly the timing of action potentials in the EMG, at least for frequencies up to 50 to 70 Hz, the frequency range their study concerned. These studies suggest that rectified composite neural signals like EMGs and neurograms provide an accurate measure of the moment-to-moment activity changes in a motoneuron pool. This suggestion is also supported by comparisons of coherence spectra computed for neurogram pairs vs. combinations of neurogram and locomotor drive potentials during fictive locomotion and scratching, as discussed below (6.5.3.2.1).

6.4.3 COMPARISON OF COHERENCE BETWEEN UNITARY AND COMPOSITE RECORDINGS

Christakos has compared coherence functions based on unit and composite, or aggregate, recordings.[82,83] Coherence functions between single-unit activities and aggregate signals, like EMG, are affected by the number of correlated units as well as by the strength of correlation in these units. The phase distribution of units in the aggregate signal also influences this form of coherence (unit-to-aggregate, or UTA), and may result in cancellations that lower the estimate of correlation. For a large, partially correlated population of neurons, the UTA coherence function is almost zero at all frequencies when the single unit used for analysis is uncorrelated. When the single unit is one of the correlated units, unless the synchrony is very restricted, the value of the UTA coherence is statistically significant at each frequency of correlation. Moreover, this value is indicative of the strength of correlation. The extent of correlation within the population of units can be estimated as the fraction of units with significant UTA coherences. The coherence function between pairs of aggregate signals (ATA coherence) is generally significant at the frequencies where there are correlations between members of two large populations. Consequently, the ATA coherence can be used for the easy detection of correlations within the two populations of neurons, such as determining the presence of correlations between motor pool activities during fictive locomotion and scratching (see 6.5.3.). This function is a very sensitive index of synchrony and may exhibit saturation effects if the correlations are very strong and widespread. In view of this work, both UTA and ATA coherence appear to be useful tools in detecting correlations among neurons. Both forms of coherence have been used recently to investigate mechanisms involved in the production of physiological tremor.[84]

6.5 USING CORRELATION TO STUDY SPINAL PATTERN GENERATION

We have used correlations in both time and frequency domains to study fictive locomotion and scratching, using mainly the coherence function.[85–87] Some of our findings are presented below to illustrate the application of correlational techniques to the study of spinal pattern generation. Note should be made of a study conducted by Baev.[88] He observed significant correlations between neurograms of coactive motor nuclei during fictive locomotion. The cross-correlation peaks were broad, on the order of ± 100 ms, and may reflect mainly modulatory processes shared by motoneuron pools. The correlations did appear to be specific for locomotion, however, since their strength varied with the strength of locomotion.

6.5.1 BASIC CONCEPTS IN SPINAL PATTERN GENERATION

Some of the basic concepts regarding spinal pattern generation should be mentioned to provide a framework for interpreting some of the findings presented below. Clearly, review of this extensive area of investigation is far beyond the scope of the present chapter, but this topic has been subject to numerous reviews to which the reader is referred.[89–92]

Graham Brown[93] proposed the half-center model for locomotion following his observations on locomotion in spinal, deafferented cats. This simple model consists of "half centers" that are mutually inhibitory and produce the pattern of activity for flexor and extensor motor pools, respectively. This model has remained an important concept in pattern generation following its revival by Lundberg, Jankowska, and colleagues.[94] Despite its simplicity and robustness, the motor patterns observed in deafferented cats and fictive locomotion,[95–97] in which afferent feedback is not modulated in a fashion that would help shape these patterns, are more complex than can easily be accounted for by a half-center model. This discrepancy has prompted more complex models, such as the unit burst generator of Grillner,[89] and models that can be adjusted to produce both locomotion and scratching.[98] Based on observations of the motor activity under various experimental conditions, several conceptual models of spinal rhythm generators have been proposed.[99,100]

Although progress has been sufficient in the study of some simpler vertebrates to provide rather detailed models,[101,102] many models are conceptual descriptions of CPG organization rather than specific proposals of neuronal connectivity. For example, in the unit-burst generator model, Grillner proposed a paired set of oscillators capable of producing the patterns of activity for the motor nuclei whose muscles act at different joints. This level of model description reflects the complexity of vertebrate, and particularly mammalian, spinal motor circuits and the difficulty of developing and testing models with greater detail and specificity. Consequently, the goals in applying correlational methods to the analysis of mammalian spinal CPGs must remain relatively modest and focus, for the present at least, on determining which motor pools are likely to share input from CPGs so that inferences may be drawn concerning the organization of the interneuronal networks that provide their synaptic drive during rhythmic activity.

Jordan[103] has proposed the concept of the module, in which the output signals of the CPG are directed to sets of agonist motor pools and to a set of inhibitory interneurons that projects to their antagonists as well. Thus, each component of the drive from the CPG to a set of motor nuclei produces inhibition in the antagonistic motor nuclei. This concept is supported by intracellular recordings showing that inhibitory components of locomotor drive potentials are absent during aberrant cycles in which the agonist burst of activity is absent, and by correlations between excitatory and inhibitory PSP amplitudes in agonist and antagonist motoneurons, respectively.

Several investigators have favored a two-stage organization of spinal pattern generators in which the first stage consists of an oscillator that provides the fundamental rhythm for motor activity and a second stage that generates the different patterns of muscle activity needed to accomplish movement. Lennard[104] found that stimulation of cutaneous and muscle afferents during monopodal swimming in the turtle produced different effects in changing the pattern of muscle activity and resetting the swim cycle; he suggested a two-stage organization for the swimming CPG. Other investigators also have argued for a two-stage organization for spinal locomotor CPGs,[105] and evidence exists for a similar organization for the respiratory CPG.[38] If a two-stage organization adequately represents the CPG for locomotion and scratching, the two components must be intermixed and distributed throughout the lumbosacral cord, since evidence from several studies indicates that these rhythms can be produced at several levels of the cord.[106,107] The application of coherence analysis should be considered in regard to a two-stage CPG. Motoneuron pools would receive presynaptic drive from the pattern-shaping components and be subject to the influences of the rhythm-generating component in the first stage of the CPG only indirectly, depending on the filtering applied by transmission through the pattern-generating network. In this case, any significant correlations or peaks in the coherent functions should reflect the influences on motoneuron pools from the pattern-shaping components. However, if the first, rhythm-generating component produces strongly correlated patterns of discharge in its neurons, then these frequencies could produce correlations at these frequencies in the second-stage components of the CPG and in the activities of the motoneuron pools. This possibility should be considered when interpreting the results of correlational analyses.

Many models of pattern generation have described components in relation to the musculoskeletal system, with outputs directed to specific groups of muscles, such as extensors and flexors, or to the muscles that act at each joint. However, outputs from elements of the pattern generator could possibly be combined to determine the activity pattern of each motoneuron pool. Patla et al.[108] considered this concept in modeling EMG activity during locomotion of decerebrate cats. Similarly, arguments have been made for a modular organization for spinal motor networks (distinct from the modules described above), in which patterns of motor activity and movement are produced by the appropriate combination of a relatively small number of "modules," which essentially form a set of basis functions for

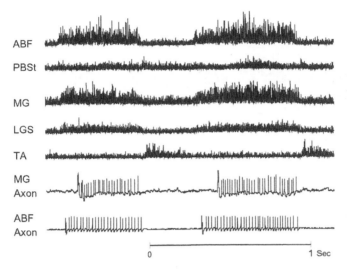

FIGURE 6.1 Data segment recorded during fictive locomotion in a decerebrate cat produced by stimulation of the mesencephalic locomotor region.[128] Movement was prevented by administration of a neuromuscular blocking agent, gallamine triethiodide. The top five traces show rectified neurograms from muscle nerves to a hip extensor, anterior and middle biceps femoris (ABF); a bifunctional knee flexor, posterior biceps femoris-semitendinosus (PBSt); an ankle flexor, tibialis anterior (TA); and two ankle extensors, medial gastrocnemius (MG) and lateral gastrocnemius-soleus (LGS). The two bottom traces show spike trains (intramyelin recordings[129]) made with glass microelectrodes from motor axons of ABF and MG in ventral-root filaments.

constructing the movement to be produced.[109–112] If the signals from different units of a pattern generator combine to produce individual motor pool activities, then correlations between different pools may occur to the extent that they receive some of the same signals, even though their overall patterns may differ.

6.5.2 Correlations during Fictive Locomotion

Correlations between the activities of different motoneuron pools can be readily determined during fictive locomotion with a set of recordings like those illustrated in Fig. 6.1. This figure shows rectified recordings of several muscle nerve neurograms obtained during an episode of fictive locomotion in a decerebrate cat. The lower traces show the discharge of single motor axons recorded in ventral root filaments. From sets of recordings like these, we have looked for correlations associated with locomotor activity between single motor axons and the motoneuron pool activity represented in rectified neurograms, and between pairs of motoneuron pools.

6.5.2.1 Spike-Triggered Averages

Figure 6.2 shows sets of spike-triggered averages of rectified neurograms (top row), triggered from the discharge of a motor axon, as shown in Fig. 6.1. These averages were taken from a single episode of fictive locomotion in which the correlations

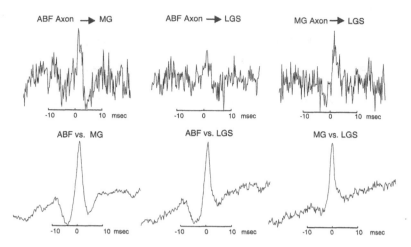

FIGURE 6.2 Correlations of motor activity during fictive locomotion were determined using data like those shown in Fig. 6.1. The top row shows spike-triggered averages of MG- or LGS-rectified neurograms, using the spike train of an ABF (left and center) or MG axon (right) as trigger. The peaks after "0" on the time axis (the time of spike occurrence) demonstrate correlations between each trigger spike train and the set of active motor axons in each muscle nerve. The bottom row shows cross-correlation functions computed from pairs of neurograms, which also exhibit correlations between the active motor axons in each muscle nerve.

were sufficiently strong that they were evident in single trials, with correlation peaks on the order of 3.5 to 4 msec in width. This was not usually the case; averages must be computed based on several trials of locomotion, each lasting 60 to 90 sec, in order to clearly resolve the central peak. In the example shown, 1777 and 397 triggers were available for the ABF- and MG-triggered averages, respectively. This should be contrasted with the number of triggers used for compiling cross-correlation histograms, which often exceeds 10,000.[8] While two motor axon spike trains can usually be recorded in such experiments, the number of spikes that can be collected, even in multiple trials of locomotion, is usually insufficient to provide histograms with sufficient resolution and clarity to be useful. However, they provide an alternative method of assessing correlations between motoneurons using spike-triggered averages.

Dispersion in the arrival of action potentials at the muscle nerve produced by differences in conduction velocity will widen the correlation peak. The correlation peaks shown in these averages may be presumed primarily due to alpha motoneurons, since gamma motoneurons, with their slower conduction velocities and smaller signal-to-noise ratios, make much smaller contributions to the rectified average (see 6.4.2). Assuming a range of conduction velocities of 60 to 110 m/s, and conduction distances of 145 and 150 mm for the MG and LGS recording sites, respectively, dispersion should widen the width of the correlation peak by a maximum of 1.2 msec. Adjusting for this dispersion, the widths of these correlations appear to be roughly 2 to 2.5 msec wide, within the range that common input via a monosynaptic connection could be considered. However, the correlation peaks are too noisy for firm conclusions to be drawn on this issue. For this purpose, averages based on larger numbers of triggers or an alternative approach would be needed, such as use of neurogram correlations.

6.5.2.2 Neurogram Correlations

The lower row of Fig. 6.2 shows correlations between pairs of rectified neurograms for the same data used in determining the spike-triggered averages shown in this figure. The improvement in the signal-to-noise ratio of the correlation peak is immediately evident. A second advantage provided by the neurogram correlation is that it provides a sampling advantage, since the majority of active, correlated motoneurons in each pool make a measurable contribution to the activity of the rectified neurogram and contribute to the correlation peak. The slope in the baselines of these correlation functions arises from the varying activity level during each cycle of locomotion. This feature suggests the need for caution, since slow common changes in neuron activity can produce spurious correlation peaks when episodes of spike activity are brief relative to the slow changes.[113] The narrowness of the primary correlation peaks in relation to the length of the step cycle and the duration of motor axon discharge (Fig. 6.1) indicates that these peaks derive from synaptic inputs.

Both the averages and correlations shown in Fig. 6.2 illustrate a consistent finding in our studies. Correlations are often found between different motor pools with extensor activity, even though the muscles of these pools may act at different joints. Thus, correlations are evident among the hip extensor, ABF, and the ankle extensors, MG and LGS. The narrowness of the correlation peaks suggests that common monosynaptic input from last-order interneurons may be a factor in these correlations, but considerable caution is warranted on this point. A feature revealed in the correlations (suggested, but not entirely clear in the averages) is the presence of troughs on either side of the correlation peak. Considering that the amplitude of the rectified neurogram represents the level of activity in the motoneuron pools at each moment, the troughs indicate reduced motor activity before and after the central peak, i.e., the probability of discharge in the population is less before and after the increase in probability of discharge in the population. This effect is likely caused by a tendency for the activities of these motoneuron populations to be modulated at rather high frequencies (on the order of 100 Hz), albeit with considerable dispersion in the frequency of modulation, since secondary peaks are not evident. It should be understood that these high frequencies are present in the discharge of the populations of the motoneurons rather than individual motoneurons; for example, the mean rates of discharge of the motor axons recorded in this experiment were 49 and 56 Hz. As a result of these troughs and the modulation in the correlated pool activity that is presumed to contribute to their presence, little confidence can be placed in the exact widths of the correlation peaks in this example. In fact, spike-triggered averages and correlation functions from other experiments without these peaks display broader correlation peaks (on the order of 4 to 5 msec), more consistent with presynaptic synchronization as a correlating mechanism, possibly in addition to common input (McCurdy and Hamm, unpublished observations).

These results suggest some of the difficulties inherent in interpreting spike-triggered averages and correlation functions. Principal among these is the fact that periodicities in the activities of the two correlated signals may affect the profile of the average or correlation in ways that may be difficult to interpret. Moreover, the effects of additional correlating factors, like the MLR stimulation used in these experiments, are not easily handled in the time domain. The use of coherence functions provides a complementary approach that helps resolve some of these difficulties.

6.5.3   COHERENCE FUNCTIONS DURING FICTIVE LOCOMOTION AND SCRATCHING

We have used coherence functions to demonstrate the correlations between motor pool activities during both fictive scratching and locomotion. In these studies, rectified neurograms have been used in most cases as indicators of motor pool activity, but locomotor drive potentials (LDPs) and scratching drive potentials (SDPs) have also been used to obtain direct measures of synaptic drive. Illustrations from both types of studies will be presented.

6.5.3.1   Coherence Functions between Rectified Neurograms

As already indicated, advantages of using rectified neurograms include the ability to sample large portions of motoneuron pools and sensitivity to small levels of correlation. Neurogram (or EMG) recordings also provide readily accessible signals for determining coherence functions in experimental preparations. EMG signals can be recorded in human subjects or in chronic behavior studies with laboratory animals, though the motor activity will reflect the effects of reflex synaptic input as well as central drive.

6.5.3.1.1   Comparison with Results from Time-Domain Correlations

Figure 6.3 shows a set of partial coherence functions obtained in the same trial used to determine the averages and correlation functions shown in Fig. 6.2. Partial coherence functions were computed to remove the correlating effect of the MLR stimulus. These functions were determined from fast Fourier transforms of data segments selected from the periods of increased neurogram activity. They are somewhat noisy; clearer functions can be obtained using several trials from an experiment (cf. top trace with Figure 1 in Reference 85). Nevertheless, broad, significant peaks are evident between 50 and 150 Hz, in addition to low-frequency peaks probably produced by modulation of activity during each burst. The broad coherence peaks in this figure start at the upper end of the range of typical motoneuron discharge. Although high-frequency doublets are often seen in this preparation, typical rates are more often in the 40 to 60 Hz range. The broad peak is more consistent with synaptic inputs at higher frequencies, a conclusion consistent with analysis of the correlation functions discussed above. These coherence functions are consistent with the correlation functions, suggest that the correlations between motor pool activities

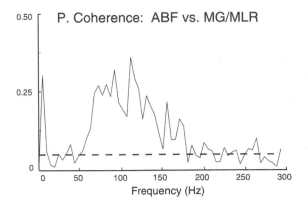

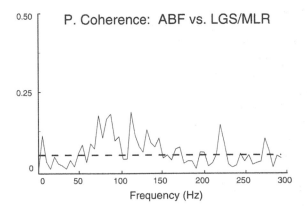

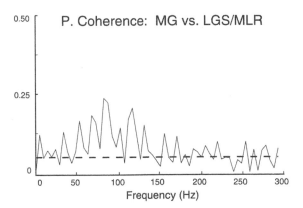

FIGURE 6.3 Partial coherence functions are shown between pairs of rectified muscle–nerve neurograms during fictive locomotion, determined using data from the same trial represented in Fig. 6.2. These functions were computed from data during epochs when each pair of muscle nerves was active. The correlating effect of stimulating the mesencephalic locomotor region (MLR) has been removed. The dashed lines indicate 99% confidence limits, showing the upper bound for coherence values that is not significantly different from 0. Broad significant peaks from roughly 50 to 150 Hz demonstrate correlations between the activities of these pools, indicating that these motor pools receive correlating inputs at these frequencies.

are caused by synaptic inputs other than those directly produced by MLR stimulation, and indicate that the frequency content of correlating synaptic input occurs from 50 to 150 Hz. The last statement must be accompanied by the caveat that using rectified signals may introduce harmonics that distort this estimation of frequency content. This issue can be addressed by considering coherence functions between neurograms and locomotor drive potentials, as discussed below (6.5.3.2).

The strength of correlation shown by these coherence functions is fairly strong, particularly compared to coherence functions determined from pairs of spike trains.[44] In part, this strength may reflect the sensitivity of coherence functions determined from pairs of composite signals.[83] Considering the greater strength of correlations produced by correlated synaptic inputs[63] and the width of many correlation functions during locomotion, discussed above, this strength may also indicate the presence of some presynaptic synchronization in the inputs to these motoneuron pools.

The use of partial coherence functions in these studies is critical, since MLR stimulation itself has a correlating influence on the discharge of motoneurons. This effect is from PSPs produced by MLR stimulation[114] and can often be observed directly in neurogram records during fictive locomotion (e.g., Figure 6.6). Partial coherence functions can be used to remove this effect, but there are several potential sites of nonlinearity in the processes carrying information from the presynaptic input to the motoneurons pools to the neurogram recording. The overall effect of these is not easily assessed. However, we have made comparisons between coherence functions and partial coherence functions determined from records obtained during spontaneous fictive locomotion and MLR-evoked fictive locomotion, respectively.[85] Similar comparisons have been made in experiments in which locomotion was induced by injection of bicuculline into the MLR (Turkin and Hamm, unpublished observations). The partial coherence functions obtained during MLR-evoked locomotion are similar to those obtained during locomotion that occurs without electrical stimulation.

6.5.3.1.2 Coherence Functions for Different Functional Groups of Motor Nuclei

Coherence functions have demonstrated consistently that the activities in the motor pools of hip extensor and ankle extensors are correlated,[85,87] consistent with results from use of spike-triggered averages and cross-correlations, as described above. Correlations between extensors are also observed during fictive scratching. Figure 6.4 shows an example of fictive scratching obtained from a decerebrate cat, with coherence functions determined from rectified neurograms from pairs of muscle nerves active during the extensor phase of fictive scratching. Correlations are evident between the hip extensor, ABF, and the ankle extensor, MG. Peaks in the coherence function are observed at lower frequencies (around 30 Hz) and over a higher frequency range extending from 60 to more than 200 Hz. Resolution on the frequency axis is limited since the extensor phase of scratching is typically rather brief, as evident from the figure. The low-frequency peak may represent modulation of the activity level during the burst. The significant coherence at higher frequencies indicates that these pools receive correlating inputs over a frequency range similar to that observed during fictive locomotion. A similar pattern is observed in the coherence function

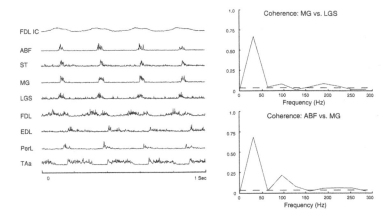

FIGURE 6.4 (Left) Episode of fictive scratching and (right) coherence functions computed for rectified muscle–nerve neurograms. The coherence functions demonstrate correlations at low frequencies and at frequencies in excess of 50 Hz. The dashed lines are 99% confidence limits. The example of fictive scratching shows an intracellularly recorded scratching drive potential from a flexor digitorum longus (FDL) motoneuron in addition to several muscle–nerve neurograms. These include ABF, semitendinosus (St), MG, LGS, flexor hallucis longus (FHL), FDL, extensor digitorum longus (EDL), peroneus longus (PerL), and the anterior part of tibialis anterior (TAa). Fictive scratching was produced in a decerebrate cat by application of bicuculline solution (1 to 2 mg/ml) to the dorsum of the C1–C2 segments of the spinal cord and gently rubbing the pinna.

between MG and LGS. Our results indicate the presence of similar excitatory drives to many extensor motor nuclei in both scratching and locomotion.

Coherence functions for motoneuron pools active during the flexion phase of fictive locomotion also demonstrate significant peaks, indicating significant correlations at both low frequencies and at frequencies greater than 50 Hz.[87] An example of coherence between pools with flexor activity is illustrated below (Fig. 6.6). Thus, both flexor and extensor motoneuron pools receive sets of common synaptic inputs (or correlated inputs) during locomotion.

Correlations within sets of both flexor and extensor pools acting at different joints suggest that signals are broadly distributed to these motor nuclei, consistent with simple models of pattern generation like the half-center hypothesis. Examination of the coherence functions involving the activity of motor nuclei with individualized or mutable patterns of activity provides evidence of a more complex CPG. A notable example of a motor nucleus with mutable patterns of activity is St, which may produce bursts of activity during either the flexion or extension phase of locomotion or in both.[115] Despite this flexibility in its use, St activity is correlated with both flexor and extensor activity during fictive locomotion when this motor nucleus exhibits flexor or extensor activity, respectively.[85,86] This finding is consistent with the suggestion that bifunctional motor nuclei, like St, can receive input from either flexor or extensor components of the locomotor CPG to produce different patterns of activity.[116]

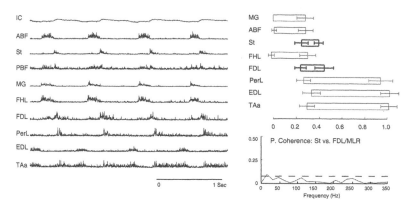

FIGURE 6.5 (Left) Pattern of fictive locomotion, including an intracellular record of the locomotor drive potential (LDP) in an unidentified motoneuron that was depolarized during the flexion phase of locomotion (IC). Spike activity in this motoneuron was blocked by injection of a sodium channel blocker, QX314. The remaining traces are rectified muscle–nerve neurograms, recorded from posterior biceps femoris (PBF) and other muscles nerves as indicated (see previous figures for abbreviations). (Upper right) Phase relations between different motor pools during fictive locomotion. The beginning of the normalized step cycle is aligned with the start of MG activity. Each bar represents the mean and standard deviation of the start and end of each burst. Bars with heavy outlines show that the timing of St and FDL activities within the step cycle do not differ significantly. Nevertheless, their activities are not correlated, as shown by the partial coherence function (lower right). The dashed line indicates 99% confidence limits.

Other muscles like extensor digitorum longus (EDL) and flexor digitorum longus (FDL) have mutable or individualized and facultative patterns of activity during locomotion.[117,118] Coherence functions involving EDL are typically weaker than those involving other motor nuclei in the same experiment, and the coherence functions for FDL usually contain no significant peaks.[87] The weaker coherence functions indicate that the FDL and EDL motor nuclei are subject to command signals that are differentiated from those received by other motor nuclei. The contrasting coherence functions of St, EDL, and FDL indicate that the CPG for locomotion may use any of several methods to produce mutable and individualized activity patterns.

6.5.3.1.3   Comparison of Coherence Functions to Phase Relations among Motor Pool Activities

Comparison of the coherence functions among the activity of two motor nuclei with their phase relation, i.e., their relative timing within the step cycle, provides additional information regarding the organization of central pattern generators not provided by either alone. Figure 6.5 shows an example of fictive locomotion accompanied by the corresponding coherence function between St and FDL. Also shown is a diagram showing the relative phases of the periods of activity within the step cycle. Each step cycle was aligned on the start of the MG burst, and the average start and end of activity for each motor pool (± standard deviation) is expressed normalized to the mean step cycle. As shown in this diagram, the timing of the St and FDL

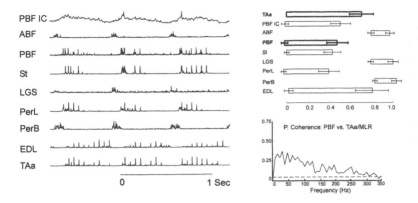

FIGURE 6.6 Episode of fictive locomotion, using the same format as Fig. 6.5. The LDP (PBF IC) shown at top left was obtained from a PBF motoneuron. Most spike activity in this motoneuron was blocked by injection of QX314. The remaining traces are rectified muscle–nerve neurograms (PerB: peroneus brevis; other abbreviations are the same as in previous figures). The phase diagram shows that the activities of TA and PBF overlap, but PBF ends earlier. Despite these distinct phases of activity, the activities of these motor pools are correlated, as shown by the partial coherence function (lower right). The dashed lines show 99% confidence limits.

bursts does not differ significantly. However, the St-FDL coherence function gives no indication of significant shared synaptic drive. Despite the similarity in timing, these motor nuclei are evidently activated by largely separate and distinct commands.

Figure 6.6 shows an example of fictive locomotion, with the accompanying phase diagram and coherence function for posterior biceps femoris (PBF) and tibialis anterior (TA). In this case, TA and PBF are recruited simultaneously, but activity in PBF ends before that in TA. Despite these different patterns, the coherence between these motor nuclei is fairly strong. Similar examples have been observed between different motor nuclei in both locomotion and scratching (Turkin and Hamm, unpublished observations). One explanation for this observation is that the variety of patterns observed during locomotion and scratching is produced by combining several independent signals produced by the pattern generator, as suggested by Patla et al.[108] The activity of different motor pools could then be correlated despite being expressed in somewhat varied patterns.

6.5.3.2 Coherence Functions between LDPs and Neurograms

Rectified neurograms provide convenient, sensitive measures of population activity, but using rectified composite signals introduces uncertainties, as indicated above (6.4.2). This limitation can be addressed through studies of single-unit activity, although at the price of less sensitivity and the need for much longer segments of data, which are impractical in many cases. An alternative we have used is to record intracellular locomotor drive potentials (LDPs) and scratching drive potentials (SDPs) during fictive locomotion and scratching, respectively, which reflect the synaptic drive to individual motoneurons.[119–121] Coherence functions between LDPs or SDPs and rectified neurograms provide measures of the correlation between recordings of the synaptic input to a motoneuron and the population activity represented in the neurograms of several motoneuron pools. These functions provide a useful basis for comparison with coherence functions computed for neurogram pairs.

6.5.3.2.1   Comparison of LDP-Ng to Ng-Ng Coherence Functions

Coherence functions between LDPs and rectified neurograms obtained during fictive locomotion are in agreement with the coherence functions computed for neurogram pairs.[87] An example of a coherence function determined for a LDP from a MG motoneuron and a rectified neurogram is shown in Fig. 6.7B. SDP-neurogram coherence functions obtained during fictive scratching also confirm the neurogram–neurogram correlations found in these studies (Turkin and Hamm, unpublished observations). The principal difference between the two forms of coherence function is the range of frequencies over which the coherence function is significant. The range is usually more restricted for the coherence between drive potential and neurogram activity than between neurograms, with correlations typically observed up to 100 to 120 Hz for the former. The correlations at greater frequencies (> 120 to 150 Hz) in neurogram–neurogram coherence functions may reflect the presence of harmonics produced by rectification. Also, the greater sensitivity expected of coherence functions based on a pair of composite signals, like the neurogram–neurogram coherences, may reveal weak correlations between high-frequency components of the spectra that the LDP-neurogram coherence functions do not. In general, the correlations between motor pool activities are somewhat weaker in LDP–neurogram coherence functions than in neurogram–neurogram coherence functions.

6.5.3.2.2   Frequency Content of LDPs

The correlating inputs between 50 and 120 Hz suggested by coherence functions should be represented directly within the synaptic potentials of the LDP. Figure 6.7F shows examples of the power spectral densities of LDPs, using both the depolarizing and hyperpolarizing phases of the LDP of the MG motoneuron used for this figure. As noted previously, the frequency content of the synaptic potentials is filtered by the passive properties of the motoneuron. For comparison, this figure also shows the effect this filtering would have on synaptic input to the dendrites of a motoneuron, as determined using a compartmental model of a motoneuron from a set whose morphology and electrophysiology have both been described.[122,123] This filtering will vary depending on the electrotonic properties of each neuron, the dendritic locations of the synaptic inputs, and changes produced in the electrotonic structure by conductance changes associated with locomotion. Nevertheless, it provides an approximate outline for gauging the frequency content of the LDP. Accordingly, this plot shows that both the depolarizing and hyperpolarizing LDP decrease roughly in parallel to the curve describing the passive filtering, perhaps falling more rapidly at higher frequencies. This comparison indicates that the synaptic noise of the LDP contains significant components within the frequency range (50 to 120 Hz) in which correlations occur between LDPs and neurograms. These frequencies are compatible with rates recorded from spinal neurons during locomotion and scratching in decerebrate cats.

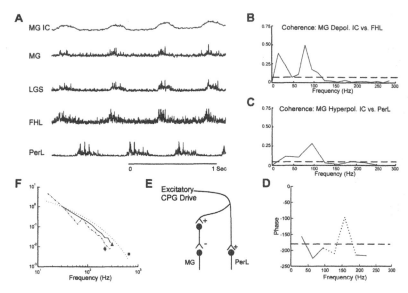

FIGURE 6.7 Data from fictive locomotion is illustrated. (A) An episode of fictive locomotion represented by a LDP from a MG motoneuron and several rectified muscle–nerve neurograms. (B) and (C) Coherence functions demonstrating correlations between the depolarizing phase of the MG LDP and activity in FHL and between hyperpolarizing phase of the MG LDP and rectified neurogram activity in PerL, respectively. These coherence functions were similar in form and magnitude to the corresponding partial coherence functions (see Figure 3 in Reference 87). (D) The corresponding phase relation between the hyperpolarizing MG LDP and the PerL neurogram. The dotted part of this curve corresponds to sections of the coherence function well below the 99% confidence limits, where phase values no longer describe the relation between correlated signals. The phase shift between hyperpolarizing LDP and PerL neurogram activity is approximately 180° (dashed line), consistent with the MG motoneuron and the PerL motor pool receiving correlated inhibition and excitation, respectively. (E) A simple neuronal circuit sufficient to explain this finding. (F) The power spectra of the depolarizing (star) and hyperpolarizing (triangle) LDPs. The effect of passive membrane properties on synaptic input is also shown (square). This curve is the squared, absolute value of the Fourier transform of an EPSP produced by a brief conductance change in a dendritic compartment 0.45 length constants from the soma (determined using a compartmental model based on the parameters of FR motoneuron 42/4 of Fleshman et al.[123]). All power spectra are normalized to the value at 32 Hz, the lowest frequency available for the hyperpolarizing LDP.

Orlovsky and Feldman[124] found that most interneurons with modulated discharge during decerebrate locomotion had rates between 25 and 150 Hz, with a mean rate of 88 Hz. Similarly, Berkinblit et al.[125] found interneurons that were modulated during the scratch cycle had mean rates of 82 to 84 Hz, with similarly wide ranges.

6.5.3.2.3 Support for Module Concept

Recording LDPs or SDPs broadens the possibilities for investigating the organization of rhythmic activities since the synaptic drive to a motoneuron pool can be recorded during the inhibitory phase of the cycle, when motor activity in the neurogram is absent, as well as during the excitatory phase. Consequently, the synaptic drive to a motoneuron can be compared with the activity in the neurogram of its antagonist. An example of this type of coherence function is provided in Fig. 6.7C, showing the correlation between the hyperpolarizing phase of the LDP in this MG motoneuron and the activity in the PerL neurogram. The significant peak in this coherence function indicates that these two motoneuron pools receive similar signals while one is excited and the other inhibited. Presumably, the signal to the active pool (PerL) is excitatory and the signal to the inactive pool (MG) is inhibitory, since the hyper-polarizing phase of the LDP is a synaptic inhibition, rather than the absence of excitation.[119,120] This is confirmed by the phase plot of the coherence function vs. frequency in Fig. 6.7D, showing that the hyperpolarizing LDP of MG and the neurogram activity of PerL are 180° out of phase. The schematic in Fig. 6.7E shows the simplest circuit consistent with this finding, in which the locomotor CPG sends excitatory drive to the PerL motoneuron pools and to a set of interneurons that concurrently inhibit the MG motoneuron pool.

6.6 SUMMARY AND CONCLUSIONS

Correlational methods have provided means in many studies for indirectly assessing the organization of neuronal circuits. Cross-correlations and coherence functions provide sensitive, complementary information on correlations between the activities of individual neurons or neuron populations. Application of these methods to inves-tigate the activities of motoneuron pools demonstrates correlations produced by their synaptic inputs. Several lines of evidence suggest that the use of coherence functions provides information on the rates of discharge in these synaptic inputs and frequen-cies at which these rates are modulated.

Our application of these methods to fictive locomotion and scratching demon-strates correlations between the activities of many motoneurons. These correlations most likely originate in the synaptic drive provided by spinal pattern generators since no movement occurs in the immobilized preparations used for these experi-ments, and common inputs from muscle afferents are often limited by extensive denervation. The strength and temporal profiles of correlations found in some exper-iments suggest that part of the coherence observed between different motor pools is derived from the synchronization of inputs to the motoneuron pools during fictive locomotion and scratching, and that the discharge of these inputs occurs at rates in excess of 50 Hz. Such synchronization would support the suggestion that correlated activities at these rates may be a general characteristic of mammalian pattern-generating circuits.[126] However, additional work is needed on the strength of corre-lations produced by common inputs in composite measures of motoneuron activity in addition to recordings of interneuronal activity in areas associated with spinal pattern generation[107,124,127] to substantiate this suggestion.

The distribution of correlations between many motoneuron pools indicates that many motor nuclei receive the same central commands during locomotion and scratching, including pools that innervate muscles with disparate mechanical actions. Comparison of coherence functions with the patterns of activity expressed by these motor nuclei suggests that some motor nuclei receive more than one command generated by the CPG in a weighting that determines the pattern of activity. Individualized and mutable patterns of activity may be produced by commands shared by many motor nuclei, possibly using some form of gating mechanism, as seems to be the case with semitendinosus, or by individualized commands, as seems to be the case with the motor nuclei of some digit muscles, like flexor digitorum longus. The correlations revealed between the inhibitory synaptic activity in locomotor drive potentials and the activity of antagonists provide additional support for a modular organization of the locomotor CPG.[103] These observations show that correlational techniques may provide substantial information about the organization of the neuronal networks responsible for spinal pattern generation.

ACKNOWLEDGMENTS

We thank Ms. Tracy Fleming for her help in figure preparation, and Ms. Fleming, Mr. Michael Burroughs, and Ms. Nancy Heter for assistance in the experiments. This work was supported by USPHS grants NS22454 (to T.M.H.), NS08773 (to M.L.M.) and NS07309 (to the Univ. Arizona-Barrow Neurological Inst., Arizona State Univ. Training Program in Motor Control Neurobiology).

REFERENCES

1. Moore, G.P., Perkel, D.H., and Segundo, J.P., Statistical analysis and functional interpretation of neuronal spike data, *Annu. Rev. Physiol.*, 28, 493, 1966.
2. Kirkwood, P.A., On the use and interpretation of cross-correlations measurements in the mammalian central nervous system, *J. Neurosci. Meth.*, 1, 107, 1979.
3. Perkel, D.H., Gerstein, G.L., and Moore, G.P., Neuronal spike trains and stochastic point processes. II. Simultaneous spike trains, *Biophys. J.*, 7, 419, 1967.
4. Moore, G.P., Segundo, J.P., Perkel, D.H., and Levitan, H., Statistical signs of synaptic interaction in neurons, *Biophys. J.*, 10, 876, 1970.
5. Gerstein, G.L. and Perkel, D.H., Mutual temporal relationships among neuronal spike trains. Statistical techniques for display and analysis, *Biophys. J.*, 12, 453, 1972.
6. Mendell, L.M. and Henneman, E., Terminals of single Ia fibers: location, density, and distribution within a pool of 300 homonymous motoneurons, *J. Neurophysiol.*, 34, 171, 1971.
7. Calvin, W.H. and Stevens, C.F., Synaptic noise and other sources of randomness in motoneuron interspike intervals, *J. Neurophysiol.*, 31, 574, 1968.
8. Sears, T.A. and Stagg, D., Short-term synchronization of intercostal motoneurone activity, *J. Physiol. (Lond.)*, 263, 357, 1976.
9. Kirkwood, P.A. and Sears, T.A., The synaptic connexions to intercostal motoneurones as revealed by the average common excitation potential, *J. Physiol. (Lond.)*, 275, 103, 1978.
10. Kirkwood, P.A., Sears, T.A., Tuck, D.L., and Westgaard, R.H., Variations in the time course of the synchronization of intercostal motoneurones in the cat, *J. Physiol. (Lond.)*, 327, 105, 1982.
11. Knox, C.K., Cross-correlation functions for a neuronal model, *Biophys. J.*, 14, 567, 1974.
12. Datta, A.K. and Stephens, J.A., Synchronization of motor unit activity during voluntary contraction in man, *J. Physiol. (Lond.)*, 422, 397, 1990.

13. Datta, A.K., Farmer, S.F., and Stephens, J.A., Central nervous pathways underlying synchronization of human motor unit firing studied during voluntary contractions, *J. Physiol. (Lond.)*, 432, 401, 1991.

14. Bremner, F.D., Baker, J.R., and Stephens, J.A., Correlation between the discharges of motor units recorded from the same and from different finger muscles in man, *J. Physiol. (Lond.)*, 432, 355, 1991.

15. Bremner, F.D., Baker, J.R., and Stephens, J.A., Effect of task on the degree of synchronization of intrinsic hand muscle motor units in man, *J. Neurophysiol.*, 66, 2072, 1991.

16. Bremner, F.D., Baker, J.R., and Stephens, J.A., Variation in the degree of synchronization exhibited by motor units lying in different finger muscles in man, *J. Physiol. (Lond.)*, 432, 381, 1991.

17. Fetz, E.E. and Gustafsson, B., Relation between shapes of post-synaptic potentials and changes in firing probability of cat motoneurones, *J. Physiol. (Lond.)*, 341, 387, 1983.

18. Gustafsson, B. and McCrea, D., Influence of stretch-evoked synaptic potentials on firing probability of cat spinal motoneurones, *J. Physiol. (Lond.)*, 347, 431, 1984.

19. Cope, T.C., Fetz, E.E., and Matsumura, M., Cross-correlation assessment of synaptic strength of single Ia fiber connections with triceps surae motoneurones in cats, *J. Physiol. (Lond.)*, 390, 161, 1987.

20. Poliakov, A.V., Powers, R.K., Sawczuk, A., and Binder, M.D., Effects of background noise on the response of rat and cat motoneurones to excitatory current transients, *J. Physiol. (Lond.)*, 495, 143, 1996.

21. Kirkwood, P.A. and Sears, T.A., Cross-correlation analyses of motoneuron inputs in a coordinated motor act., in *Neural Cooperativity*, Krüger, J., Ed., Springer-Verlag, Berlin, 1991, 225.

22. Vaughan, C.W. and Kirkwood, P.A., Evidence from motoneurone synchronization for disynaptic pathways in the control of inspiratory motoneurones in the cat, *J. Physiol. (Lond.)*, 503, 673, 1997.

23. Poliakov, A.V., Powers, R.K., and Binder, M.D., Functional identification of the input-output transforms of motoneurones in the rat and cat, *J. Physiol. (Lond.)*, 504, 401, 1997.

24. Powers, R.K. and Binder, M.D., Models of spike encoding and their use in the interpretation of motor unit recordings in man, *Prog. Brain Res.*, 123, 83, 1999.

25. Nordstrom, M.A., Fuglevand, A.J., and Enoka, R.M., Estimating the strength of common input to human motoneurons from the cross-correlogram, *J. Physiol. (Lond.)*, 453, 547, 1992.

26. Bendat, J.S. and Piersol, A.G., *Random Data. Analysis and Measurements Procedures*, 2nd ed., John Wiley & Sons, New York, 1986.

27. Marmarelis, P.Z. and Marmarelis, V.Z., *Analysis of Physiological Systems: The White Noise Approach*, Plenum Press, New York, 1978.

28. Rosenberg, J.R., Amjad, A.M., Breeze, P., Brillinger, D.R., and Halliday, D.M., The Fourier approach to the identification of functional coupling between neuronal spike trains, *Prog. Biophys. Mol. Biol.*, 53, 1, 1989.

29. Halliday, D.M., Rosenberg, J.R., Amjad, A.M., Breeze, P., Conway, B.A., and Farmer, S.F., A framework for the analysis of mixed time series/point process data — theory and application to the study of physiological tremor, single motor unit discharges and electromyograms, *Prog. Biophys. Mol. Biol.*, 64, 237, 1995.

30. Press, W.H., Teukolsky, S.A., Vetterling, W.T., and Flannery, B.P., *Numerical Recipes in C: The Art of Scientific Computing*, 2nd ed., Cambridge University Press, New York, 1992.

31. Elble, R.J. and Randall, J.E., Motor-unit activity responsible for 8- to 12-Hz component of human physiological finger tremor, *J. Neurophysiol.*, 39, 370, 1976.
32. Clark, F.J., Matthews, P.B.C., and Muir, R.B., Response of soleus Ia afferents to vibration in the presence of the tonic vibration reflex in the decerebrate cat, *J. Physiol. (Lond.)*, 311, 97, 1981.
33. Houk, J.C., Dessem, D.A., Miller, L.E., and Sybirska, H., Correlation and spectral analysis of relations between single unit discharge and muscle activities, *J. Neurosci. Meth.*, 21, 201, 1987.
34. Wallin, B.G., Burke, D., and Gandevia, S.C., Coherence between the sympathetic drives to relaxed and contracting muscles of different limbs of human subjects, *J. Physiol. (Lond.)*, 455, 219, 1992.
35. Contreras, D., Destexhe, A., Sejnowski, T.J., and Steriade, M., Control of spatiotemporal coherence of a thalamic oscillation by corticothalamic feedback, *Science,* 274, 771, 1996.
36. Cohen, M.I., Synchronization of discharge, spontaneous and evoked, between inspiratory neurons, *Acta Neurobiol. Exp.*, 33, 189, 1973.
37. Mitchell, R.A. and Herbert, D.A., Synchronized high frequency synaptic potentials in medullary respiratory neurons, *Brain Res.*, 75, 350, 1974.
38. Feldman, J.L., Neurophysiology of breathing in animals, in *Handbook of Physiology: The Nervous System IV. Intrinsic Regulatory Systems of the Brain,* Bloom, F.E., Ed., American Physiological Society, Bethesda, 1986, 463.
39. Christakos, C.N., Cohen, M.I., See, W.R., and Barnhardt, R., Changes in frequency content of inspiratory neuron and nerve activities in the course of inspiration, *Brain Res.*, 482, 376, 1989.
40. Christakos, C.N., Cohen, M.I., Sica, A.L., Huang, W.X., See, W.R., and Barnhardt, R., Analysis of recurrent laryngeal inspiratory discharges in relation to fast rhythms, *J. Neurophysiol.*, 72, 1304, 1994.
41. Huang, W.-X., Cohen, M.I., Yu, Q., See, W.R., and He, Q., High-frequency oscillations in membrane potentials of medullary inspiratory and expiratory neurons (including laryngeal motoneurons), *J. Neurophysiol.*, 76, 1405, 1996.
42. Bruce, E.N. and Ackerson, L.M., High-frequency oscillations in human electromyograms during voluntary contractions, *J. Neurophysiol.*, 56, 542, 1986.
43. Smith, A. and Denny, M., High-frequency oscillations as indicators of neural control mechanisms in human respiration, mastication, and speech, *J. Neurophysiol.*, 63, 745, 1990.
44. Farmer, S.F., Bremner, F.D., Halliday, D.M., Rosenberg, J.R., and Stephens, J.A., The frequency content of common synaptic inputs to motoneurones studied during voluntary isometric contraction in man, *J. Physiol. (Lond.)*, 470, 127, 1993.
45. Conway, B.A., Halliday, D.M., Farmer, S.F., Shahani, U., Maas, P., Weir, A.I., and Rosenberg, J.R., Synchronization between motor cortex and spinal motoneuronal pool during the performance of a maintained motor task in man, *J. Physiol. (Lond.)*, 489, 917, 1995.
46. Brown, P., Farmer, S.F., Halliday, D.M., Marsden, J., and Rosenberg, J.R., Coherent cortical and muscle discharge in cortical myoclonus, *Brain,* 122, 461, 1999.
47. Kilner, J.M., Baker, S.N., Salenius, S., Jousmaki, V., Hari, R., and Lemon, R.N., Task-dependent modulation of 15-30 Hz coherence between rectified EMGs from human hand and forearm muscles, *J. Physiol. (Lond.)*, 516, 559, 1999.
48. Kakuda, N., Nagaoka, M., and Wessberg, J., Common modulation of motor unit pairs during slow wrist movement in man, *J. Physiol. (Lond.)*, 520, 929, 1999.

49. Wessberg, J. and Kakuda, N., Single motor unit activity in relation to pulsatile motor output in human finger movements, *J. Physiol. (Lond.)*, 517, 273, 1999.

50. Davey, N.J., Ellaway, P.H., Baker, J.R., and Friedland, C.L., Rhythmicity associated with a high degree of short-term synchrony of motor unit discharge in man, *Exp. Physiol.*, 78, 649, 1993.

51. Kuipers, U., Laouris, Y., Kokkoroyiannis, T., Meyer-Lohmann, J., and Windhorst, U., Relations between time-and frequency-domain measures of signal transmission from cutaneous afferents to dorsal horn neurons, *Brain Res.*, 462, 154, 1988.

52. Bayly, E.J., Spectral analysis of pulse frequency modulation in the nervous systems, *IEEE Trans. Biomed. Eng.*, 15, 257, 1968.

53. Finkel, A.S. and Redman, S.J., The synaptic current evoked in cat spinal motoneurones by impulses in single group Ia axons, *J. Physiol. (Lond.)*, 342, 615, 1983.

54. Stuart, G.J. and Redman, S.J., Voltage dependence of Ia reciprocal inhibitory currents in cat spinal motoneurones, *J. Physiol. (Lond.)*, 420, 111, 1990.

55. Rall, W., Distinguishing theoretical synaptic potentials computed for different soma-dendritic distributions of synaptic inputs, *J. Neurophysiol.*, 30, 1138, 1967.

56. Jack, J.J., Miller, S., Porter, R., and Redman, S.J., The time course of minimal excitatory post-synaptic potentials evoked in spinal motoneurones by group Ia afferent fibers, *J. Physiol. (Lond.)*, 215, 353, 1971.

57. Burke, R.E., Composite nature of the monosynaptic excitatory postsynaptic potential, *J. Neurophysiol.*, 30, 1114, 1967.

58. Burke, R.E., Fedina, L., and Lundberg, A., Spatial synaptic distribution of recurrent and group Ia inhibitory systems in cat spinal motoneurones, *J. Physiol. (Lond.)*, 214, 305, 1971.

59. Powers, R.K. and Binder, M.D., Summation of effective synaptic currents and firing rate modulation in cat spinal motoneurons, *J. Neurophysiol.*, 83, 483, 2000.

60. Boskov, D., Jocic, M., Jovanovic, K., Ljubisavljevic, M., and Anastasijevic, R., Spike discharges of skeletomotor neurons during random noise modulated transmembrane current stimulation and muscle stretch, *Biol. Cybern.*, 71, 341, 1994.

61. Brownstone, R.M., Gossard, J.-P., and Hultborn, H., Voltage-dependent excitation of motoneurones from spinal locomotor centres in the cat, *Exp. Brain Res.*, 102, 34, 1994.

62. Rosenberg, J.R., Halliday, D.M., Breeze, P., and Conway, B.A., Identification of patterns of neuronal connectivity — partial spectra, partial coherence, and neuronal interactions, *J. Neurosci. Meth.*, 83, 57, 1998.

63. Halliday, D.M., Weak, stochastic temporal correlation of large scale synaptic input is a major determinant of neuronal bandwidth, *Neural Comput.*, 12, 693, 2000.

64. DeLuca, C.J., LeFever, R.S., McCue, M.P., and Xenakis, A.P., Control scheme governing concurrently active human motor units during voluntary contractions, *J. Physiol. (Lond.)*, 329, 129, 1982.

65. Henneman, E. and Mendell, L.W., Functional organization of the motoneuron pool and its inputs, in *Handbook of Physiology: The Nervous System II, Pt. 1*, Brooks, V.B., Ed., American Physiological Society, Bethesda, 1981, 423.

66. Stein, R.B. and Lee, R.G., Tremor and clonus, in *Handbook of Physiology: The Nervous System II. Motor Control, Pt. 1*, Brooks, V.B., Ed., American Physiological Society, Bethesda, 1981, 325.

67. Halliday, D.M., Conway, B.A., Farmer, S.F., and Rosenberg, J.R., Load-independent contributions from motor-unit synchronization to human physiological tremor, *J. Neurophysiol.*, 82, 664, 1999.

68. Nicolelis, M.A.L., Baccala, L.A., Lin, R.C.S., and Chapin, J.K., Sensorimotor encoding by synchronous neural ensemble activity at multiple levels of the somatosensory system, *Science,* 268, 1353, 1995.

69. Chrobak, J.J. and Buzsaki, G., High-frequency oscillations in the output networks of the hippocampal-entorhinal axis of the freely behaving rat, *J. Neurosci.,* 16, 3056, 1996.

70. Gothard, K.M., Skaggs, W.E., Moore, K.M., and McNaughton, B.L., Binding of hippocampal CA1 neural activity to multiple reference frames in a landmark-based navigation task, *J. Neurosci.,* 16, 823, 1996.

71. Tresch, M.C. and Kiehn, O., Coding of locomotor phase in populations of neurons in rostral and caudal segments of the neonatal rat lumbar spinal cord, *J. Neurophysiol.,* 82, 3563, 1999.

72. Milner-Brown, H.S., Stein, R.B., and Yemm, R., The contractile properties of human motor units during voluntary isometric contractions, *J. Physiol. (Lond.),* 228, 285, 1973.

73. Hamm, T.M., Reinking, R.M., Roscoe, D.D., and Stuart, D.G., Synchronous afferent discharge from a passive muscle of the cat: significance for interpreting spike-triggered averages, *J. Physiol. (Lond.),* 365, 77, 1985.

74. Hamm, T.M., Roscoe, D.D., Reinking, R.M., and Stuart, D.G., Detection of synchrony in the discharge of a population of neurons. I. Development of a synchronization index, *J. Neurosci. Meth.,* 13, 37, 1985.

75. Fetz, E.E. and Cheney, P.D., Postspike facilitation of forelimb muscle activity by primate corticomotoneuronal cells, *J. Neurophysiol.,* 44, 751, 1980.

76. Lemon, R.N., Mantel, G.W., and Muir, R.B., Corticospinal facilitation of hand muscles during voluntary movement in the conscious monkey, *J. Physiol. (Lond.),* 381, 497, 1986.

77. Perlmutter, S.I., Maier, M.A., and Fetz, E.E., Activity of spinal interneurons and their effects on forearm muscles during voluntary wrist movements in the monkey, *J. Neurophysiol.,* 80, 2475, 1998.

78. Fortier, P.A., Use of spike triggered averaging of muscle activity to quantify inputs to motoneuron pools, *J. Neurophysiol.,* 72, 248, 1994.

79. Hogan, N., A review of the methods of processing EMG for use as a proportional control signal, *Biomed. Eng.,* 11, 81, 1976.

80. Roscoe, D.D., Hamm, T.M., Reinking, R.M., and Stuart, D.G., Detection of synchrony in the discharge of a population of neurons. II. Implementation and sensitivity of a synchronization index, *J. Neurosci. Meth.,* 13, 51, 1985.

81. Hoffer, J.A., Sugano, N., Loeb, G.E., Marks, W.B., O'Donovan, M.J., and Pratt, C.A., Cat hindlimb motoneurons during locomotion. II. Normal activity patterns, *J. Neurophysiol.,* 57, 530, 1987.

82. Christakos, C.N., Analysis of synchrony (correlations) in neural populations by means of unit-to-aggregate coherence computations, *Neuroscience,* 58, 43, 1994.

83. Christakos, C.N., On the detection and measurement of synchrony in neural populations by coherence analysis, *J. Neurophysiol.,* 78, 3453, 1997.

84. Erimaki, S. and Christakos, C.N., Occurrence of widespread motor-unit firing correlations in muscle contractions: their role in the generation of tremor and time-varying voluntary force, *J. Neurophysiol.,* 82, 2839, 1999.

85. Hamm, T.M. and McCurdy, M.L., The use of coherence spectra to determine common synaptic inputs to motoneurone pools of the cat during fictive locomotion, in *Alpha and Gamma Motor Systems,* Taylor, A., Gladden, M.H., and Durbaba, R., Eds., Plenum, New York, 1995, 309.

86. Trank, T.V., Turkin, V.V., and Hamm, T.M., Coherence between locomotor drive potentials and neurograms of motor pools with variable patterns of locomotion, *Ann. N.Y. Acad. Sci.,* 860, 448, 1998.

87. Hamm, T.M., Trank, T.V., and Turkin, V.V., Correlations between neurograms and locomotor drive potentials in motoneurons during fictive locomotion: implications for the organization of locomotor commands, *Prog. Brain Res.,* 123, 331, 1999.

88. Bayev, K.V., Central locomotor program for the cat's hindlimb, *Neuroscience,* 3, 1081, 1978.

89. Grillner, S., Control of locomotion in bipeds, tetrapods, and fish, in *Handbook of Physiology, Vol. II, Pt. 2, The Nervous System: Motor Control,* Brooks, V.B., Ed., American Physiological Society, Bethesda, 1981, 1179.

90. Cohen, A.H., Rossignol, S., and Grillner, S., *Neural Control of Rhythmic Movements in Vertebrates,* John Wiley & Sons, New York, 1988.

91. Orlovsky, G.N., Deliagina, T.G., and Grillner, S., *Neural Control of Locomotion,* Oxford University Press, Oxford, 1999.

92. Kiehn, O., Harris-Warrick, R.M., Jordan, L.M., Hultborn, H., and Kudo, N., Eds., *Neural Mechanisms for Generating Locomotor Activity,* New York Academy of Sciences, New York, 1998.

93. Brown, T.G., On the nature of the fundamental activity of the nervous centres; together with an analysis of rhythmic activity, *J. Physiol. (Lond.),* 48, 18, 1914.

94. Jankowska, E., Jukes, M.G.M., Lund, S., and Lundberg, A., The effect of DOPA on the spinal cord. 5. Reciprocal organization of pathways transmitting excitatory action to alpha motoneurones of flexors and extensors, *Acta Physiol. Scand.,* 70, 369, 1967.

95. Grillner, S. and Zangger, P., On the central generation of locomotion in the low spinal cat, *Exp. Brain Res.,* 34, 241, 1979.

96. Fleshman, J.W., Lev-Tov, A., and Burke, R.E., Peripheral and central control of flexor digitorum longus and flexor hallucis longus motoneurons: the synaptic basis of functional diversity, *Exp. Brain Res.,* 54, 133, 1984.

97. Pearson, K.G. and Rossignol, S., Fictive motor patterns in chronic spinal cats, *J. Neurophysiol.,* 66, 1874, 1991.

98. Gelfand, I.M., Orlovsky, G.N., and Shik, M.L., Locomotion and scratching in tetrapods, in *Neural Control of Rhythmic Movements in Vertebrates,* Cohen, A.H., Rossignol, S., and Grillner, S., Eds., John Wiley & Sons, New York, 1988, 167.

99. Smith, J.L., Carlson-Kuhta, P., and Trank, T.V., Forms of forward quadrupedal locomotion. III. A comparison of posture, hindlimb kinematics, and motor patterns for downslope and level walking, *J. Neurophysiol.,* 79, 1702, 1998.

100. Beato, M. and Nistri, A., Interaction between disinhibited bursting and fictive locomotor patterns in the rat isolated spinal cord, *J. Neurophysiol.,* 82, 2029, 1999.

101. Roberts, A., Soffe, S.R., and Perrins, R., Spinal networks controlling swimming in hatchling *Xenopus* tadpoles, in *Neurons, Networks, and Motor Behavior,* Stein, P.S. G., Grillner, S., Selverston, A.I., and Stuart, D.G., Eds., MIT Press, Cambridge, 1997, 83.

102. Wallen, P., Spinal networks and sensory feedback in the control of undulatory swimming in lamprey, in *Neurons, Networks, and Motor Behavior,* Stein, P.S.G., Grillner, S., Selverston, A.I., and Stuart, D.G., Eds., MIT Press, Cambridge, 1997, 75.

103. Jordan, L.M., Brainstem and spinal cord mechanisms for the initiation of locomotion, in *Neurobiological Basis of Human Locomotion.,* Shimamura, M., Grillner, S., and Edgerton, V.R., Eds., Japan Scientific Societies Press, Tokyo, 1991, 3.

104. Lennard, P.R., Afferent perturbations during "monopodal" swimming movements in the turtle: phase-dependent cutaneous modulation and proprioceptive resetting of the locomotor rhythm, *J. Neurosci.*, 5, 1434, 1985.

105. Stein, P.S.G. and Smith, J.L., Neural and biomechanical control strategies for different forms of vertebrate hindlimb motor tasks, in *Neurons, Networks, and Motor Behavior,* Stein, P.S.G., Grillner, S., Selverston, A.I., and Stuart, D.G., Eds., MIT Press, Cambridge, 1997, 61.

106. Deliagina, T.G., Orlovsky, G.N., and Pavlova, G.A., The capacity for generation of rhythmic oscillations is distributed in the lumbosacral spinal cord of the cat, *Exp. Brain Res.*, 53, 81, 1983.

107. Kiehn, O. and Kjaerulff, O., Distribution of central pattern generators for rhythmic motor outputs in the spinal cord of limbed vertebrates, *Ann. N.Y. Acad. Sci.*, 860, 110, 1998.

108. Patla, A.E., Calvert, T.W., and Stein, R.B., Model of a pattern generator for locomotion in mammals, *Am. J. Physiol.*, 248, R484, 1985.

109. Giszter, S.F., Mussa-Ivaldi, F.A., and Bizzi, E., Convergent force fields organized in the frog's spinal cord, *J. Neurosci.*, 13, 467, 1993.

110. Saltiel, P., Tresch, M.C., and Bizzi, E., Spinal cord modular organization and rhythm generation: an NMDA iontophoretic study in the frog, *J. Neurophysiol.*, 80, 2323, 1998.

111. Tresch, M.C. and Bizzi, E., Responses to spinal microstimulation in the chronically spinalized rat and their relationship to spinal systems activated by low threshold cutaneous stimulation, *Exp. Brain Res.*, 129, 401, 1999.

112. Tresch, M.C., Saltiel, P., and Bizzi, E., The construction of movement by the spinal cord, *Nat. Neurosci.*, 2, 162, 1999.

113. Brody, C.D., Slow covariations in neuronal resting potentials can lead to artefactually fast cross-correlations in their spike trains, *J. Neurophysiol.*, 80, 3345, 1998.

114. Shefchyk, S.J. and Jordan, L.M., Excitatory and inhibitory postsynaptic potentials in alpha-motoneurons produced during fictive locomotion by stimulation of the mesencephalic locomotor region, *J. Neurophysiol.*, 53, 1345, 1985.

115. Engberg, I. and Lundberg, A., An electromyographic analysis of muscular activity in the hindlimb of the cat during unrestrained locomotion, *Acta Physiol. Scand.*, 75, 614, 1969.

116. Perret, C. and Cabelguen, J.M., Main characteristics of the hindlimb locomotor cycle in the decorticate cat with special reference to bifunctional muscles, *Brain Res.*, 187, 333, 1980.

117. O'Donovan, M.J., Pinter, M.J., Dum, R.P., and Burke, R.E., Actions of FDL and FHL muscles in intact cats: functional dissociation between anatomical synergists, *J. Neurophysiol.*, 47, 1126, 1982.

118. Trank, T.V., Chen, C., and Smith, J.L., Forms of forward quadrupedal locomotion. I. A comparison of posture, hindlimb kinematics, and motor patterns for normal and crouched walking, *J. Neurophysiol.*, 76, 2316, 1996.

119. Jordan, L.M., Factors determining motoneuron rhythmicity during fictive locomotion, in *Neural Origin of Rhythmic Movements. Symposia of the Society for Experimental Biology,* 37th, Roberts, A. and Roberts, B.L., Eds., Cambridge University Press, London, 1983, 423.

120. Perret, C., Centrally generated pattern of motoneuron activity during locomotion in the cat, in *Neural Origin of Rhythmic Movements. Symposia of the Society for Experimental Biology,* 37, Roberts, A. and Roberts, B.L., Eds., Cambridge University Press, London, 1983, 405.

121. Degtyarenko, A.M., Simon, E.S., Norden-Krichmar, T., and Burke, R.E., Modulation of oligosynaptic cutaneous and muscle afferent reflex pathways during fictive locomotion and scratching in the cat, *J. Neurophysiol.,* 79, 447, 1998.

122. Cullheim, S., Fleshman, J.W., Glenn, L.L., and Burke, R.E., Membrane area and dendritic structure in type-identified triceps surae alpha motoneurons, *J. Comp. Neurol.,* 255, 68, 1987.

123. Fleshman, J.W., Segev, I., and Burke, R.E., Electrotonic architecture of type-identified alpha-motoneurons in the cat spinal cord, *J. Neurophysiol.,* 60, 60, 1988.

124. Orlovsky, G.N. and Feldman, A.G., Classification of lumbosacral neurons according to their discharge patterns during evoked locomotion. (Russian), *Neirofiziologia,* 4, 410, 1972.

125. Berkinblit, M.B., Deliagina, T.G., Feldman, A.G., Gelfand, I.M., and Orlovsky, G.N., Generation of scratching. I. Activity of spinal interneurons during scratching, *J. Neurophysiol.,* 41, 1040, 1978.

126. Huang, W.-X., Christakos, C.N., Cohen, M.I., and He, Q., Possible network interactions indicated by bilaterally coherent fast rhythms in expiratory recurrent laryngeal nerve discharges, *J. Neurophysiol.,* 70, 2192, 1993.

127. Noga, B.R., Fortier, P.A., Kriellaars, D.J., Dai, X., Detillieux, G.R., and Jordan, L.M., Field potential mapping of neurons in the lumbar spinal cord activated following stimulation of the mesencephalic locomotor region, *J. Neurosci.,* 15, 2203, 1995.

128. Jordan, L.M., Initiation of locomotion in mammals, *Ann. N.Y. Acad. Sci.,* 860, 83, 1998.

129. Zealear, D.L. and Crandall, W.F., Stimulating and recording from axons within their myelin sheaths: a stable and nondamaging method for studying single motor units, *J. Neurosci. Meth.,* 5, 47, 1982.

7 Sensory–Motor Experience during the Development of Motility in Chick Embryos

Andrew A. Sharp and Anne Bekoff

CONTENTS

0-8493-0006-1/01/$0.00+$1.50
© 2001 by CRC Press LLC

7.1 INTRODUCTION

Feeling a baby kick in its mother's womb is the first experience most people have with embryonic motility. The first motor events for a human fetus occur just prior to 8 weeks of gestation.[1-4] General aversive movements to touch first occur at 8 weeks,[2,3] and plantar flexion of the toes when the sole of the foot is touched starts at 11 weeks.[5] Sensory–motor interactions are an essential component of normal postnatal locomotion and are quite well developed at birth. Great advances have been made toward understanding the mechanisms of sensory modulation of motor output in adults; however, despite the early onset of fetal motility and reflexic behavior, there is very little knowledge about the role of sensory feedback in coordinating fetal motility and it is not known whether sensory input is necessary for normal spinal-motor development.

Complete understanding of the contribution of embryonic sensory input to the development of motor circuitry requires knowledge of several factors. It is important to know when various components of sensory–motor circuitry first form functional connections. Next, it is necessary to determine when the various components of the circuitry are integrated into the spinal-motor pattern generators and how they each contribute to embryonic motor output. Finally, and perhaps most interestingly, the contribution of various forms of embryonic sensory input to the development of normal adult spinal-motor circuits needs to be determined.

Model systems have been particularly useful in gaining insights into the development of sensory–motor systems. In particular, the chick has presented numerous advantages for studying the development of motility. The most notable advantage of the chick is that it develops almost entirely within the egg, which is conveniently located outside of the mother. This allows for easy access to the chick embryo throughout embryogenesis. Also, embryonic motility and reflex behaviors begin early in embryogenesis, which is very similar to the onset of fetal human motility. Finally, most mammals used for locomotion studies (i.e., rats and cats) are not nearly as precocious in their neuromuscular development as humans and chicks and begin to move and show reflexes relatively late in embryogenesis.[6,7] While this attribute has its own set of advantages for studying developmental processes, it does not allow for easy comparison to the prenatal development of human motor behaviors.

The purpose of the present work is to review our understanding of the development of embryonic motility and the related sensory systems. Primary focus will be placed on what has been learned from studying the motor output of intact embryos. Recent studies have begun to shed some light on possible roles for sensory regulation of embryonic motility. Additionally, we will discuss some new approaches directed toward gaining a better understanding of embryonic sensory–motor interactions. Recently, we have begun to study embryonic motor output of chicks grown in an *in vitro* culture system,[8] and the effects of high doses of pyridoxine, vitamin B_6, during embryogenesis on embryonic motility and on walking.[9-11] This is particularly exciting, because pyridoxine has been shown to selectively kill proprioceptive neurons in adult mammals[12,13] and may, therefore, provide a very powerful approach to understanding the role of a single sensory modality during development.

7.2 ONTOGENY OF MOTILITY, REFLEXES, AND SENSORY SYNAPSES

Early observations of chick embryos described the neurogenic and episodic nature of embryonic motility.[14] Embryos move for a period of time, rest, and then move again. The first studies described the early movements of embryos as jerky and uncoordinated. Although this is an accurate description of the appearance of the behavior, later investigators utilizing quantitative kinematic and EMG approaches, realized that embryonic motility was not uncoordinated, but rather showed many types of organization.[15–17] The patterns of organization actually change during embryogenesis and seem to reflect developmental changes in the sensory–motor circuitry.[15,18,19] Before describing these events, it would be useful to review the general techniques used for studying embryonic motor output.

7.2.1 GENERAL METHODS

Eggs are removed from a standard incubator and candled to determine the location of the embryo within the egg. The egg is then placed in a heated and humidified recording chamber so that the egg is on its side with the embryo at the top surface. A small hole is then made in the blunt end of the egg into the air sac and a second small hole is carefully made in the lateral side of the egg above the embryo. If the second hole is made carefully, the chorioallantoic membrane separates from the shell membrane and settles deeper into the shell. This allows the lateral hole to be enlarged without damaging the blood vessels of the chorioallantoic membrane. Once the hole has been enlarged sufficiently so that the portion of the embryo to be observed is totally exposed, the chorioallantoic and amniotic membranes are carefully cut open to allow physical access to the embryo. It is usually not possible to avoid cutting some of the blood vessels, but care must be taken to selectively cut only the smallest vessels.

Once the embryo is exposed, small kinematic markers are applied to the embryo on the lateral surface of all the joints to be studied. The markers are usually small spots of paint or nail polish. It is sometimes necessary to retract some of the membranes or blood vessels in order to provide a clear view of the embryo. This is accomplished with fine wires that can be hung over the side of the shell and situated to retract the membranes and thereby allow free movement of the embryo within full view of the observer. The embryo is then typically videotaped for later analysis, the videotapes are digitized, and the coordinates of the markers are determined for the segments of movements that are of interest. Joint properties such as joint angle and velocity are then calculated from these values.

Because embryos do not normally remain in the x–y plane during motility, it is necessary to somehow correct for rotations out of the plane when calculating joint angles. Hoy et al.[20] determined that rotations that cause an apparent change of less than 10% in length of a limb segment did not present problems, but larger rotations produced errors that were significant. Two approaches have been used to address this issue. It is possible to use trigonometry to correct for the error.[21] This process uses the fact that joint segment lengths are constant to correct the measured joint angles, and works well as long as the embryo does not move its limb behind some opaque object such as another limb or a blood vessel. Since this is not an uncommon occurrence, particularly for older embryos, we have taken a somewhat different approach. We typically use an acrylate glue to attach the back of the embryo to two rigid paddles.[18] This allows the embryo to be stabilized in the x–y plane and we have not seen any alterations in normal motility patterns from this procedure between embryonic day E9 and E13. The advantage to this method is that the embryo can be placed in clear view. However, it is possible that at some stage of development after E13 the paddles may prove to alter normal motility patterns, which would then require not using them at these stages.

Electromyographic recordings can be made at the same time as kinematic recordings if care is taken to place the electrodes such that they do not block kinematic markers. If EMG recordings are to be made in the absence of kinematics, then the orientation of the embryo is less critical. In order to place the electrodes, a small incision must be made in the skin above the muscle to be recorded. Embryos usually exhibit a withdrawal reflex when cut, but seem to desensitize rapidly to the cut. Two different types of bipolar electrodes have been used for EMG recordings in chick embryos. The first method uses a suction electrode with a flexible polyethylene tip that can be pulled to a small diameter and placed onto the muscle.[16] The second method uses very fine, lacquer-coated silver wire that is inserted into the muscle.[22] The suction electrodes are somewhat easier to orient and reposition onto different locations along a muscle, but they are often knocked loose by the motion of the limb. The silver wire is somewhat more difficult to place without damaging the muscle, but provides for more stable long-term recordings. This can be quite useful if long experiments using experimental manipulation are to be conducted. Also, the fine diameter wire does not obscure joint markers.

7.2.2 DEVELOPMENT OF MOTILITY

Embryonic motility in the chick begins after 3.5 days of incubation,[23,24] with slight movements of the head and soon includes cyclical movements of the limbs. Early observations of motility characterized the movements as random with no coordination of body parts.[14] Later kinematic recordings of E9 to E13 embryos demonstrated that extension and flexion of the leg joints show coordination.[17–19,25,26] There is also coordination of extension and flexion between joints of the leg and wing.[19,26] EMG recordings from the leg of E7[15] and E9[15,16] embryos showed a high degree of coactivity between muscle synergies in the leg as well as a half-center type alternation of extensors and flexors. Figure 7.1 shows an example of synchronous kinematic and EMG recordings. The coordination of joint extension and flexion and the alternation of extensor and flexor discharge can be clearly seen. It has been suggested that the variability in the number of joints moving and the duration of movements are largely responsible for the appearance of uncoordinated motility described in the early studies.[17]

As the embryo becomes older, its activity increases to a peak around E13 and then decreases until about E18.[14,15,18] Embryos move for longer periods with shorter

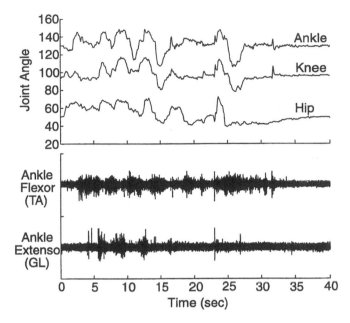

FIGURE 7.1 Simultaneous kinematic and EMG recordings from an E9 embryo. The top traces are plots of joint angles for the ankle, knee, and hip. The lower traces are simultaneous EMG recordings from the ankle extensor and flexor muscles, gastrocnemius lateralis and tibialis anterior, respectively.

rests between each motility episode. The increase in activity state is also accompanied by a decrease in the coordination of limbs.[15,18] Between E9 and E13,[18] in particular, the movements of the ankle become uncoupled from those of the knee and hip. It is possible that these changes are due to an increase in the size of the embryo. We have proposed that this causes the limbs to make more contacts within the shell and generate more sensory feedback, which needs to be incorporated into the motor patterns by the immature spinal circuitry.[18] Coordination among the joints returns by E17 when the embryo begins to exhibit pre-hatching behavior.[15]

7.2.3 SENSORY DEVELOPMENT

For motor circuitry to be modulated by sensory information, the presence of a functional sensory system that can transfer information from a sensory organ into the motor pattern-generating circuitry is required. Oppenheim[27] showed that reflex responses to flipping the limb could first be elicited on E7.5 and the first responses to limb stroking occurred on E8.5. This implies that the sensory neurons must be able to transduce sensory input and form functional synapses within the spinal cord by this time. The first sensory projections into the spinal cord are seen on E6.[28,29] Primary afferents begin to reach motor neurons on E7.5.[30,31] In fact, it is possible to record synaptic potentials in motor neurons after dorsal root stimulation at this time.[30]

The presence of functional primary afferent (Ia) input to the motor neurons and the ability to initiate reflexes on E7.5 suggest that proprioception should be available

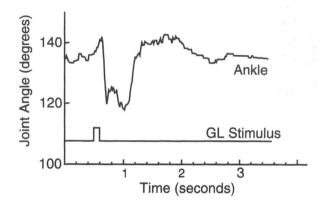

FIGURE 7.2 Ankle stretch reflex. After electrical stimulation of the ankle extensor, gastroc-nemius lateralis, the ankle first extends slightly and then shows a much larger flexion as a result of the ankle flexor having been stretched.

to modify motor patterns at this time. However, based on standard anatomical features, no muscle spindles can be observed until E13.[32] We found this curious and decided to try to elicit a stretch reflex prior to E13. By electrically stimulating the gastrocnemius muscle (ankle extensor) in an E9 embryo, we were able to generate a stretch reflex in the limb (Fig. 7.2). After stimulation, there was a very small extension of the ankle followed by a more sustained and larger flexion. The flexion of the ankle is probably the result of extensor motor neurons being activated by the brief stretch of the ankle flexors. Therefore, functional proprioceptive feedback must be available to the motor central pattern generator long before an anatomically identifiable muscle spindle is present.

The role that sensory inputs play in modulating the motor CPG is not well understood. Nevertheless, the fact that descending and sensory inputs are established concomitant with alterations in motor behaviors suggests that the integration of these inputs is responsible for altering the motor patterns. Two studies suggest that sensory input causes an increase in interjoint organization under conditions of reduced buoyancy for E9 embryos.[25,26] Persistent, phasic perturbation of the leg of the E9 embryo with a fixed paddle results in visually detectable alterations in motility,[22] but variability of kinematic and EMG records have confounded the interpretation of these results. No obvious alterations in embryonic motility occur following removal of sensory neuron precursor cells and spinal transection.[14] However, quantitative kinematic analysis was not employed and this study did not address removal of sensory information alone. A recent study used a splint to immobilize the ankle[33] and showed that immobilization of the ankle resulted in a decrease in the amplitude and duration of both leg and wing movements of E12 embryos. The movements of E9 embryos were not altered significantly.

Sensory information is clearly available to modulate motor output as early as E7.5. It also seems likely that sensory input plays a role in the generation of embryonic motility. The challenge now is to develop methods to determine directly how sensory feedback modulates embryonic motility and if this input is required for the proper structuring of the spinal motor circuitry. The following sections present two methods we are presently using to address these issues.

7.3 *IN VITRO* CULTURE SYSTEM

7.3.1 INTRODUCTION

Since experience could be an important factor in normal neuromuscular development, we were interested in determining if chicks grown in an *in vitro* culture system would display normal motor features. Numerous investigators have used a variety of techniques to grow chick embryos in artificial environments.[34–38] These techniques vary a great deal and have been used for short-term studies as well as for long-term studies that involve the maturation of a healthy chicken from a single-celled ovum. Culture systems for chicks have received sufficient attention that many factors that affect the size and survival of the animals (i.e., culture dish size and composition, gas exchange, and exogenous calcium) have been identified and characterized. Despite the fact that it is possible to grow a chick to maturation using this approach, the effect of the artificial environment on motor patterning and neuronal function of the embryo has not been examined.

In our initial study of the motility of embryos grown *in vitro,* we used a culture system that would keep the embryo in an environment that was fairly normal in shape and would be relatively simple to reproduce and manipulate in future studies. We examined the motility of E9 embryos grown in culture and used kinematic techniques to compare these movements to those of normal E9 embryos grown and recorded *in ovo* in previous studies. We wished to first test if growth in an artificial environment of similar shape to normal would alter motility at this early, well-described, stage.

7.3.2 METHODS

The method we chose for culturing embryos was a combination of several described in the literature.[34–38] We wanted an inexpensive system that could be easily replicated and altered in order to study the effects of environment on development. We also wanted a system that would provide easy access to the embryo for embryo manipulation and recording. We settled on a system employing a 3-in. diameter PVC pipe coupling as the base for a sling of plastic into which the contents of an egg were emptied. The entire chamber was covered with a 10-cm petri dish cover. These chambers were easy to manufacture, clean, transport between the incubator and recording chamber, and they provided a clear view of the developing embryo. The culturing procedure is described below.

The culturing chambers were assembled and sterilized immediately prior to use. A Glad® pleated sandwich bag was stretched over the opening of a 3-in. diameter PVC pipe coupling and held in place with a rubber band around the coupling. Several ¼-in. holes had been made into the couplings at an earlier time to provide gas exchange underneath the plastic bag. The permeability of the plastic to gas has been shown to be an important factor in the growth of the embryos,[34] so it was important to maintain gas exchange at that surface. The bag was positioned to allow sufficient space for the contents of the egg to be below the top edge of the coupling, such that the upper surface of the contents remained about a centimeter below the edge. The chamber and the lids (10-cm petri dish covers) were placed under an ultraviolet light in a laminar flow hood for about an hour prior to placing the contents of the egg into the chamber.

Embryos were placed into culture on E3. This is prior to the development of the extra-embryonic membranes. It is important to maintain the orientation of the eggs such that the embryo remains on top of the yolk. After the eggs were removed from the incubator, they were quickly wiped with alcohol and placed into the laminar flow hood. The eggs were lightly cracked on the edge of the chamber and gently decanted into the chamber. Care was taken to prevent rupturing the yolk sac and to keep the embryo on top of the yolk. Also, any fluids that collected on the edge of the dish were removed with sterile gauze to prevent contamination and wicking of the egg contents out of the chamber. The chambers were then covered and placed into a standard water-jacketed incubator. The temperature of the incubator was maintained at 37°C, but the humidity was not strictly regulated. High humidity was maintained by placing a pan of distilled water on the bottom shelf of the incubator.

Kinematic recordings were made as previously described *in ovo*.[18] We found that it was generally easier to prepare the cultured embryos for recording since the extra-embryonic vascularization formed a consistent pattern and the embryos were always on their sides. It should also be noted that it is possible to make numerous observations of the embryos as long as the membranes are not ruptured. Care must be taken to maintain temperature, humidity, and aseptic conditions during these observations.

7.3.3 RESULTS

Six embryos that passed our standard criteria for viability (a heart rate of at least 120 beats/min and at least one motility episode every 5 min) were analyzed for comparison to animals recorded *in ovo*.[18] Joint angle measurements from two representative bouts of motility are presented in Fig. 7.3. In general, the movements recorded *in vitro* resembled those recorded *in ovo* quite well. There were no statistical differences seen for the amplitude or range of angles measured at the hip, knee, and ankle; the movement episode duration and inter-episode interval were also normal. Examination of joint angle vs. time plots showed typical characteristics of movement for E9 embryos. In particular, there was normal rhythmic alternation of extension and flexion of the joints with a high level of coordination among the joints. Generally, these recordings could not be visually distinguished from those of normal embryos.

We did notice one interesting difference in recordings from some of the animals. Figure 7.3B shows an example of this phenomenon. Notice that there are 12 rapid, well-synchronized, consecutive oscillations in this example. This is about twice the typical number seen in a recording from a normal E9 embryo. Half of the embryos displayed this type of behavior in 2 to 3 of the 5 motility episodes analyzed. The frequency of leg movements also appears to increase, but this only occurs some of the time. One possible interpretation of this result is that there was some normal

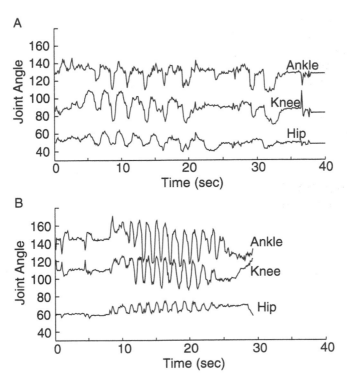

FIGURE 7.3 Two representative joint angle plots from E9 embryos grown in the *in vitro* culture system. The recording in (A) is not distinguishable from a recording done *in ovo*, but the recording in (B) shows about twice as many cycles of rhythmic motility as is normal for an *in ovo* recording.

constraint removed from the environment of these embryos that led to the ability of these particular animals to generate longer sequences of rhythmic motility.

7.3.4 SUMMARY

Our initial study indicates that growing embryos in an *in vitro* culture system may not lead to significant alterations in motor output at E9. Most of the characteristics typical of E9 embryos *in ovo* are retained. The ability of some of the animals to generate abnormally long sequences of rhythmic motor output is very intriguing and requires a larger sample size to fully validate. This finding brings to mind the recordings of long sequences of motor neuron discharge recorded from the ventral roots of isolated spinal cord preparations of this age.[39] This could indicate that the culture environment is reducing some constraint on embryonic motility that normally suppresses the ability of the animal to generate repetitive oscillatory movements of the legs. Clearly, we will need to examine this phenomenon more closely.

The *in vitro* culture system will provide a useful system for a number of experimental paradigms. We will be able to alter the shape and size of the embryonic environment by altering the chamber. It will also allow for long-term pharmacological manipulation of the embryo. Application of drugs to the chorioallantoic membrane is a standard method, but injecting substances through the shell typically results in about a 50% mortality rate. Applications to the chorioallantoic membrane in this system only require lifting the lid off the culture and should significantly increase the survival rate. Additionally, it should be possible to make long term observations of the same animal over the course of days using these cultures. It may even be possible to make kinematic recordings of these animals through the membranes if care is taken during video recording. We project that observation and manipulation of embryos in this type of *in vitro* culture system will provide many important insights into the role of the environment in structuring sensory–motor circuitry.

7.4 PYRIDOXINE: A SELECTIVE TOXIN FOR PROPRIOCEPTIVE NEURONS

7.4.1 INTRODUCTION

Selective removal of a particular type of sensory information is a useful way of studying the role of sensory inputs in organizing patterned motor behavior. It is not possible to surgically remove an individual sensory modality since sensory afferents run in mixed sensory/motor nerves from peripheral origins through the DRGs and into dorsal roots. Blocking neurotrophin pathways with antibodies would be a way to approach this issue, but to date the specificity of the neurotrophins for different sensory modalities has not always been high and only a small percentage of neurons have been killed with this approach.[40,41] Knockout mice present a number of difficulties for this type of study, ranging from the difficulty of *in utero* behavioral recording and the relatively late onset of reflex behaviors when compared to chicks and humans to the low viability of knockouts affecting sensory neurons.[42] A number of chemotherapeutic agents, e.g., capsaicin and vitamin B_{12}, can alter sensory experience, but they are either not selective for one sensory modality or their effects are not limited to sensory neurons. However, it has been known for at least 55 years that high doses of pyridoxine (vitamin B_6) cause selective large fiber neuropathy in vertebrates.[12] Pyridoxine was not utilized to understand the role of proprioception in motor function and central pattern generation until recently.[43,44]

7.4.1.1 Pyridoxine-Induced Neuropathy in Adult Mammals

Large doses of pyridoxine cause a peripheral sensory neuropathy in adult humans,[45–48] dogs,[12,49,50] rats,[13,51–53] cats,[45] and guinea pigs.[53] Dosages of 40 mg/kg/d in humans and 100 mg/kg/d in rats can result in permanent loss of proprioception, temporary loss of some cutaneous reception, and severe ataxia. There does not appear to be any effect on motor neurons, muscles, or other tissues.[13,47]

The initial stages of pyridoxine-induced neuropathy involve ataxia.[45,47,52] The first behavioral effects occur prior to observed pathological changes,[52] i.e., accumulation of neurofilaments in the large diameter axons of sensory nerves.[51] This is followed by the death of the large dorsal root ganglia cells,[51] predominantly located in the ventral-lateral portion of the DRG. Many of the ventral-laterally located cells form monosynaptic connections with motor neurons in the ventral horn and are, therefore, proprioceptive (Ia) sensory afferents.[54] Cutaneous afferents account for the majority of the neurons in the DRG,[54,55] but these are smaller, located more dorsal-medially in the DRG and project only into the dorsal horns. Since it is specifically the large proprioceptive neurons that are killed by high doses of pyridoxine, the subject is ultimately left with a permanent loss of proprioception,[48,52] but relatively intact cutaneous sensation. The mechanism of pyridoxine toxicity is unknown although the co-application of NT-3, normally required for proprioceptive neuron survival,[56] blocks the toxic effects of pyridoxine.[13]

We have begun to examine the effects of high doses of pyridoxine administered to chick embryos,[9–11] and are examining the effects on both pre- and post-hatching motility. Pyridoxine is highly soluble in physiological saline and quite easy to inject into the yolk sac at different stages of development. The following section describes the alterations we have seen in the motility of embryos and post-hatch chicks that received injections of pyridoxine during embryogenesis.

7.4.2 EMBRYONIC EFFECTS

7.4.2.1 Effects on Motility

We have begun to test the effects of pyridoxine on embryonic chicks. Pyridoxine hydrochloride in physiological saline or only saline was injected once daily into the yolk sac of eggs. Embryos were then prepared for kinematic recordings on either E9 or E13. Each animal received one, two, or three injections on the days prior to observation. Pyridoxine treatment did not cause any gross morphological changes in the embryos. Treated embryos reached the appropriate developmental stage for their age and the heart rate of the animals also was normal. The only change that was immediately obvious when the embryos were at rest was that the legs of the treated E13 embryos were more flexed than those of control animals. Duration and periodicity of activity episodes of treated embryos fell within the normal range. This is consistent with the observations made previously on embryos that had sensory precursor cells removed at E2 along with spinal transections.[14]

Nevertheless, treated embryos show significant deficits in other aspects of motor behavior. Major changes in the amplitude of motility are obvious visually in all treated embryos and can be quantified in the kinematic analysis. We have completed a behavioral study (n = 6) of embryos injected with 7.5 mg of pyridoxine on E7 and E8, then recorded on E9.[11] Figure 7.4 shows representative joint angle plots for the ankle, knee, and hip from a saline- and a pyridoxine-treated E9 animal. It is immediately apparent that the amplitude of motility is severely reduced after pyridoxine treatment. While amplitude is reduced at E9, the rest position is not significantly altered. Therefore, only the extent of movement from a normal resting position is altered by pyridoxine treatment at this stage of development.

Initial examination of treated embryos on E13 shows both similarities and differences from the effects noted on E9. Figure 7.5 shows an example of the effects of a single treatment of 15 mg of pyridoxine administered on E12. Note that the amplitude of motility is reduced, much like the E9 embryos. However, the legs of

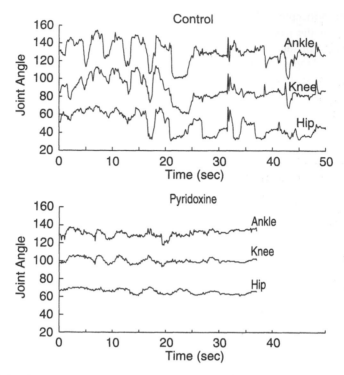

FIGURE 7.4 Joint angle recordings of the ankle, knee, and hip from a control and a pyridoxine-treated embryos recorded on E9. The pyridoxine-treated animal was injected on E7 and E8. The amplitude of motility is dramatically reduced by pyridoxine treatment.

E13 animals are more flexed both at rest and during motility. Unlike the control animals, the joints do not extend far beyond the rest position.

Despite the changes in amplitude and posture caused by pyridoxine, there is no change in the fine structure of motility at either stage examined so far. The coordination of extension/flexion between joints seen in the E9 animals appears to be the same and the period of these events also appears normal. The increase in variability of motility normally seen at E13 is also retained. For example, in Fig. 7.5, a number of events are seen in which one joint is moving in anti-phase to the other two.

7.4.2.2 Histological Analysis

We have begun the histological examination of these pyridoxine-treated animals. Three E9 embryos that received 0, 3.75, or 15 mg of pyridoxine have been examined histologically. The spinal columns were removed and fixed for 24 h in 4% paraformaldehyde. They were then rinsed in PBS, dehydrated, embedded in paraffin, sectioned at 10 μm, and stained with cresyl violet. Observations of the third lumbosacral segment were then performed. The morphology of the spinal cord and dorsal root ganglion (DRG) appear grossly normal. In particular, motor neurons appear healthy and normal. However, examination of the sensory neurons in the third lumbosacral DRGs reveals some interesting changes. Most large cells in the control DRG have

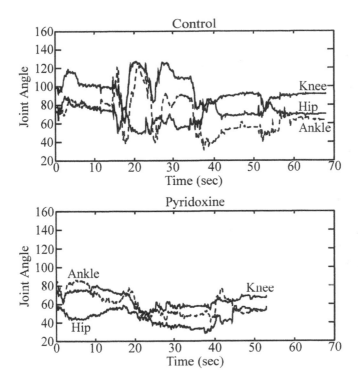

FIGURE 7.5 Joint angle recordings of the ankle, knee, and hip from a control and a pyridoxine-treated embryo recorded on E13. The pyridoxine-treated animal was injected once on E12. Notice in the pyridoxine treated animal that the amplitude of joint movements is reduced and the general posture is more flexed, but the basic characteristics are otherwise unchanged.

a clear nucleus with 1 or 2 distinct nucleoli. The cells without clear nuclei most likely represent cells that are undergoing normal cell death at this time.[55] In the DRG of the animal that received 15 mg/d, it is difficult to find any large neurons with clear nuclear profiles. This suggests that the majority of these cells are dying as a result of the pyridoxine treatment. Counts of large, "healthy" neurons in every fourth section through the DRGs suggest that this may be a dose-dependent effect. Pyridoxine treatment with 3.75 mg/d caused about a 50% reduction and 15 mg/d caused a 90% reduction in the large DRG neurons with clear nuclei, respectively. It is possible that the animal that received the highest dose also may have had damage to the small DRG neurons. However, this was not quantified in the preliminary survey.

7.4.3 POST-HATCH EFFECTS

7.4.3.1 Effects on Motility

We have begun to study the effects of embryonic pyridoxine administration on post-hatch behavior. We have tried a variety of concentrations and injection ages. From 50 to 75% of the treated animals did not hatch despite the fact that they had clearly reached E20 developmentally. Only about 25% of saline-injected animals did not hatch. All of the treated animals that hatched showed signs of behavioral deficit. These deficits ranged from a slight difficulty balancing and walking with a general crouched stance to severe cases where the animal could not get up from its back or side. Some of the more severely damaged animals were never able to walk at all. Animals with only minor deficits appeared to substantially recover after several days. Interestingly, pyridoxine-treated animals that initially appeared to have no deficit in behavior, refused to walk when blindfolded and had difficulty getting up when placed on their backs. Normal chicks will walk when blindfolded and have no difficulty standing when placed on their backs.

We have completed a kinematic study of walking on six animals that were injected on E12 with 15 mg of pyridoxine.[10,11] Animals were prepared for kinematic recordings and analyzed as previously described.[57] Figure 7.6 shows joint angle vs. time plots from a control and pyridoxine-treated animal 1 day after hatching (P1). Notice that the pattern of joint angle changes in the treated animal shows a higher degree of variability and that the chick is walking more slowly. These animals showed a hesitancy to walk and took shorter steps than normal animals. Additionally, treated animals spent a greater portion of each walking cycle in the stance phase of walking than in the swing phase (when the leg is in the air). Interestingly, we found that we could not find statistical differences in any of these variables on P3 or later. An example of walking from a control and pyridoxine-treated animal on P3 is shown in Fig. 7.7. However, these animals did not develop the ability to compensate for a rapid perturbation of position such as a rapid translocation on a movable platform.[58]

7.4.3.2 Histological Analysis

Initial histological examination of these animals (one control and one pyridoxine-treated animal) is consistent with findings for pyridoxine toxicity in adult mammals. There were no obvious changes in motor neurons, but we found a 15% decrease in the number of neurons in the lumbosacral DRGs. This loss was seen only in the medium and large cell classes within the ganglia and likely represents a loss of proprioceptive neurons. This indicates that a single dose of pyridoxine on E12 was sufficient to cause proprioceptive damage that resulted in behavioral deficits after hatching.

7.4.4 SUMMARY

The ability to selectively remove proprioception or part of the proprioceptive neuronal pool starting at a given developmental stage would be a very useful tool in understanding the role of proprioception during development. Our preliminary results suggest that pyridoxine application to embryonic chicks results in a selective loss of proprioceptive neurons as it does in adult mammals. It is clear that we must conduct additional anatomical and physiological experiments to test the selectivity of pyridoxine toxicity for proprioceptive neurons. Toward this end, it would be extremely useful to know the mechanism of pyridoxine toxicity.

The effects of pyridoxine on the motility of chick embryos have some interesting implications for the role of proprioception during development. It would seem that sensory modulation from proprioceptive neurons acts to amplify movements that are otherwise organized by central mechanisms. The loss of proprioceptive feedback,

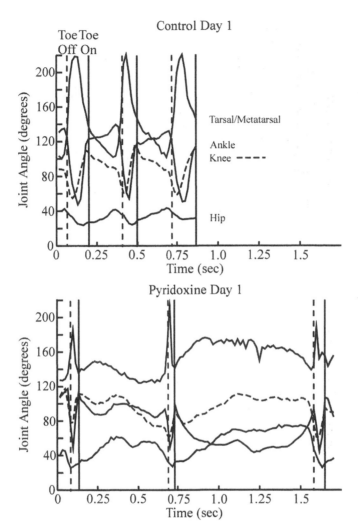

FIGURE 7.6 Joint angle recordings from the tarsal/metatarsal, ankle, knee, and hip of a control and a pyridoxine-treated chick 1 day after hatching. The pyridoxine-treated animal was injected on E12. Vertical lines denote when the right toe first contacted or left the ground as indicated in the top panel.

therefore, reduces the amplitude of movements as can be seen in E9 and E13 embryos that received pyridoxine treatment. This supports the idea that proprioception acts as a positive feedback mechanism during locomotion as has previously been suggested.[59]

We had previously postulated that the increase in variability of behavior seen at E11 and E13 is the result of sensory feedback as the embryo becomes large enough to be limited in its free space by the confines of the egg.[18] Bradley and Sebelski[33] have shown that limiting ankle movements with a splint reduces the amplitude and duration of motility on E13 thus supporting the idea that sensory feedback is important during motility on E13. Our preliminary results after pyridoxine treatment

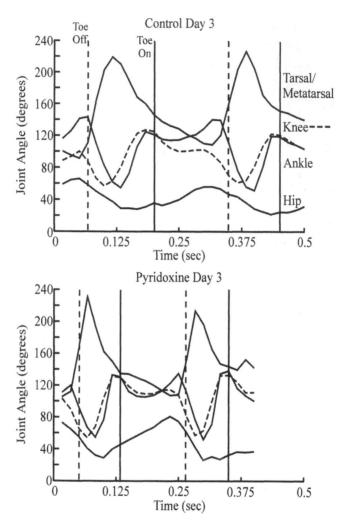

FIGURE 7.7 Joint angle recordings from the same chicks as in Fig. 7.6 recorded 3 days after hatching. Notice that the motor patterns are now much more similar.

suggest that the change in organization of the motor pattern seen at E13 may be mediated by cutaneous receptors. Cutaneous receptors appear to still be functioning after pyridoxine treatment (embryos retract their legs after pinching or stroking a foot). One possible explanation for the increased flexion seen on E13 is that the loss of proprioception results in a hypersensitivity to touch together with a loss of movement-generated proprioceptive positive feedback. This could result in the general retraction of the leg without altering other characteristics of the motor pattern. This would, therefore, suggest that proprioception acts in conjunction with cutaneous feedback to regulate the strength and extent of motor output. This is an extremely important role for the developing sensory–motor nervous system, because an embryo must prevent itself from damaging its environment during motor activity.

Our results show that embryonic administration of pyridoxine causes neuronal damage that persists after hatching. The fact that fewer animals hatch after pyridoxine injection than after saline injection suggests that proprioception plays an important role during hatching. Previous studies[60,61] indicate that sensory input from the neck is required to initiate hatching behavior and it is quite possible that pyridoxine may disrupt the ability of animals to perform this necessary motor activity. The requirement for proprioception for the initiation of hatching may explain why many of the animals appear to have only minor motor deficits. If the dosage of pyridoxine is sufficiently low to allow hatching to occur, it may not kill enough lumbosacral proprioceptive neurons to severely affect walking. If the one animal examined histologically is an indication of normal neuronal loss, it is interesting that a 15% loss of proprioceptive neurons is sufficient to generate a demonstrable motor deficit.

The alterations in walking seen in treated animals are what one might expect for animals that are uncertain of their foot placement. They take short, small steps and they try to keep their feet in contact with the ground as much as possible. The delayed onset of swing is consistent with experiments that have been done in cats. It has been shown that proprioception in cats is involved in the initiation of swing.[59] The deficits displayed by the chicks are, therefore, consistent with a spinal deficit in proprioception as well as a higher order compensatory strategy that could be applied to many situations when motor capacity is diminished. We found it quite interesting that these animals learned how to mask their sensory deficit after only 2 days of walking. It should be noticed that these animals did not develop the ability to compensate for an unexpected perturbation such as a sudden push. This suggests that the recovery of the ability to walk may be due to compensation by higher centers of the nervous system or due to plasticity of the spinal circuits.

7.5 CONCLUDING REMARKS

The chick is an excellent model system for studying the development of the neural circuitry that controls locomotion. The ability to observe and perturb motor activity during embryogenesis is a fundamental advantage of this system. The early onset of motility and incorporation of sensory feedback into the spinal circuitry provides an advantage over most mammalian systems when drawing correlations to sensory–motor development in humans. Recent experiments[9,11,33] have shown that the sensory information available to spinal-motor circuitry is actively used during the generation of embryonic motility. While the details of these interactions have not been described, they are clearly important components of the embryonic nervous system.

The *in vitro* culture system presented here should prove very useful for understanding the role of sensory information during development. It allows for a wide range of manipulation of the environmental conditions. It also simplifies access so that the same embryo can be observed over multiple days. This will allow for examination of changes in a single individual as a result of physical or pharmacological manipulations.

The ability to selectively alter a specific sensory modality is essential to fully understand the role of sensation during the development of the nervous system. It is likely that pyridoxine will prove to be selective for killing proprioceptive neurons, but we still lack selective tools for various types of cutaneous feedback. Transgenic techniques will undoubtedly be applied to this issue and provide some useful tools. Ultimately, we hope to discover methods that will allow for reversible blockade of a specific sensory modality. By applying substances that disrupt specific sensory modalities, reversibly or irreversibly, at different stages of development we expect to be able to determine if there are critical periods during which the motor circuitry requires specific types of sensory input to develop normally.

REFERENCES

1. Strassmann, P., Das Leben vor der Geburt, *Samml. klin. Vortr. 1900-1903, Gynak.*, 132, 947, 1903.
2. Hooker, D., Early fetal activity in mammals, *Yale J. Biol. Med.*, 8, 579, 1936.
3. Fitzgerald, J.E. and Windle, W.F., Some observations on early human fetal movements, *J. Comp. Neurol.*, 76, 159, 1942.
4. de Vries, J.I.P., Visser, G.H., A. and Prechtl, H.F.R., The emergence of fetal behaviour. I. Qualitative aspects, *Early Hum. Dev.*, 7, 301, 1982.
5. Humphrey, T. and Hooker, D., Double simultaneous stimulation of human fetuses and the anatomical patterns underlying the reflexes elicited, *J. Comp. Neurol.*, 112, 75, 1959.
6. Kudo, N. and Yamada, T., Morphological and physiological studies of development of the monsynaptic reflex pathway in the rat lumbar spinal cord, *J. Physiol.*, 389, 441, 1987.
7. Windle, W.F. and Baxter, R.E., Development of reflex mechanisms in the spinal cord of albino rat embryos. Correlations between structure and function, and comparisons with the cat and the chick, *J. Comp. Neurol.*, 63, 189, 1936.
8. Bekoff, A., Sharp, A.A., Koster, M., and Tahja, S., Embryonic motility of cultured chicks, *Soc. Neurosci. Abstr.*, 26, 454, 2000.
9. Sharp, A.A., Boyle, C.A., and Bekoff, A., Pyridoxine induced proprioceptive neuronal loss during embryogenesis alters both embryonic and post-hatch motility, *Soc. Neurosci. Abstr.*, 24, 1666, 1998.
10. Sharp, A.A., Jasiewicz, J., Woollacott, M.H., and Bekoff, A., Pre-hatch injection of pyridoxine (vitamin B$_6$) alters post-hatch walking in chick, *Gait and Posture*, 9(1),S54, 1999.
11. Sharp, A.A. and Bekoff, A., High doses of pyridoxine administered during embryogenesis alter embryonic motility and walking in chicks, *Gait and Posture*, 9(1)S16, 1999.
12. Antopol, W. and Tarlov, I.M., Experimental study of the effects produced by large doses of vitamin B$_6$, *J. Neuropathol. Exp. Neurol.*, 1, 330, 1942.
13. Helgren, M.E., Cliffer, K.D., Torrento, K., Cavnor, C., Curtis, R., DiStefano, P.S., Wiegand, S.J., and Lindsay, R.M., Neurotrophin-3 administration attenuates deficits of pyridoxine-induced large-fiber sensory neuropathy, *J. Neurosci.*, 17, 372, 1997.
14. Hamburger, V., Wenger, E., and Oppenheim, R., Motility in the absence of sensory input, *J. Exp. Zool.*, 162, 133, 1966.
15. Bekoff, A., Ontogeny of leg motor output in the chick embryo: a neural analysis, *Brain Res.*, 106, 271, 1976.
16. Bradley, N.S. and Bekoff, A., Development of coordinated movement in chicks: I. Temporal analysis of hindlimb muscle synergies at embryonic days 9 and 10, *Dev. Psychobiol.*, 23, 763, 1990.

17. Watson, S.J. and Bekoff, A., A kinematic analysis of hindlimb motility in 9- and 10-day old chick embryos, *J. Neurobiol.*, 21, 651, 1990.

18. Sharp, A.A., Ma, E., and Bekoff, A., Developmental changes in leg coordination of the chick at embryonic days 9, 11 and 13: Uncoupling of ankle movements, *J. Neurophysiol.*, 82, 2406, 1999.

19. Bradley, N.S., Transformations in embryonic motility in chick: Kinematic correlates of Type I and II motility at E9 and E12, *J. Neurophysiol.*, 81, 1486, 1999.

20. Hoy, M.G., Zernicke, R.F., and Smith, J.C., Contrasting roles of inertial and muscle moments at knee and ankle during paw-shake responses, *J. Neurophysiol.*, 54, 1282, 1985.

21. Orosz, M.D., Bradley, N.S., and Chambers, S.H., Correcting two-dimensional kinematic errors for chick embryonic movements *in ovo*, *Comput. Biol. Med.*, 24, 305, 1994.

22. Sharp, A.A. and Bekoff, A., Effect of sensory input during rhythmic embryonic motility, *Soc. Neurosci. Abst.*, 22, 1641, 1996.

23. Hamburger, V., Some aspects of the embryology of behavior, *Quart. Rev. Biol.*, 38, 342, 1963.

24. Hamburger, V. and Balaban, M., Observations and experiments on spontaneous rhythmical behavior in the chick embryo, *Devel. Biol.*, 7, 533, 1963.

25. Chambers, S.H., Bradley, N.S., and Orosz, M.D., Kinematic analysis of wing and leg movements for type I motility in E9 chick embryos, *Exp. Brain. Res.*, 103, 218, 1995.

26. Bradley, N.S., Reduction in buoyancy alters parameters of motility in E9 chick embryos, *Physiol. Behav.*, 62, 591, 1997.

27. Oppenheim, R.W., An experimental investigation of the possible role of tactile and proprioceptive stimulation in certain aspects of embryonic behavior in the chick, *Dev. Psychobiol.*, 5, 71, 1972.

28. Windle, W.F. and Orr, S.W., The development of behavior in chick embryos: spinal cord structure correlated with early somatic motility, *J. Comp. Neurol.*, 60, 287, 1934.

29. Mendelson, B., Koerber, H.R., and Frank, E., Development of cutaneous and proprioceptive afferent projections in the chick spinal cord, *Neurosci. Lett.*, 138, 72, 1992.

30. Lee, M.T., Koebbe M.J., and O'Donovan, M.J., The development of sensorimotor synaptic connections in the lumbosacral spinal cord of the chick embryo, *J. Neurosci.*, 8, 2530, 1988.

31. Davis, B.M., Frank, E., Johnson, F.A., and Scott, S.A., Development of central projections of lumbosacral sensory neurons in the chick, *J. Comp. Neurol.*, 279, 556, 1989.

32. Toutant, M., Bourgeois, J.P., Rouaud, R., and Toutant, J.P., Morphological and histochemical differentiation of intrafusal fibers in the posterior latissimus dorsi muscle of the developing chick, *Anat. Embryol.*, 162, 325, 1981.

33. Bradley, N.S. and Sebelski, C., Ankle restraint modifies motility at E12 in chick embryos, *J. Neurophysiol.*, 83, 431, 2000.

34. Dunn, B.E., Fitzharris, T.P., and Barnett, B.D., Effects of varying chamber construction and embryo pre-incubation age on survival and growth of chick embryos in shell-less culture, *Anat. Rec.*, 199, 33, 1981.

35. Perry, M.M., A complete culture system for the chick embryo, *Nature*, 331, 70, 1988.

36. Jakobson, A.M., Hahnenberger, R., and Magnusson, A., A simple method for shell-less cultivation of chick embryos, *Pharmacol. Toxicol.*, 64, 193, 1989.

37. Ono, T., Murakami, T., Mochii, M., Agata, K., Kino, K., Otsuka, K., Ohta, M., Mizutani, M., Yoshida, M., and Eguchi, G., A complete culture system for avian transgenesis, supporting quail embryos from the single-cell stage to hatching, *Devel. Biol.*, 161, 126, 1994.

38. Selleck, M.A.J., Culture and microsurgical manipulation of the early avian embryo, *Meth. Cell Biol.*, 51, 1, 1996.

39. Landmesser, L.T. and O'Donovan, M.J., Activation patterns of embryonic chick hind limb muscles recorded *in ovo* and in an isolated spinal cord preparation, *J. Physiol.*, 347, 189, 1984.

40. Gaese, F., Kolbeck, R., and Barde, Y.A., Sensory ganglia require neurotrophin-3 early in development, *Development*, 120, 1613, 1994.

41. Lefcort, F.B., Clary, D.O., Rusoff, A.C., and Reichardt, F., Inhibition of the NT-3 receptor trkC, early in chick embryogenesis, results in severe reductions in multiple neuronal subpopulations in the dorsal root ganglia, *J. Neurosci.*, 16, 3704, 1996.

42. Ernfors, P., Lee, K-F., Kucera, J., and Jaenisch, R., Lack of neurotrophin-3 leads to deficiencies in the peripheral nervous system and loss of limb proprioceptive afferents, *Cell*, 77, 503, 1994.

43. Bishop, G.M., Hulliger, M., Djupsjobacka, M., Wojciechowski, A., and O'Callaghan, I., Motor deficits following large-fiber deafferentation in the cat, *Soc. Neurosci. Abstr.*, 23, 1567, 1997.

44. Bishop, G.M., Hulliger, M., and Foweraker, J.P.A., Partial recovery from motor deficits due to large-fiber deafferentation by pyridoxine, *Soc. Neurosci. Abstr.*, 24, 1413, 1998.

45. Schaumburg, H., Kaplan, J., Windebank, A., Vick, N., Rasmus, S., Pleasure, D., and Brown, M.J., Sensory neuropathy from pyridoxine abuse, *N. Engl. J. Med.*, 309, 445, 1983.

46. Parry, G.J. and Bredesen, D.E., Sensory neuropathy with low-dose pyridoxine, *Neurology*, 35, 1466, 1985.

47. Albin, R.L., Albers, J.W., Greenberg, H.S., Townsend, J.B., Lynn, R.B., Burke, J.M., and Alessi, A.G., Acute sensory neuropathy-neuronopathy from pyridoxine overdose, *Neurology*, 37, 1729, 1987.

48. Albin, R.L. and Albers, J.W., Long-term follow-up of pyridoxine-induced acute sensory neuropathy-neuronopathy, *Neurology*, 40, 1319, 1990.

49. Schaeppi, U. and Krinke, G., Pyridoxine neuropathy: correlation of functional tests and neuropathology in beagle dogs treated with large doses of vitamin B_6, *Agents Actions*, 12, 575, 1982.

50. Schaeppi, U. and Krinke, G., Differential vulnerability of 3 rapidly conducting somatosensory pathways in the dog with vitamin B_6 neuropathy, *Agents Actions*, 16, 567, 1985.

51. Krinke, G., Naylor, D.C., and Skorpil, V., Pyridoxine megavitaminosis: an analysis of the early changes induced with massive doses of vitamin B_6 in rat primary sensory neurons, *J. Neuropathol. Exp. Neurol.*, 44, 117, 1985.

52. Windebank, A.J., Low, P.A., Blexred, M.D., Schmelzer, J.D., and Schaumburg, H.H., Pyridoxine neuropathy in rats: specific degeneration of sensory axons, *Neuorology*, 35, 1617, 1985.

53. Xu, Y., Sladky, J.T., and Brown, M.J., Dose-dependent expression of neuronopathy after experimental pyridoxine intoxication, *Neurology*, 39, 1077, 1989.

54. Willis, W.D. and Coggeshall, R.E., *Sensory Mechanisms of the Spinal Cord*, Plenum, New York, 1991.

55. Hamburger, V., Brunso-Bechtold, J.K., and Yip, J.W., Neuronal death in the spinal ganglia of the chick embryo and its reduction by nerve growth factor, *J. Neurosci.*, 1, 60, 1981.

56. Snider, W.D., Functions of the neurotrophins during nervous system development: what the knockouts are teaching us, *Cell*, 77, 627, 1994.

57. Johnston, R.M. and Bekoff, A., Constrained and flexible features of rhythmical hindlimb movements in chicks: kinematic profiles of walking, swimming and airstepping, *J. Exp. Biol.*, 171, 43, 1992.

58. Jasiewicz, J., Sharp, A.A., Bekoff, A., and Woolacott, M.H., Pre-hatch injection of pyridoxine (vitamin B_6) causes postural instability in post-hatch chicks, *Soc. Neurosci. Abstr.*, 25, 2182, 1999.

59. Pearson, K.G., Misiaszek, J.E., and Fouad, K., Enhancement and resetting of locomotor activity by muscle afferents, *Ann. N.Y. Acad. Sci.*, 860, 203, 1998.

60. Bekoff, A. and Kauer, J.A., Neural control of hatching: role of neck position in turning on hatching leg movements in post-hatching chicks, *J. Comp. Physiol.*, 145, 497, 1982.

61. Bekoff, A. and Sabichi A.L., Sensory control of the injection of hatching in chicks: effects of a local anesthetic injected into the neck, *Dev. Psychobiol.*, 20, 489, 1987.

8 Transformation of Descending Commands into Muscle Activity by Spinal Interneurons in Behaving Primates

Steve I. Perlmutter and Yifat Prut

CONTENTS

8.1   INTRODUCTION

Ever since Sherrington's pioneering experiments led him to conclude that reflexes were "the unit reaction in nervous integration,"[1] physiologists have conceived of descending systems recruiting spinal circuitry to produce voluntary movements. This insight has evolved to the present view that transmission through spinal pathways, which execute the stereotyped, stimulus-driven motor behaviors referred to as reflexes, is mutable, dynamically modulated, and under differential control by supraspinal structures.[2] By using spinal pathways to specify motoneuron activity, the job of the motor cortices is presumably simplified, and sensory information can be employed rapidly and "on-the-fly" to guide movements and correct errors.

Sherrington believed spinal reflexes were anatomical and functional elements that could be isolated and that operate in a highly interactive and combinative manner. He inferred that cortical systems also take advantage of this organization, and his discussion of behavioral control by the cerebral hemispheres ("nervous organs of control") is very much in accord with the modern view:

> The way in which we ourselves acquire a new skilled movement, the means by which we get more precision and speed in the use of a tool, the handling of an instrument, or marksmanship with a weapon, is by a process of learning in which nervous organs of control modify the activities of reflex centres, themselves already perfected for other though kindred actions.[1]

The development of these ideas originated in the early appreciation of the flexibility of spinal reflexes, as discussed by Goldstein.[3] He described "reflex reversals" and the dependence of the stretch reflex "on the position of the limb, on the behavior of the rest of the organism, and on whether or not attention is paid to it." The neural substrates for this state-dependence were elucidated in the second half of the 20th century by elegant, meticulous experiments that revealed the extensive convergence of information from multiple afferent and descending sources onto individual spinal interneurons.[4-7] More recent work has demonstrated that the activation of particular cutaneous or proprioceptive receptors can produce different motor outputs during different phases of real or fictive movements, and that the excitability of motoneurons and interneurons can be modulated by monoamines and neuropeptides.

Our conceptual framework of spinal function during movement has progressed significantly as these studies have ascertained the functional organization of spinal interneurons.[8,9] However, it has been difficult to verify and elaborate these concepts in action, during natural movements, because of the inaccessibility of spinal circuits to direct study in awake, behaving animals. Preparations exhibiting fictive behaviors have enabled the direct investigation of the neural mechanisms of locomotion and scratching,[10-12] but other types of movement have been studied only in anesthetized or decerebrate animals, or with indirect measurements of neural activity in moving animals or human subjects. We believe that information on the properties of spinal interneurons during normal behaviors is needed to fully explicate the recruitment and modulation of spinal pathways by descending systems. Accordingly, we have been recording the activity of spinal neurons during voluntary wrist movements in monkeys, using techniques developed in the laboratory of Dr. Eberhard Fetz.[13-15]

In our initial studies, we have examined the activity of spinal interneurons during, and in preparation for, normal hand movements, and have compared these results to data from motor cortex, red nucleus, and peripheral afferents during a similar task.[15-17] Our efforts to classify interneurons have focused on identifying their output linkages to motoneurons with spike-triggered averaging of electromyographic activity (EMG), and we have characterized the distribution of connections from premotor interneurons to synergistic and antagonistic muscles of the forearm.[18]

We believe our experimental technique provides a new approach to studying spinal control of movements. It enables the direct measurement of the interactions between descending commands and proprioceptive signals that generate voluntary muscle activity. This approach complements the extensive data from previous studies on the wiring and flexibility of spinal pathways. In addition, information on the properties of spinal interneurons during normal behavior will help interpret data on descending signals, and advance hypotheses about information processing in supraspinal motor structures. For example, current perspectives on the computational organization of the motor system envision cortical commands in terms of abstract features, such as movement direction referenced to a head- or shoulder-centered coordinate frame.[19,20] The task of completing the transformation into joint- or muscle-centered representations, patterns of muscle activities that execute the desired movement, is often ascribed to spinal circuits. We will address this hypothesis in this chapter by summarizing our results on the features of interneuronal activity that do, and do not, relate to movement parameters, and on the temporal properties of firing of spinal neurons.

8.2 METHODOLOGY

To study the properties of individual spinal cord neurons during voluntary movements, we have applied classical, chronic recording techniques developed in studies on the brain during the last 30 to 40 years. These techniques allow us to measure the activity of single spinal neurons in awake, trained macaque monkeys performing natural behaviors.[18] A laminectomy exposes the dura mater overlying three segments in the lower cervical cord and bone screws are inserted into the lateral masses of the vertebrae overlying these, and adjacent, segments. A stainless steel chamber with a removable cap is cemented to the screws with dental acrylic, providing long-term access to the cord for daily recording sessions. Monkeys exhibit a stiffened posture of the upper back with this implant, which fuses several vertebrae together, but are otherwise undisturbed and behave normally. While the monkeys work at trained hand and arm tasks, the head and spinal column are immobilized by fixing the skull and vertebral implants to the apparatus. Glass-coated tungsten electrodes are introduced through the dura with a hydraulic microdrive mounted to the chamber. To date, we have recorded spinal neurons during single-joint wrist movements, a power grip, and small amplitude, free-form reaching movements. We are able to maintain stable recordings of single, well-isolated neurons for more than 30 min if the monkey refrains from making large postural shifts. At the end of the recording session, the electrode is removed, the chamber is re-sealed, and the monkey is returned to his home cage as in brain-recording studies.

Our electrodes encounter many spinal neurons with spontaneous and task-related activity in the awake monkey. We have taken two approaches to classifying these neurons. First, input and output connectivity can be characterized in the awake animal using well-developed criteria from earlier studies. Motoneurons and premotor interneurons produce characteristic post-spike effects in spike-triggered averages of EMG[21] from arm muscles (Fig. 8.1). Consequently, we simultaneously record the EMG of multiple forearm muscles and neuron activity. Most interneurons with post-spike effects in muscles are probably last-order cells, but some may influence motoneurons through oligosynaptic pathways.[18] Inputs from peripheral afferents can be identified by responses to electrical stimulation of peripheral nerves or muscles and by responses to passive displacements of the wrist and mechanical stimulation of the skin. These techniques provide tests for inputs from large-diameter muscle and cutaneous afferents. However, in the awake animal inputs from groups I and II, muscle afferents can be difficult to distinguish, and tests for inputs from high-threshold group III and IV fibers are not feasible. We have not focused on identifying

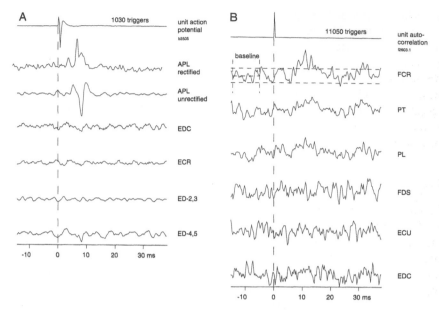

FIGURE 8.1 Spike-triggered averages of EMG for a motoneuron (A) and a spinal premotor interneuron (B). EMG of multiple forearm muscles was averaged for 15 ms before and 35 ms after the occurrence of action potentials of well-isolated neurons. Top traces show average waveform of the action potential (A) or the autocorrelation of firing (B) for the recorded neurons. Bottom traces show average unrectified (A, except APL rectified) or rectified (B) EMG aligned on the time of spike occurrence for independently recorded forearm muscles that were co-active with the neuron. Spike-triggered averages of the motoneuron show a motor unit action potential in APL (A). Premotor interneuron produced a post-spike facilitation in FCR, and possibly in PL (B). The short, dashed horizontal line on the spike-triggered average of FCR shows the mean EMG level during the baseline, pre-spike period (identified by the short, dashed vertical lines). Post-spike effects that were sustained increases or decreases in average EMG above or below the baseline mean ± 2 standard deviations (long, dashed horizontal lines) were considered significant. Note that post-spike effects of cells classified as motoneurons and premotor interneurons were noticeably different. Cells were classified as motoneurons only if they also were recorded at an appropriate depth in the cord, had a low peak firing rate and unidirectional activity (see 8.3, Interneuronal activity related to the parameters of movement). Muscles are APL, abductor pollicis longus; EDC, extensor digitorum communis; ECR, extensor carpi radialis; ED-2,3, extensor digitorum 2,3; ED-4,5, extensor digitorum 4,5; FCR, flexor carpi radialis; PT, pronator teres; PL, palmaris longus; FDS, flexor digitorum superficialis; ECU, extensor carpi ulnaris.

descending inputs to interneurons, but this is possible with electrical stimulation of supraspinal structures, such as the pyramidal tract, motor or sensory cortex, red nucleus, or reticulospinal centers.

Second, we foresee our studies developing a new classification scheme based on the response properties of interneurons during normal behavior. Our hope is that this new classification scheme will augment rather than parallel the well-established organizational framework developed by previous studies, and that the comparison of the two will provide new insights into interneuronal function.

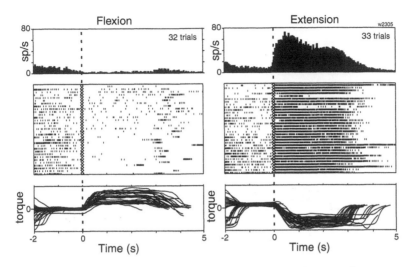

FIGURE 8.2 C6 premotor interneuron with phasic-tonic activity for extension torques. The monkey performed isometric, ramp-and-hold flexion (left) and extension (right) torques starting from rest. Torque profiles for all trials are superimposed (bottom). Rasters (middle) indicate timing of action potentials (small vertical lines) and torque onset (diamonds) in individual trials (rows). Histograms (top) show the average activity of the neuron. All traces are aligned on torque onset (time = 0). Average firing rate was 11 sp/s when the monkey exerted no torque at the wrist (baseline). During extension, the average rate peaked at 71 sp/s during dynamic torques and then decreased to a steady level of 43 sp/s during the static hold period; this response was termed phasic-tonic activity. Firing rate decreased during flexion relative to baseline. The neuron produced a post-spike facilitation in the spike-triggered average of rectified EMG of one forearm muscle, EDC.

This chapter will discuss primarily data on spinal interneurons recorded in the C6-T1 segments as monkeys generated isometric or auxotonic (against an elastic load) flexion and extension torques about the wrist. Torque controlled the position of a cursor on a CRT screen in front of the animal. The monkey was required to move the cursor into target boxes displayed on the screen. The position of each box specified a fixed level of wrist torque in flexion or extension. The monkey received an applesauce reward when he produced a ramp-and-hold torque that met velocity and amplitude criteria.

8.3 INTERNEURONAL ACTIVITY RELATED TO THE PARAMETERS OF MOVEMENT

The activity of many C6-T1 interneurons was related to components of the torque generated during extension and flexion of the wrist.[22] The responses of interneurons with and without effects on muscle activity, identified by spike-triggered averages of EMG, were similar. Figure 8.2 shows the activity of a premotor interneuron recorded in the C6 segment as the monkey generated isometric torques. The neuron produced a post-spike facilitation of activity in the extensor digitorum communis

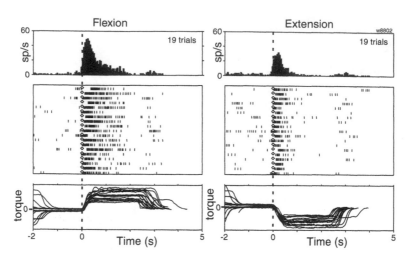

FIGURE 8.3 C7 interneuron with phasic activity for flexion and extension torques. Format as in Fig. 8.2. Neuron had little activity when no torque was generated at the wrist, and fired a transient burst at the onset of flexion (peak rate, 48 sp/s) and extension (peak rate, 31 sp/s). After the burst, firing rate declined to near 0 during the static hold period. The neuron produced no observable effects on forearm muscle activity in spike-triggered averages of EMG.

muscle (not shown) and had a steady baseline discharge rate when the monkey exerted no torque at the wrist. The firing rate of the cell increased dramatically at the onset of torque (Fig. 8.2, right), after which it plateaued at a lower level significantly above the baseline rate. This type of activity was termed phasic-tonic, in relation to the ramp-and-hold torques generated during the task. The cell had very little activity during flexion torques. Figure 8.3 shows a C7 interneuron that exhibited phasic activity during dynamic torques in both directions. This neuron, which had no observable effects on forearm muscle activity, fired at a very low rate during the active hold period.

Ninety-three percent (470/503) of interneurons with activity modulated during the task exhibited tonic and/or phasic components of firing (Fig. 8.4). Similar response types were seen for premotor neurons in the motor cortex and dorsal root ganglia, in different proportions. In particular, corticomotoneuronal cells rarely had purely phasic activity, and premotor peripheral afferents had a higher percentage of purely tonic responses. Phasic activity is also less common for motor units, and many fired in a decrementing, or adapting, pattern during ramp-and-hold torques, which few spinal interneurons exhibited. Phasic activity in spinal premotor circuits helps bring motoneurons to firing threshold, perhaps overcoming strong inhibition. This could account for the relative inability of premotor neurons to relay phasic activity to motor units at the onset of movement. Sustained activity contributes to the maintenance of a steady level of muscle activity during the hold period.

The firing rate of motoneurons of forearm flexor and extensor muscles is tightly coupled to the amplitude of wrist flexor and extensor torque, respectively, within the motoneurons' dynamic range.[23] In addition, there is evidence that peak motoneuron firing rate is correlated with movement speed.[24,25] The phasic and tonic

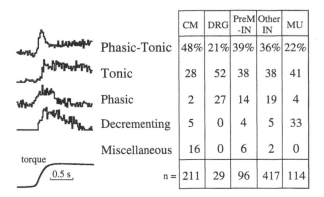

	CM	DRG	PreM-IN	Other IN	MU
Phasic-Tonic	48%	21%	39%	36%	22%
Tonic	28	52	38	38	41
Phasic	2	27	14	19	4
Decrementing	5	0	4	5	33
Miscellaneous	16	0	6	2	0
n =	211	29	96	417	114

FIGURE 8.4 Summary of activity patterns for different populations of neurons during generation of flexion and extension torques at the wrist. Examples of each pattern are illustrated on the left, above corresponding torque trajectory. Proportions are given for corticomotoneuronal cells (CM),[17] premotor afferents in dorsal root ganglia (DRG),[15] spinal premotor interneurons (PreM-IN) and spinal interneurons without post-spike effects in spike-triggered averages of forearm muscle EMG (Other IN),[22] and motor units from forearm muscles (MN, combined data).[22,23] Total number of neurons in each population given at bottom (n). Miscellaneous includes cells with ramp, phasic-ramp, and unmodulated activity. Note similar proportions of each activity pattern for PreM-IN and Other IN.

response components of the majority of interneurons also were related to movement parameters. The discharge rate of 80% of interneurons with a tonic firing component during the static hold period was linearly related to the torque level (Fig. 8.5). Similarly, the peak firing rate of 69% of cells with phasic activity during dynamic torques was linearly related to the maximum rate of change of torque during individual trials (Fig. 8.6).

The parametric relation of firing to active torque suggests that the activity of many spinal interneurons encodes movement amplitude or speed. Many premotor neurons in motor cortex and red nucleus exhibit similar properties.[16] In this regard, spinal circuits reinforce supraspinal signals that convey information about static and dynamic parameters of movement to motoneurons. Parametric features of interneuronal activity could also be related to sensory feedback from proprioceptive afferents, which contributes in turn to the ongoing generation of muscle activity during movement.[26-30] Afferent input may modify the movement metrics specified by descending signals, and the correlation of interneuronal activity to movement parameters may be a manifestation of this fine tuning.

8.4 NON-PARAMETRIC FEATURES OF INTERNEURONAL FIRING

Spinal interneurons commonly exhibit other properties that do not resemble those of motoneurons. Motoneurons of the long flexor and extensor muscles of the forearm are active for wrist flexion and extension, respectively, and are silent for movements in the opposite direction and when no force is exerted at the wrist. This directionality

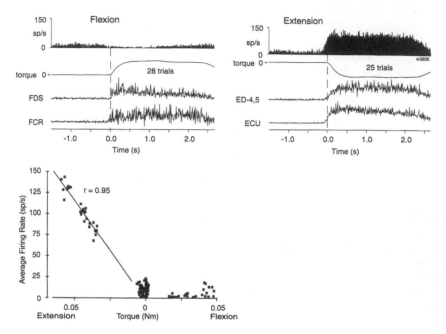

FIGURE 8.5 Interneuron with activity correlated with static torque in one direction. Histograms (top) show average activity during flexion (left) and extension (right) torques at the wrist. Averaged isometric torque trajectory (middle) and averaged rectified EMG of coactive muscles (bottom) shown below. All traces are aligned on torque onset (time = 0). Neuron exhibited tonic activity for extension and a phasic decrease in activity for flexion, relative to baseline activity. Scatter diagram shows average firing rate in the last second of the hold period plotted against static torque level for all individual trials. Cluster of points near 0 torque (baseline) corresponds to the zero-torque target box that initiated each trial. Regression line fitted to data from extension hold period only. No effects on muscle activity were measured for this neuron.

is not exhibited by the majority of premotor and other interneurons in the spinal cord. Seventy-seven percent of spinal interneurons were bidirectionally active (Fig. 8.7), including one third of the cells that had increased discharge relative to baseline for both flexion and extension torques (Fig. 8.8). Furthermore, the firing rate of 15% of the interneurons with tonic and/or phasic response components was correlated with movement parameters for both directions of torque (Fig. 8.8). Most interneurons also had some baseline activity when the forearm muscles were silent.

Bidirectional activity in spinal interneurons may originate in descending or peripheral inputs, or both. Most premotor neurons in dorsal root ganglia and the motor cortex, like motoneurons, are silent for one direction of torque.[15,31] Branches of reciprocally firing neurons may converge on spinal interneurons to generate bidirectional activity, or other supraspinal cells that discharge during both flexion and extension may project to interneurons.[32] Alternatively, bidirectional activity in interneurons may be driven by the sensory responses of cutaneous or joint receptors in the arm that are stimulated by both directions of movement, or may be related to

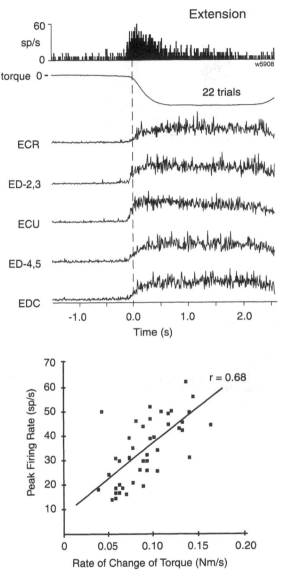

FIGURE 8.6 Premotor interneuron with peak firing rate correlated with maximum rate of change of torque at the wrist. Format as in Fig. 8.5. Neuron exhibited phasic burst of activity during dynamic extension torques. Scatter diagram shows the peak firing rate in the burst plotted against maximum rate of change of torque during dynamic extension for all individual trials. The neuron produced a post-spike facilitation in the ED-2,3 muscle. Note decrementing pattern of EMG in ECU muscle, which was characteristic of many single motor units.[23]

activity in non-prime movers, such as intrinsic hand muscles or upper arm or back muscles that act to stabilize the limb. Regardless of its source, bidirectionally active premotor interneurons produce competing EPSPs and IPSPs in motoneurons of the

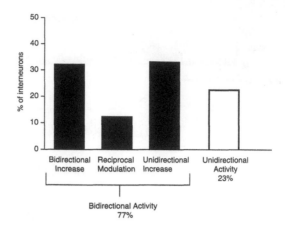

FIGURE 8.7 Directionality of movement-related activity of spinal interneurons. Histogram shows percentage of all interneurons with bidirectional and unidirectional activity for flexion and extension torques. Bidirectional activity includes bidirectional increases in activity, and tonic activity with similar (Unidirectional Increase) or lower (Reciprocal Modulation) average firing rates for torques in the non-preferred direction compared to baseline. Percentages were approximately the same for premotor interneurons and interneurons with no identified linkages to forearm muscles (not shown).

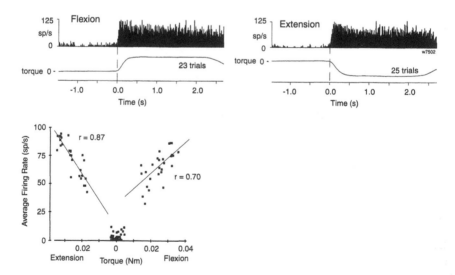

FIGURE 8.8 Interneuron with activity correlated with static torque in both directions. Format as in Fig. 8.5. Neuron exhibited tonic activity with similar average firing rates for extension (72 sp/s) and flexion (65 sp/s) torques. Regression lines fitted separately to data from extension hold and flexion hold. This neuron had no correlation with muscle activity in spike-triggered averages of EMG.

long flexor and extensor muscles of the forearm at times when their target muscles are silent and active, respectively. Despite the strong parametric relation between interneuronal firing and movement, the activity of the majority of interneurons is not governed exclusively by the activation patterns of primary wrist movers. Instead, interneuron activity reflects functionally broader inputs. Bidirectional increases in activity had latencies before torque onset for some interneurons and after torque onset for other interneurons, suggesting that both descending and feedback systems are involved.

Our data suggest that the excitability of forearm motoneurons is regulated by adjusting the balance of excitatory and inhibitory synaptic inputs, even during behaviors in which they might be expected to alternate. Periods of overlap between excitatory and inhibitory drive regulate activity in other types of motoneurons,[33–35] and in premotor pathways.[36–39] Inhibition during the active phase can produce a significant reduction in the strength of motoneuron activity.[40] The fine adjustment of overlapping excitation and inhibition may serve to control gain,[41] to maintain a sensitivity to sensory inputs or the ability to respond quickly to changing motor commands, or to control movements other than reciprocal wrist flexion/extension. The integration of the excitatory and inhibitory inputs that serve these functions shape the discharge patterns of spinal interneurons during voluntary movements. It will be our goal in future studies to determine the contribution of interneuron activity to each of these functions.

8.5 SPATIAL TUNING OF SPINAL INTERNEURONS

We have begun studying the spatial tuning of spinal interneurons in a multidirectional wrist task. Our observations again indicate that the activity of spinal interneurons is related to motoneuron activity and to functions other than the specification of movement parameters. Monkeys were trained to generate isometric torques in flexion/extension (FE), radial/ulnar deviation (RU), and pronation/supination (PS), and to execute a power grip (G) that co-contracted wrist flexor and extensor muscles. The activity of many interneurons was cosine-tuned to torque exerted in the FE-RU plane, but was also modulated strongly during PS and/or G. Many interneurons were modulated over a wider range of movements than were individual forearm muscles. Figure 8.9 shows data from a premotor interneuron that was tuned more broadly than EMG in its target muscle. Other interneurons were modulated strongly by PS or G but negligibly with FE-RU, exhibiting specificity for certain movements, rather than specific muscle contractions.

Although our sample is still small, the preliminary evidence suggests that spinal interneurons do not have spatial properties that are closer to those of motoneurons than neurons in the motor cortex.[42] Inputs from spinal interneurons with competing spatial, task-dependent, and probably other, properties contribute to the generation of motoneuron activity. These inputs represent cortical commands for movement or torque direction combined with other types of descending and peripheral signals.

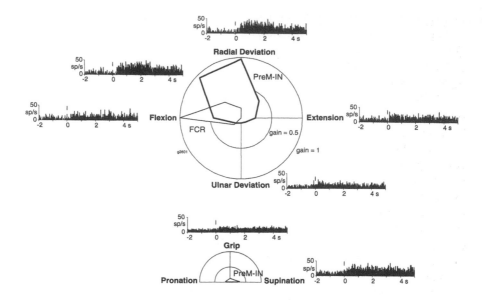

FIGURE 8.9 Spatial tuning of a spinal premotor interneuron for a multidimensional wrist task. Neuron produced post-spike facilitation of FCR muscle, and had tonic activity for isometric torques in several directions. Polar plots show response gains of neuron (PreM-IN) and target muscle EMG (FCR) for different directions of torque generated at the wrist. Gain was taken as the difference between the mean firing rate or rectified EMG level during the last second of the static hold and the baseline (when no torque was exerted at the wrist) periods, divided by the baseline value. The neuron's gain was well approximated as a cosine function of torque direction in the flexion/extension–radial/ulnar deviation plane (i.e., torque direction taken as an independent variable with extension = $0°$, radial deviation = $90°$, flexion = $180°$, ulnar deviation = $270°$). Vertices of polygons in upper plot show average gain from separate trials of (counterclockwise from right) extension, extension + radial deviation, radial deviation, flexion + radial deviation, flexion, flexion + ulnar deviation, ulnar deviation, and extension + ulnar deviation. Vertices of polygons in lower plot show data from supination, grip, and pronation trials. Neuron and FCR gains were normalized separately to their maximum responses (radial deviation for the neuron; flexion for FCR). Each histogram shows the average activity of the neuron for ramp-and-hold torques in the direction indicated by its position relative to the polar plots. Histograms were aligned on target onset (time = 0). Note the broader tuning of the neuron's activity than EMG in its target muscle (i.e., relative size of polygons).

8.6 ACTIVITY DURING AN INSTRUCTED DELAY PERIOD

Spinal interneurons appear to be involved in preparing the motor system for an upcoming movement.[43] Monkeys were trained to perform isometric wrist flexion/extension with an instructed delay period. This epoch begins after a visual cue that specifies the next required movement and is prior to a "go" signal that instructs the monkey to execute that movement. About one third of the interneurons (133/397)

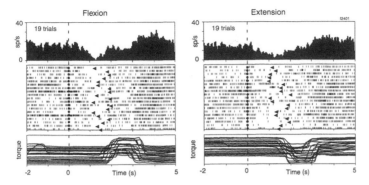

FIGURE 8.10 Spinal interneuron with significant decrease in activity during instructed delay period. Format as in Fig. 8.2, except all traces are aligned on cue onset and torque traces are stacked (i.e., not superimposed) for clarity. As in standard flexion/extension task, trials begin with the monkey relaxing his forearm muscles to keep the cursor in the zero-torque target box for a variable hold period. A visual cue (filled circles) then informs the monkey of the position on the screen of the next target, but the monkey is required to keep the cursor in the zero-torque box. After a variable delay period, the center target box is extinguished (filled triangles), signaling the monkey to execute the cued movement. The interneuron had an average discharge of 18 sp/s during the baseline period. Firing rate decreased gradually to near 0 during the delay period before both flexion (left) and extension (right). Activity returned to pre-cue levels during maintenance of static torque and increased during release of torque. No effects on muscle activity were observed in spike-triggered averages of EMG. Only 3% of interneurons with delay period modulation had no movement-related activity, as did this cell.

recorded in this task exhibited significant modulation of activity during the delay period, when there was no EMG in forearm muscles. Firing rate decreased during the delay period relative to baseline for 60% of the interneurons (Fig. 8.10), and increased for 40% (Fig. 8.11). Many interneurons were modulated prior to both flexion and extension trials. The vast majority of interneurons with delay activity also exhibited movement-related activity, which was facilitation more often than suppression.

The visual cue specified both the direction and amplitude of torque for the next target box. Some interneurons exhibited delay activity that was correlated with one or both of these parameters; however, delay activity usually did not predict either the direction or amplitude of the upcoming movement. The average firing rates before flexion and extension trials were significantly different for only 21% of the interneurons with delay activity. There was a significant correlation between delay activity and torque magnitude of the upcoming movement for only 10% of the cells. Interneuronal activity during the delay period was much less related to movement parameters than activity during the generation of active torque.

Furthermore, delay activity was not related to the subsequent response during active torque for many interneurons. As shown in Fig. 8.12, the change in firing rate during the delay period had a different polarity (facilitation or suppression) than the subsequent modulation during active torque for 39% of the cases (delay modulations before flexion and extension torques for the same interneuron, when present, were considered separately). Most often these neurons were inhibited relative to baseline during the delay period and facilitated during active torque (upper left quadrant, Fig. 8.12).

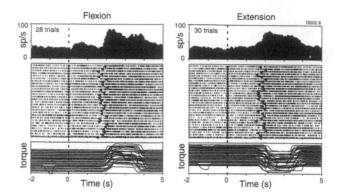

FIGURE 8.11 Spinal interneuron with significant increase in activity during instructed delay period. Format as in Fig. 8.10. Interneuron had a baseline firing rate of 30 sp/s. During the delay period prior to flexion torques, discharge increased to an average rate of 46 sp/s. During the generation of active torque the neuron exhibited a phasic-tonic pattern of activity; firing rate plateaued at 69 sp/s. No effects on muscle activity were observed in spike-triggered averages of EMG.

    Two independent spinal processes appear to operate during the preparation for movement and generate modulated activity during the delay period. First, as exemplified by the neuron of Fig. 8.11, a priming of the activity that will be exhibited during movement execution occurs during the delay period. From the point of view of agonist motoneurons, this response represents a subthreshold build-up of facilitatory input that may shorten reaction times. The paucity of correlated activity with torque direction or amplitude suggests that this priming is independent of the parameters of the upcoming movement. Even for neurons in motor cortical regions, the question of whether delay activity is well correlated with movement parameters remains unresolved.[44] Second, as exemplified by the neuron of Fig. 8.10, a general inhibition occurs during the delay period that may suppress the tendency to initiate any movement, including those elicited by sensory stimuli.[45,46] In fact, premotor interneurons were significantly more likely to exhibit modulated activity during the delay period than interneurons with no functional linkages to muscles, and this response was more often inhibitory. The latencies of inhibitory responses during the delay, relative to cue onset, tended to be significantly shorter than those of facilitatory responses (median latencies of 170 and 230 ms, respectively), supporting the hypothesis of two independent spinal processes. In addition, facilitatory delay activity was much more tightly locked in time to cue onset than inhibitory delay activity.

8.7 TEMPORAL PROPERTIES OF FIRING

Underlying information processing in the spinal cord, embedded within the highly convergent and divergent connectivity of spinal circuits, are the dynamic input–output transformations of individual spinal interneurons. These transformations are a function of the cells' intrinsic biophysical properties and the labile temporal sequence, spatial distribution, and strength of synaptic inputs. Information about these factors, and consequently about the computational properties of the spinal network as a

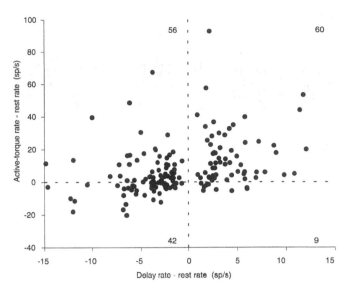

FIGURE 8.12 Relation between the modulation of activity during the delay and the active hold periods for interneurons with significant delay period modulation. Change in firing rate relative to baseline during the delay period is plotted against change in rate during the active hold period. The values were computed by averaging for each cell the single-trial difference in mean firing rate during the delay and baseline periods, and between the static hold and baseline periods. Each of the 167 cases of significant delay modulation is represented by a single data point (from 133 neurons; 34 cells contributed values for both flexion and extension). The numbers of points in each quadrant are given in the corners. Neurons in upper left and lower right quadrants have delay period modulation with polarity (facilitation or suppression) opposite that during active torque period. Note there are more cells with inhibitory (left quadrants) than excitatory (right quadrants) responses during the delay period. (From Prut, Y. and Fetz, E.E., *Nature*, 401, 590, 1999. With permission.)

whole, can be obtained by examining the temporal firing properties of the neurons.[47,48] Based on this rationale, we have examined the firing properties of single neurons, expressed by the regularity of their discharge, and the functional interactions between pairs of simultaneously recorded interneurons, measured by cross-correlations of their spike trains, to provide additional clues to the nature of spinal integration.[49]

Auto-correlations of firing were used to document the rhythmic components of discharge in individual neurons. The extent of periodicity was quantified using the coefficient of variation of interspike intervals (CV) in individual trials, and correlated with the neuron's mean firing rate during different phases of the flexion/extension task. Interneuronal variability often depended on the phase of the task: baseline, instructed delay, or movement execution (Fig. 8.13A). This dependence was not always a decrease in variability with increased firing rate, as expected from the properties of cell repolarization and refractoriness.[50] The firing of more than 15% of the interneurons became more irregular as mean firing rate increased, and the CV-rate relationship often depended on the direction of active torque (Fig. 8.13B). These results suggest that the types of synaptic inputs that act on interneurons in

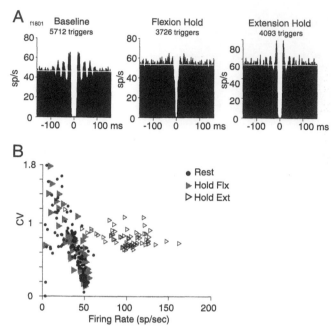

FIGURE 8.13 Task-dependent regularity of discharge for two interneurons. (A) Autocorrelations for an interneuron compiled separately during baseline (no torque) and static hold periods for flexion and extension torques. Bin at time 0 is not shown for clarity. White horizontal lines show mean firing rates. Periodicity of firing is indicated by side peaks around time 0. The neuron exhibited increased activity and firing became less regular during flexion and extension torques relative to baseline. However, discharge was much more irregular during flexion than during extension torques, even though the mean firing rate was very similar. (B) Coefficient of variation of interspike intervals (CV) vs. mean firing rate for the last second of the baseline and static hold periods of individual trials for another interneuron, plotted separately for flexion and extension. Rate did not change significantly between baseline and flexion, and the inverse relation between CV and mean rate was similar. Firing rate increased for extension torques and the relation between CV and mean rate was very different than in other phases of the task.

different behavioral contexts can be inferred from the cells' regularity of discharge. For example, the firing of interneurons with modulated delay period activity tended to be more irregular during the delay than during baseline. Since delay activity is probably due to cortical, and not feedback, input, this increased variability reflects the statistics of cortical inputs that are active during the instructed delay period.

The variability of spinal interneurons tended to be significantly lower than that reported for neurons in the cerebral cortex,[51–54] and higher than that of primary afferents.[55,56] Furthermore, premotor interneurons fired, on average, more regularly than interneurons without functional linkages to muscles, and motoneurons fired even more regularly (Fig. 8.14). Interneurons change convergent descending and sensory inputs with very different discharge variability to spike trains with intermediate temporal properties, creating a continuum of increasingly regular discharge from motor cortex to motoneurons.

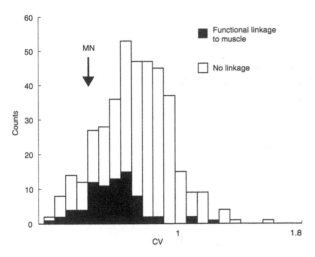

FIGURE 8.14 Histogram of CVs for spinal interneurons with (filled) and without (open) functional linkages to forearm muscles. Arrow shows mean CV for motoneurons from our data. CVs calculated across all phases of the task. For comparison, a Poisson process has a CV of 1.0.

We believe this continuum of regularity indicates a function of spinal processing that is not related to the coding of movement parameters. This hypothesis is based on two additional results. First, models of neuronal firing suggest that the temporal properties of a neuron's discharge reflect those of its inputs under certain conditions. One case is the presence of inputs with synchronous firing,[50] which may reflect the nature of corticospinal[57] and muscle afferent signals[58] projecting to interneurons. Second, we have found only a few cases of correlated firing between pairs of simultaneously recorded spinal interneurons.[49] The association of regular discharge with the lack of synchronous firing between cells also has been demonstrated for gamma motoneurons.[59] In light of these results, one interpretation of the lower CV of premotor interneurons compared to cortical cells and other interneurons is that spinal premotor circuits transform cortical motor commands by decorrelating descending and feedback signals.[60,61] This may be necessary given the extensive convergence in the projection from a large population of spinal interneurons to a smaller population of motoneurons, which may tend to induce excess synchrony and produce undesirable tremor.[62]

8.8 CONCLUDING REMARKS

In the Introduction, we expressed a belief that studies of spinal interneurons in behaving animals will be necessary to understand the spinal cord's role in motor control. Do our data to date justify this claim? We think our initial examination of sensorimotor transformations in the spinal cord show the advantage of this approach.

In many respects, interneuron activity is well correlated with motor output. Premotor interneurons exhibit temporal patterns of discharge (e.g., tonic, phasic activity) that match features of the torque trajectory, and their firing rate is well correlated with the amplitude and speed of movement. These properties are expected if interneurons execute the transformation of a motor command into muscle-centered coordinates. However, many supraspinal cells exhibit the same properties, and we do not have enough data to distinguish between representations in different coordinate frames. Our studies on the spatial tuning of interneurons for three-dimensional hand movements and grip are designed to address this issue. The tuning of interneuronal activity to movement direction and force, and the posture- and task-specificity of this tuning, should elucidate what is coded by spinal interneurons and how this compares with signals in motor cortical regions.

Aspects of interneuron activity attest to other functions mediated by spinal circuits. Some of these could be predicted from earlier studies. For example, bidirectional activity may be related to the distribution of afferent feedback to the cervical segments and the mechanical requirement of stabilizing the limb during wrist movements. Other results, such as the widespread suppression of activity during an instructed delay period, and differences in discharge variability during various phases of the task and between premotor and other interneurons, could not be predicted from other types of experiments. The ability to study the transformation of descending commands into muscle activity during behavior provides opportunities to address questions of spinal function that are difficult to answer with other methods. This ability should prove to be a useful tool to unravel the function of spinal circuits during voluntary movements.

ACKNOWLEDGMENTS

We thank Dr. Eberhard Fetz for his valuable comments on the manuscript. This work was supported by NIH grants NS36781, NS12542, and RR00166, and American Paralysis Association grants PB1-9402-1 and PBR2-9502.

REFERENCES

1. Sherrington, C.S., *The Integrative Action of the Nervous System*, Yale University Press, New Haven, 1906.
2. McCrea, D.A., Supraspinal and segmental interactions, *Can. J. Physiol. Pharmacol.*, 74, 513, 1996.
3. Goldstein, K., *The Organism. A Holistic Approach to Biology Derived from Pathological Data in Man*, American Book, New York, 1939.
4. Hongo, T., Jankowska, E., and Lundberg, A., Convergence of excitatory and inhibitory action on interneurones in the lumbosacral cord, *Exp. Brain Res.*, 1, 338, 1966.
5. Hultborn, H., Illert, M., and Santini, M., Convergence on interneurones mediating the reciprocal Ia inhibition of motoneurones, *Acta Physiol. Scand.*, 96, 193, 1976.
6. Jankowska, E. and Tanaka, R., Neuronal mechanism of the disynaptic inhibition evoked in primate spinal motoneurones from the corticospinal tract, *Brain Res.*, 75, 163, 1974.
7. Lundberg, A., Multisensory control of spinal reflex pathways, *Prog. Brain Res.*, 50, 11, 1979.

8. Baldissera, F., Hultborn, H., and Illert, M., Integration in spinal neuronal systems, in *Handbook of Physiology, The Nervous System, Vol. II: Motor Control,* Brooks, V.B., Ed., American Physiological Society, Bethesda, MD, 1981, 509.

9. Jankowska, E., Interneuronal relay in spinal pathways from proprioceptors, *Prog. Neurobiol.,* 38, 335, 1992.

10. Grillner, S., Bridging the gap — from ion channels to networks and behaviour, *Curr. Opin. Neurobiol.,* 9, 663, 1999.

11. Kiehn, O., Harris-Warrick, R.M., Jordan, L.M., Hultborn, H., and Kudo, N., Eds., Neuronal Mechanisms for Generating Locomotor Activity, *Ann. NY Acad. Sci.,* 860, 110, 1998.

12. Rossignol, S., Neural control of stereotypic limb movements, in *Handbook of Physiology, Exercise: Regulation and Integration of Multiple Systems,* Rowell, L.B. and Shepherd, J.T., Eds., Oxford University Press, New York, 1996, 173.

13. Courtney, K.R. and Fetz, E.E., Unit responses recorded from cervical spinal cord of awake monkey, *Brain Res.,* 53, 445, 1973.

14. Fetz, E.E., Perlmutter, S.I., Maier, M.A., Flament, D., and Fortier, P..A., Response patterns and postspike effects of premotor neurons in cervical spinal cord of behaving monkeys, *Can. J. Physiol. Pharmacol.,* 74, 531, 1996.

15. Flament, D., Fortier, P.A., and Fetz, E.E., Response patterns and postspike effects of peripheral afferents in dorsal root ganglia of behaving monkeys, *J. Neurophysiol.,* 67, 875, 1992.

16. Cheney, P.D., Fetz, E.E., and Mewes, K., Neural mechanisms underlying corticospinal and rubrospinal control of limb movements, *Prog. Brain Res.,* 87, 213, 1991.

17. Fetz, E.E., Cheney, P.D., Mewes, K., and Palmer, S., Control of forelimb muscle activity by populations of corticomotoneuronal and rubromotoneuronal cells, *Prog. Brain Res.,* 80, 437, 1989.

18. Perlmutter, S.I., Maier, M.A., and Fetz, E.E., Activity of spinal interneurons and their effects on forearm muscles during voluntary wrist movements in the monkey, *J. Neurophysiol.,* 80, 2475, 1998.

19. Kalaska, J.F., Scott, S.H., Cisek, P., and Sergio, L.E., Cortical control of reaching movements, *Curr. Opin. Neurobiol.,* 7, 849, 1997.

20. Soechting, J.F. and Flanders, M., Psychophysical approaches to motor control, *Curr. Opin. Neurobiol.,* 5, 742, 1995.

21. Fetz, E.E. and Cheney, P.D., Postspike facilitation of forelimb muscle activity by primate corticomotoneuronal cells, *J. Neurophysiol.,* 44, 751, 1980.

22. Maier, M.A., Perlmutter, S.I., and Fetz, E.E., Response patterns and force relations of monkey spinal interneurons during active wrist movement, *J. Neurophysiol.,* 80, 2495, 1998.

23. Palmer, S.S. and Fetz, E.E., Discharge properties of primate forearm motor units during isometric muscle activity, *J. Neurophysiol.,* 54, 1178, 1985.

24. Desmedt, J.E. and Godaux, E., Ballistic contractions in man: characteristic recruitment pattern of single motor units of the tibialis anterior muscle, *J. Physiol.,* 264, 673, 1977.

25. Van Cutsem, M., Duchateau, J., and Hainaut, K., Changes in single motor unit behaviour contribute to the increase in contraction speed after dynamic training in humans, *J. Physiol.,* 513, 295, 1998.

26. Hiebert, G.W. and Pearson, K.G., Contribution of sensory feedback to the generation of extensor activity during walking in the decerebrate cat, *J. Neurophysiol.,* 81, 758, 1999.

27. Lundberg, A., Malmgren, K., and Schomburg, E.D., Reflex pathways from group II muscle afferents. 3. Secondary spindle afferents and the FRA: A new hypothesis, *Exp. Brain Res.*, 65, 294, 1987.

28. Severin, F.V., Role of the gamma-motor system in activation of extensor alpha-motor neurons during controlled locomotion, *Biofizika*, 15, 1096, 1970.

29. Sinkjaer, T., Andersen, J.B., Ladouceur, M., Christensen, L.O., and Nielsen, J.B., Major role for sensory feedback in soleus EMG activity in the stance phase of walking in man, *J. Physiol.*, 523, 817, 2000.

30. Yang, J.F., Stein, R.B., and James, K.B., Contribution of peripheral afferents to the activation of the soleus muscle during walking in humans, *Exp. Brain Res.*, 87, 679, 1991.

31. Cheney, P.D. and Fetz, E.E., Functional classes of primate corticomotoneuronal cells and their relation to active force, *J. Neurophysiol.*, 44, 773, 1980.

32. Mewes, K. and Cheney, P.D., Primate rubromotoneuronal cells: parametric relations and contribution to wrist movement, *J. Neurophysiol.*, 72, 14, 1994.

33. Woch, G. and Kubin, L., Non-reciprocal control of rhythmic activity in respiratory-modulated XII motoneurons, *NeuroReport*, 6, 2085, 1995.

34. Orsal, D., Perret, C., and Cabelguen, J.M., Evidence of rhythmic inhibitory synaptic influences in hindlimb motoneurons during fictive locomotion in the thalamic cat, *Exp. Brain Res.*, 64, 217, 1986.

35. Robertson, G.A. and Stein, P.S., Synaptic control of hindlimb motoneurones during three forms of the fictive scratch reflex in the turtle, *J. Physiol.*, 404, 101, 1988.

36. Miyazaki, M., Tanaka, I., and Ezure, K., Excitatory and inhibitory synaptic inputs shape the discharge pattern of pump neurons of the nucleus tractus solitarii in the rat, *Exp. Brain Res.*, 129, 191, 1999.

37. Ballantyne, D. and Richter, D.W., Post-synaptic inhibition of bulbar inspiratory neurones in the cat, *J. Physiol.*, 348, 67, 1984.

38. Buschges, A. and El Manira, A., Sensory pathways and their modulation in the control of locomotion, *Curr. Opin. Neurobiol.*, 8, 733, 1998.

39. Pearson, K.G., Proprioceptive regulation of locomotion, *Curr. Opin. Neurobiol.*, 5, 786, 1995.

40. Parkis, M.A., Dong, X., Feldman, J.L., and Funk, G.D., Concurrent inhibition and excitation of phrenic motoneurons during inspiration: phase-specific control of excitability, *J. Neurosci.*, 19, 2368, 1999.

41. McCrimmon, D.R., Zuperku, E.J., Hayashi, F., Dogas, Z., Hinrichsen, C.F., Stuth, E.A., Tonkovic-Capin, M., Krolo, M., and Hopp, F.A., Modulation of the synaptic drive to respiratory premotor and motor neurons, *Respir. Physiol.*, 110, 161, 1997.

42. Georgopoulos, A.P., Kalaska, J.F., Caminiti, R., and Massey, J.T., On the relations between the direction of two-dimensional arm movements and cell discharge in primate motor cortex, *J. Neurosci.*, 2, 1527, 1982.

43. Prut, Y. and Fetz, E.E., Primate spinal interneurons show pre-movement instructed delay activity, *Nature*, 401, 590, 1999.

44. Messier, J. and Kalaska, J.F., Covariation of primate dorsal premotor cell activity with direction and amplitude during a memorized-delay reaching task, *J. Neurophysiol.*, 84, 152, 2000.

45. Bonnet, M. and Requin, J., Long loop and spinal reflexes in man during preparation for intended directional hand movements, *J. Neurosci.*, 2, 90, 1982.

46. Requin, J., Bonnet, M., and Semjen, A., Is there a specificity in the supraspinal control of motor structure during preparation?, in *Attention and Performance IV*, Dornic, S., Ed., Lawrence Erlbaum, Hillsdale, NJ, 1977, 139.

47. Bergman, H., Wichmann, T., Karmon, B., and DeLong, M.R., The primate subthalamic nucleus. II. Neuronal activity in the MPTP model of parkinsonism, *J. Neurophysiol.*, 72, 507, 1994.

48. Sun, T.Y., Chen, J.J., and Lin, T.S., Analysis of motor unit firing patterns in patients with central or peripheral lesions using singular-value decomposition, *Muscle Nerve*, 23, 1057, 2000.

49. Prut, Y., Perlmutter, S.I., and Fetz, E.E., Distributed processing in the motor system: Spinal cord perspective, *Prog. Brain Res.*, in press.

50. Segundo, J.P., Perkel, D.H., Wyman, H., Hegstad, H., and Moore, G.P., Input-output relations in computer-simulated nerve cells, *Kybernetik*, 4, 157, 1968.

51. Lee, D., Port, N.L., Kruse, W., and Georgopoulos, A.P., Variability and correlated noise in the discharge of neurons in motor and parietal areas of the primate cortex, *J. Neurosci.*, 18, 1161, 1998.

52. Shadlen, M.N. and Newsome, W.T., The variable discharge of cortical neurons: implications for connectivity, computation, and information coding, *J. Neurosci.*, 18, 3870, 1998.

53. Softky, W.R. and Koch, C., The highly irregular firing of cortical cells is inconsistent with temporal integration of random EPSPs, *J. Neurosci.*, 13, 334, 1993.

54. Stevens, C.F. and Zador, A.M., Input synchrony and the irregular firing of cortical neurons, *Nat. Neurosci.*, 1, 210, 1998.

55. Matthews, P.B. and Stein, R.B., The regularity of primary and secondary muscle spindle afferent discharges, *J. Physiol.*, 202, 59, 1969.

56. Nordh, E., Hulliger, M., and Vallbo, A.B., The variability of inter-spike intervals of human spindle afferents in relaxed muscles, *Brain Res.*, 271, 89, 1983.

57. Hatsopoulos, N.G., Ojakangas, C.L., Paninski, L., and Donoghue, J.P., Information about movement direction obtained from synchronous activity of motor cortical neurons, *Proc. Natl. Acad. Sci.*, 95, 15706, 1998.

58. Hamm, T.M., Reinking, R.M., Roscoe, D.D., and Stuart, D.G., Synchronous afferent discharge from a passive muscle of the cat: significance for interpreting spike-triggered averages, *J. Physiol.*, 365, 77, 1985.

59. Baker, J.R., Catley, M.C., Davey, N.J., and Ellaway, P.H., Influence of the pontine and medullary reticular formation on synchrony of gamma motoneurone discharge in the cat, *Exp. Brain Res.*, 87, 604, 1991.

60. Maltenfort, M.G., Heckman, C.J., and Rymer, W.Z., Decorrelating actions of Renshaw interneurons on the firing of spinal motoneurons within a motor nucleus: a simulation study, *J. Neurophysiol.*, 80, 309, 1998.

61. Windhorst, U., Adam, D., and Inbar, G.F., The effects of recurrent inhibitory feedback in shaping discharge patterns of motoneurones excited by phasic muscle stretches, *Biol. Cybern.*, 29, 221, 1978.

62. Dietz, V., Bischofberger, E., Wita, C., and Freund, H.J., Correlation between the discharges of two simultaneously recorded motor units and physiological tremor, *EEG Clin. Neurophysiol.*, 40, 97, 1976.

9 Muscle Afferent Feedback during Human Walking

Thomas Sinkjær, Jens B. Nielsen,
Michael Voigt, Michel Ladouceur,
Michael Grey, and Jacob B. Andersen

CONTENTS

9.1 INTRODUCTION

In cat and other quadrupeds, the basic walking pattern is generated by a spinal network under the control of supraspinal structures.[1,2] In addition, sensory feedback from skin and moving muscles plays a significant role in the regulation of the network activity and the locomotor movements. In humans, it is still unclear to what extent a spinal network is involved in the generation of walking and whether or not sensory feedback to the spinal cord plays a similarly significant role. In large parts of the stance phase of human walking, the ankle extensors undergo eccentric contractions, which make the large and fast conducting muscle afferents from these muscles strongly increase their discharge.[3] Through monosynaptic or polysynaptic projections, muscle afferents might, therefore, be expected to make a significant contribution to the activation of the muscle ankle extensors in the stance phase of walking. Several H-reflex studies have examined the importance of muscle (Ia) afferent feedback from the ankle extensors during walking. However, interpretation of such studies can be difficult when trying to quantify the actual contribution of the afferent feedback to the muscle activity. Consequently, several groups have attempted to evaluate this contribution by applying a mechanical stretch to the muscle(s) of interest during different phases of the walking cycle.[4-7] Force measurements provide evidence for the significance of the muscle afferents in the generation of the correction of unexpected external perturbations during gait, but they do not necessarily reveal information about the involvement of the muscle afferent activity in generating the muscle activity during unperturbed movements.

In this chapter, we review some of the recent studies investigating muscle responses to unexpected stretches. Using studies of the different muscle afferent pathways, we then set up a framework for the discussion of how muscle afferents might contribute to the muscle control in disturbed as well as undisturbed human gait. We would like to point out that we do not believe that spinal muscle afferent pathways are the only important sensory pathways in the control of walking. For a review on the importance of cutaneous afferents see, for example, Zehr and Stein,[8] and on other transcortical pathways see, for example, Christensen et al.[9]

9.2 EVOKED MUSCLE AFFERENT ACTIVITY IS AN IMPORTANT ADDITION TO MUSCLE FORCE WITHIN THE SAME STEP CYCLE DURING WALKING

Whereas electrophysiological investigations are relevant in probing different neural pathways, mechanical measures are required to investigate the function of such pathways. For example, by applying a well-defined stretch to a muscle, the force elicited by the stretch reflex can provide information about the mechanical importance of the muscle afferent feedback mediating the stretch reflex. This method has shown that reflex responses mediate from muscle afferents during tonic contractions in reduced and intact animal studies[10-12] and during tonic contractions in human subjects[13-16] more than double the stiffness of the stretched muscles.[17] Due to methodological difficulties, stretch reflex responses have not been studied in intact free-walking animals; however, Akazawa et al.[18] were able to elicit well-defined stretches of the soleus muscle during the entire step cycle in a decerebrated cat model and at the same time measure the evoked stretch reflex. Due to the experimental set-up, where the soleus muscle was isolated from the hindlimb during treadmill walking, Akazawa et al.[18] were able to measure the mechanical reflex response. They showed that the mechanical importance of the reflex reached its maximum in early stance just after foot contact. During locomotion in the spinal cats treated with clonidine, Bennett et al.[19] showed that afferent feedback from imposed low-frequency ankle movements, similar to those occurring during the normal step cycle, produced, on average, 23% of the total stretch-related force modulation. The 23% mechanical reflex response is probably an underestimation because clonidine itself depresses the group II afferent-mediated component of the stretch reflex (see later). As only the triceps surae muscles were stretched, the importance of heteronymous reflexes was not included.[20,21] Despite these limitations, the afferent feedback was responsible for half of the stretch-induced force in some cats. A similar estimate is obtained during a maintained contraction in intact humans.[14,16]

In human subjects, Yang et al.[5] used a pneumatic system to stretch the ankle extensors early in the stance phase at velocities comparable to those observed during the normal step cycle. From their measurements, they predicted that the short latency stretch reflex added 30 to 60% to the background soleus electromyogram (EMG). Using a stretch device capable of imposing well-defined mechanical perturbations to the ankle joint during all phases of the step cycle, Sinkjær et al.[6] found that in the stance phase the amplitude of the afferent-mediated soleus EMG response to a stretch of the ankle extensors is similar to the one found during standing at matched soleus background EMG. This implies an important afferent-mediated muscle activity during walking as also suggested by Yang et al.[5] However, the afferent-mediated EMG-measured activity during walking cannot be translated into reflex torque because of the highly nonlinear relation between EMG stretch reflexes and mechanical reflexes.[16,22]

Kearney et al.[23] recognize these controversies and quantified the reflex-mediated ankle extensor torque contribution during "walking like" ankle joint rotations while subjects were laying supine. Assuming that the central activation was held constant, the torque contribution from muscle afferents was between 40 and 60% of the peak ankle extensor torque during the imposed walking movements. However, because the loading on the body and the processing of the afferent input from the ankle extensor muscles in the spinal cord are modulated by supraspinal and other spinal influences,[24] the reflex contribution to the ankle extensor torque and, consequently, its functional significance may be different during real walking.

When ankle extensor torque is measured, it is generally assumed that the triceps surae dominates while the contribution from other ankle extensor muscles is negligible. Therefore, direct measurement of the Achilles tendon force *in vivo* would seem to be a method by which more direct information about the functional significance of muscle afferent feedback from the ankle extensors following a stretch could be obtained. Voigt et al.[25] used the mildly invasive optic fiber technique recently developed by Komi et al.[26] to measure Achilles tendon force in humans during walking was applied in combination with the established methods to study stretch reflex responses.[27] The perturbations of the ankle joint were elicited during treadmill walking by a portable stretch device (Fig. 9.1).

During walking, the optic fiber technique provided force profiles comparable to those reported from other experiments, including *in vivo* methods used to measure Achilles tendon force.[28] These measures typically show a decrease in Achilles tendon force shortly after heel contact while the foot is plantar-flexing and unloading the Achilles tendon, followed by a generally monotonous increase during the dorsiflexion movement and an abrupt decrease after the push off (Fig. 9.2, heavy line).

In Fig. 9.2 stretch reflex responses were elicited by ankle joint perturbations in mid-stance during walking together with the control steps in one subject. The reflex-mediated response in soleus EMG and tendon force was quantified as detailed in Voigt et al.[25] In eight able-bodied subjects the average increment in the reflex mediated soleus EMG was 49%, while the average increment in the reflex-mediated

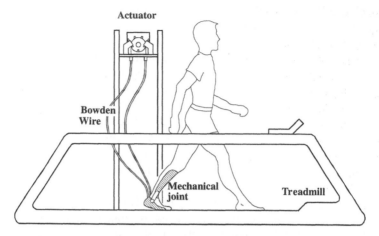

FIGURE 9.1 A schematic presentation of the experimental set-up for studying the importance of muscle afferent feedback during walking. The system consisted of a mechanical joint attached to the subject's ankle joint and a motor system placed next to the treadmill. Using position feedback from the joint, the motor was regulated in such a way that it followed the movement of the ankle joint without influencing the pattern of gait, and at any time of the gait cycle, it was possible to evoke a well-defined muscle stretch of the ankle extensors or dorsiflexors by rotating the ankle joint. The weight of the total system attached to the subject's leg was approximately 1 kg. The mechanical importance of the perturbation was measured through changes in the joint torque or muscle forces. Muscle electrical activity was recorded through bipolar surface EMG electrodes from soleus and tibialis anterior muscles.

tendon force was 59%. There was no systematic relationship between the soleus EMG changes and the force changes.

In summary, studies where the mechanical effect of the stretch reflex from the ankle extensors has been measured clearly indicate that muscle afferents contribute significantly to the stabilization of the limb in connection with unexpected perturbations during the stance phase of walking. This might be of particular importance in stabilizing body posture over the base of support in the case of an uneven surface.[8]

9.3 WHICH AFFERENTS CONTRIBUTE TO THE STRONG STRETCH-EVOKED REFLEX DURING WALKING?

In the able-bodied sitting human subject, an imposed dorsiflexion of the ankle joint causes a series of distinct responses in the EMG of the stretched ankle extensors.[13] The first response is the short-latency stretch reflex (labeled "M1" in this chapter) with an onset latency at 40 to 50 ms and a peak latency at 50 to 60 ms. During an isometric contraction of the ankle extensors, the M1 reflex is typically followed by a medium-latency reflex response (M2) with a peak latency at 70 to 90 ms.[16,29] In some subjects, a long-latency stretch reflex (M3) appears.[30,31]

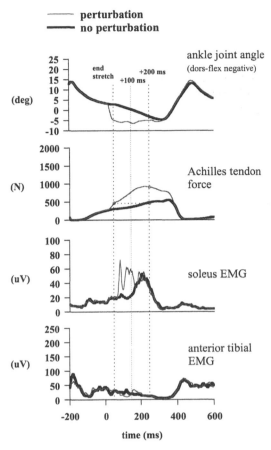

FIGURE 9.2 Stretch reflex responses recorded from one subject walking 4 km/h^{-1} on a treadmill. The EMG signals were from the left soleus and tibialis anterior muscles, and the Achilles tendon force was obtained with optical fiber technique. The responses were elicited in mid-stance by 8° perturbations in dorsiflexion (rise time 25 ms and hold time 250 ms). Each trace represents an average of 10 steps. Time zero indicates the time of mid-stance when both the perturbator and the data acquisition were triggered. The thick traces are from the control steps, i.e., steps without perturbation, while the thin lines are the traces from the perturbed steps. The vertical lines indicate (left to right) the timing of the end of the perturbation as well as 100 and 200 ms later. (Adapted from Voigt et al., *J. Neurophysiol.*, 2001 (provisionally accepted).)

The afferents primarily responsible for the onset of the M1 response are the stretch velocity sensitive group Ia-afferents from muscle spindles.[32,33] The latency of the M1 response is so short that its reflex pathway is certainly spinal and very likely monosynaptic. The origin and pathways of the M2 and M3 responses are, however, still a matter of dispute.[24,29,34–36] Several observations support the view that the M2 response in the soleus muscle is mainly mediated by the conduction of the slower spindle group II afferent fibers through an oligosynaptic spinal pathway.[24,37]

Dietz and co-workers showed an enhancement of the M2 during walking compared with a tonic contraction during standing, when a mechanical perturbation is applied by a sudden acceleration or deceleration of a treadmill.[38]

Together with the latency, this led them to suggest that the M2 response is a compensatory polysynaptic spinal reflex mediated mainly by muscle proprioceptive input from group II afferents.[4] Others have argued that the physiological properties of the medium latency M2 reflex are similar to those of the short-latency reflex. This makes them represent responses of the motoneuron pool to successive Ia bursts[34] or responses transmitted over a more complex spinal pathway.[29]

The functional importance of the long-latency reflexes has been addressed in several studies.[9,24] Evidence for involvement from group Ib force-sensitive afferents has also been shown in the cat[39,40] and may contribute to the regulation of human stance[41,42] and gait.[43]

The studies referred to above give an indication of which afferents are likely candidates to elicit the strong increase in force generation that occurs when an unexpected perturbation is imposed onto the ankle joint during human walking (Fig. 9.2). However, several of the studies were conducted under conditions other than walking. In order to show which afferents are important during walking, it is important to investigate these pathways while the subject is actually performing this task.

Figure 9.3 shows a set of averaged soleus EMG data when a stretch is applied to the ankle extensors in mid-stance of walking. In this case, the subject was walking at 3.5 km h^{-1}, and a stretch was applied 200 ms following heel contact. Prior to the stretch, the soleus EMG for the control and perturbed steps was similar, and the onset of the stretch reflex at 40 ms was clearly evident (Fig. 9.3, top). A second (M2) burst and a third (M3) burst of activity were also noticeable in this trace. M1 and M2 are present in nearly all subjects, whereas M3 is less often visible in the EMG and seems to a larger extent to depend on the stretch profile.

Grey et al.[44] found that whereas the M1 response was velocity sensitive, this was not the case for the medium M2 response. Nerve cooling increased the delay of the medium M2 latency component to a greater extent than that of the early latency M1 component. Two hours after the ingestion of tizanidine, an ($\propto_2$-adrenergic receptor agonist known to selectively depress the group II afferent pathway), the medium M2 latency reflex was strongly depressed whereas the short-latency component was unchanged. Figure 9.4 shows a soleus EMG record from a single subject together with the corresponding ankle position records when an ischemic block was applied to investigate if the large diameter afferents contribute to the medium-latency response. For clarity, only the records for the perturbed steps are shown in Fig. 9.4. The figure shows a depression of the short-latency reflex response in the ischemia condition (thick line, top trace) with only a small change in the medium-latency component. In all subjects, the ischemia strongly decreased the early latency component, whereas the medium component was only slightly and insignificantly reduced.

The results from Grey et al.[44] support the hypothesis that during walking the short-latency M1 reflex is mediated by group Ia afferents (monosynaptic pathway), while the medium-latency M2 reflex is most likely mediated through a polysynaptic group II afferent pathway. Interestingly, the group II pathway seems to be the dominant contributor to the muscle force generation at stretch velocities within the

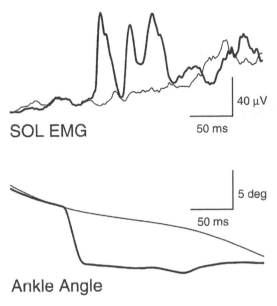

FIGURE 9.3 Example of short-, medium-, and long-latency stretch reflexes during walking. The onset of the stretch occurs at 200 ms after heel contact. The thin line is an average of 8 control steps. Top curve shows averaged soleus EMG reflexes to the imposed dorsiflexion movement. The thick line shows the rectified and filtered soleus EMG with a short-latency reflex (labeled M1) followed by medium-latency (M2) and long-latency (M3) reflexes. The soleus EMG activity is superimposed on the EMG activity from a control step.

range of normal unperturbed walking whereas the group Ia afferents seem to be more important the faster the applied stretch is.[44]

In the subject shown in Fig. 9.4, the short-latency M1 response as well as the late M3 response were reduced during ischemia, which is consistent with an observation made by Gottlieb et al.[31] and Nielsen et al.[45] This implies that the long-latency M3 response is, at least partly, mediated by the same Ia afferents as the short-latency M1. Sinkjær et al.[7] showed that the three stretch reflex responses in the soleus muscle (M1, M2, and M3) were modulated in a similar fashion and with a similar amplitude that functionally will add to the torque at the ankle joint during a step. A recent study showed that during isometric contractions, M3 recorded from the dorsiflexors is part of a transcortical reflex loop through motor cortex,[47] most likely evoked by muscle proprioceptive input from group Ia. The peak latency of M3 (120 ms) is not significantly different than the one found in the dorsiflexors.[22,47]

Interestingly, M3 is rarely present in isometric contractions during sitting and standing.[13,34,48] In contrast, the M3 responses in the preactivated tibialis anterior muscle are seen consistently during sitting[22] and walking.[9] Whether this indicates that a transcortical reflex pathway plays a more important and integrated part in the control of dorsiflexors than a transcortical reflex pathway does for the plantar flexors still remains to be investigated.

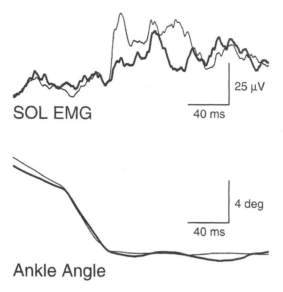

FIGURE 9.4 The effect of an ischemic block on the stretch reflex responses. During ischemia the short-latency response (M1) was reduced nearly to the level of the background EMG determined just prior to the stretch. The medium response decreased, but the decrease was not significant. Top trace: Soleus (SOL) EMG. Bottom trace: Ankle angular angle for a single subject during perturbed steps before (thin) and after (thick) the ischemic block.

The existence of transcortical stretch reflexes in the tibialis anterior and soleus muscles might have evolved to help integrate strong muscle afferent feedback with strong visual input at a site where internally generated influences may most easily use this information to generate an adequate reaction.

In summary, the results referred to in this chapter show that during the stance phase of walking, a strong stretch reflex is elicited when the ankle extensors are unexpectedly stretched. The findings suggest that the short-latency M1 stretch reflex is mediated by group Ia afferents while the medium-latency M2 stretch reflex is at least partly mediated by group II afferents from the stretched muscles. The onset latencies of these responses suggest that both responses are mediated through spinal pathways. The long-latency M3 stretch reflex is at least partly a transcortical group Ia afferent-mediated response.

9.4 DOES MUSCLE AFFERENT FEEDBACK CONTRIBUTE TO THE MUSCLE ACTIVITY DURING NORMAL HUMAN WALKING?

The studies presented so far provide evidence for the significance of muscle afferent contributions to the corrective responses to unexpected external perturbations of the gait, but do not reveal much about the involvement of the muscle afferent activity in generating muscle activity during unperturbed movements. In Sinkjær et al.,[46] the

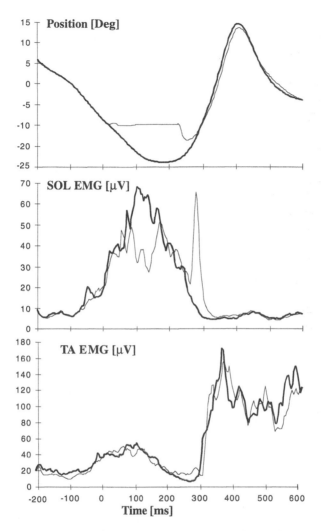

FIGURE 9.5 Example of averaged data during control steps (heavy lines) and steps during an arrest input (thin lines) to the ankle extensors in the stance phase. (Top) Ankle angle positions. (Middle) Rectified and filtered soleus muscle EMG. (Bottom) Rectified and filtered tibialis anterior muscle EMG. 0° equals standing position. Positive degrees are plantar flexion direction.

portable device in Fig. 9.1 was used to "arrest" the ankle joint in the stance phase of walking, i.e., the ankle extensors (instead of being stretched as they normally do in the stance phase of walking), and the ankle flexors were both kept constant in muscle length. The idea was that if the muscle afferents contributed importantly to the background EMG, arresting the ankle extensors would diminish the firing of the muscle afferents from the ankle extensors and thereby reduce the background EMG. Figure 9.5 shows an example from a subject for whom the ankle movement in midstance was arrested for approximately 200 ms. In each graph, the EMG and ankle joint position recorded in the control situation (heavy lines) and with the arrest input (thin lines) are superimposed. At time zero, the steps in which the arrest was imposed deflected from the position of the control steps (Fig. 9.5 top). When the ankle was released, it returned to the control trajectory within 100 ms (Fig. 9.5 top).

In this subject, the soleus EMG decreased in amplitude at a latency of 60 ms and lasted until 40 ms after the release of the arrest where a marked short-latency M1 response occurred. Due to the actuator properties of the perturbation system, the release after the arrest input caused a stretch of the ankle extensors. This explains the marked short-latency stretch reflex in soleus at this time. Unloading of the ankle extensors, which caused a real shortening of ankle extensors, gave results similar to arresting the ankle joint. During the stance phase of walking, unloading or arresting the ankle extensors on average reduced the soleus activity by 50% in early and mid-stance at an average onset latency of 64 ms.

The reduction of EMG activity was still present when transmission in Ia afferents was blocked by ischemia. This implies that sensory feedback from afferents other than group Ia plays an important role in the generation of the soleus EMG background activity during human gait, as previously suggested by Dietz et al.[4,38]

On this basis, group Ib and/or group II afferents were thought to make a significant contribution to the extensor EMG activity in the stance phase of human walking. In this respect, it is interesting that group II afferents in the cat activate a group of interneurons in the midlumbar region, which is believed to be closely integrated into the spinal locomotor circuitry and thereby to add significantly to the generation of the locomotor activity.[49]

9.5 DIFFERENT SPINAL MUSCLE AFFERENT PATHWAYS ADD TO THE MUSCLE ACTIVITY DURING NORMAL AND UNEXPECTED PERTURBED WALKING

Sinkjær et al.[46] raised the question: "Why would the Ia short latency reflex pathway contribute importantly when the muscle is unexpectedly lengthened during walking as demonstrated by Yang et al.[5] and Sinkjær et al.,[6] but less so when it is unexpectedly shortened?" There is good evidence to suggest that the monosynaptic input to the motoneurons is depressed by presynaptic inhibition during normal human walking.[50,51] This may partially explain why the Ia afferent feedback generated during normal walking seems to make only a small contribution to the soleus EMG activity (see Fig. 9.4). When a strong external force perturbs the ankle during the stance phase of walking, however, the Ia afferents respond with discharges at a very high rate. As shown by Morita et al.[52] presynaptic inhibition seems to have very little effect in depressing the synaptic input from Ia afferents to the spinal motoneurons. Therefore, a stretch reflex may be elicited in spite of the presynaptic inhibition. This means that the strength of the presynaptic inhibition of the monosynaptic Ia afferent input to the motoneurons may result in the Ia afferents making little or no contribution to the background EMG during normal walking. The presynaptic inhibition may, however, be too weak to prevent a mechanically strong compensatory short-latency stretch reflex acting in response to a large disturbance.

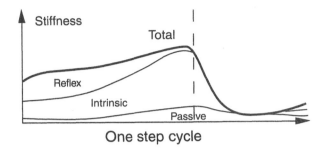

FIGURE 9.6 A sketch of the passive stiffness, intrinsic stiffness, and reflex stiffness during walking. The intrinsic stiffness in this case is related to the centrally mediated drive of the muscle.

Not only does sensory feedback add to the activity level of a muscle, but as shown in the past, sensory feedback seems very important in the timing of individual muscle activity. For example, Grillner and Rossignol[53] demonstrated in spinalised cats that changes in the hip position have a significant effect on the timing and amplitude of the locomotor bursts. Several recent studies have demonstrated a resetting of the locomotion movements in the cat by stimulation of different afferents such as group Ib afferents[54] and the afferents involved in flexor reflexes (FRA afferents[55]). This indicates that the sensory feedback mediated by these afferents at least in cats is closely integrated into the activity of the spinal network generating the locomotion. Whether a similar integration of sensory input into the spinal network also exists in humans is not known.

9.6 SUMMARY

In this chapter, we have focused on how muscle afferent feedback contributes to the control of the ankle extensors during stance phase when these muscles are normally active. The mechanical importance of the findings is illustrated in Fig. 9.6. This is a sketch of the ankle joint stiffness during a full step cycle in an able-bodied person. The total stiffness is composed of passive, intrinsic, and afferent-mediated (reflex) components. The total stiffness in the stance phase will increase as the intrinsic stiffness increases throughout the stance (due to more active cross-bridges from increased central input to the muscle), and as the afferent-mediated muscle stiffness and passive stiffness increase when the ankle extensors are being naturally stretched. During normal walking, we suggest that the group II/Ib muscle afferents contribute importantly to the reflex component. Regardless of which afferents and which pathways are responsible, our data signify that sensory feedback from ankle extensors contributes importantly to the ongoing muscle activity during human walking. One possibility is that it provides a background input to spinal interneurons and motoneurons that may be integrated with central motor commands or used by the central nervous system to achieve an optimal activation of the muscles and adjust to the constraints of the supporting surface. On top of this integrated afferent input during normal walking, an added afferent-mediated response is elicited when a strong unexpected stretch of the ankle extensors takes place (for example, when stepping on a stone with the forefoot). Such a disturbance brings the Ia afferent firing up to a level where it exceeds the presynaptic inhibition, and within the same step cycle the Ia afferent feedback (together with the increased activities in the group II and possibly group Ib afferents) importantly adds to the muscle forces to prevent a fall. This added afferent-mediated response will happen via a fast conducting monosynaptic pathway and under some circumstances through a transcortical pathway. The transcortical pathway may integrate muscle afferent feedback from the leg with other sensory inputs to generate the adequate reactions.

Over the last few decades, two extreme views have emerged regarding the control of muscle stiffness by the nervous system during a natural motor task. One view claimed that the neuromuscular system is under the exclusive control of suspraspinal mechanisms because the reflexes were considered too weak to be functionally significant. The other extreme view claimed that the stretch reflex system formed the very basis of models of motor organization.[56,57] One reason for such extreme views has been the lack of quantitative documentation of the importance of peripheral and central components in human motor tasks. As new methods have developed in many motor control laboratories, researchers have being able to separate and quantitate the functional importance of the various components that control a movement such as walking. This has, in our opinion, merged the two views and showed a potentially important role for both "simple" spinal reflex pathways and supraspinal control systems. These findings not only have an impact on our understanding of normal CNS motor programs, but are as important in understanding the basis of pathophysiological conditions of the central nervous system.

ACKNOWLEDGMENT

The Danish National Research Foundation is acknowledged for financial support.

REFERENCES

1. Grillner, S., Control of locomotion in bipeds, tetrapeds and fish. In *Handbook of Physiology, The Nervous System,* Brooks, V.B., Ed., American Physiological Society, Bethesda, MD, 1981, 1179.
2. Armstrong, D.M., The supraspinal control of mammalian locomotion, review lecture, *J. Physiol.*, 405, 1, 1988.
3. Prochazka, A., Proprioceptive feedback and movement regulation, integration of motor, circulatory, respiratory and metabolic control during exercise, *American Handbook of Physiology,* Rowell, L. and Shepard, J., Eds., Oxford University Press, New York, 1995, 1.
4. Dietz, V., Quintern, J., and Sillem, M., Stumbling reactions in man: significance of proprioceptive and pre-programmed mechanisms, *J. Physiol. (Lond.)*, 368, 149, 1987.
5. Yang, J.F., Stein, R.B., and James, K.B., Contribution of peripheral afferents to the activation of the soleus muscle during walking in humans, *Exp. Brain Res.*, 87, 679, 1991.
6. Sinkjær, T., Andersen, J.B., and Larsen, B., Soleus stretch reflex modulation during gait in man, *J. Neurophysiol.*, 76(2), 1112, 1996.

7. Sinkjær, T., Andersen, J.B., Nielsen, J.F., and Hansen, H.J., Soleus long-latency stretch reflexes during walking in healthy and spastic humans, *Clin. Neurophysiol.*, 110, 951, 1999.

8. Zehr, E.P. and Stein, R.B., What functions do reflexes serve during human locomotion? *Prog. Neurobiol.*, 58, 185, 1999.

9. Christensen, L.O.D., Petersen, N., Andersen, J.B., Sinkjær, T., and Nielsen, J., Evidence for transcortical reflexes in the lower limb in man, *Progr. Neurobiol.* 62, 251, 2000.

10. Nichols, T.R. and Houk, J.C., Improvement in linearity and regulation of stiffness that results from actions of stretch reflex, *J. Neurophysiol.*, 39, 119, 1976.

11. Hoffer, J.A. and Andreassen, S., Regulation of soleus muscle stiffness in premammillary cats: intrinsic and reflex components, *J. Neurophysiol.*, 45, 267, 1981.

12. Sinkjær, T. and Hoffer, J.A., Factors determining segmental reflex action in normal and decerebrate cats, *J. Neurophysiol.*, 64, 1625, 1991.

13. Gottlieb, G.L. and Agarwall, G.C., Response to sudden torques about ankle in man: myotactic reflex, *J. Neurophysiol.*, 42, 91, 1979.

14. Allum, J.H.J. and Mauritz, K.H., Compensation for intrinsic muscle stiffness by short-latency reflexes in human triceps surae muscles, *J. Neurophysiol.*, 52, 797, 1984.

15. Sinkjær, T., Toft, E., Andreassen, S., and Hornemann, B.C., Muscle stiffness in human ankle dorsiflexors: intrinsic and reflex components, *J. Neurophysiol.*, 60, 1110, 1988.

16. Toft, E., Sinkjær, T., Andreassen, S., and Larsen, K., Mechanical and electromyographic responses to stretch of the human ankle extensors, *J. Neurophysiol.* 65, 1402, 1991.

17. Sinkjær, T., Muscle, reflex and central components in the control of the ankle joint in healthy and spastic man, Doctoral thesis, *Acta Neurol. Scand. Suppl.*, 96(170), 1, 1997.

18. Akazawa, K., Aldridge, J.W., Steeves, J.D., and Stein, R.B., Modulation of stretch reflexes during locomotion in the mesencephalic cat, *J. Physiol.*, 329, 553, 1982.

19. Bennett, D.J., DeSerres, S.J., and Stein, R.B., Gain of the triceps surae stretch reflex in decerebrate and spinal cats during postural and locomotor activities, *J. Physiol.*, 496, 837, 1996.

20. Nichols, T.R., The organization of heterogenic reflexes among muscles crossing the ankle joint in the decerebrate cat, *J. Physiol.*, 410, 463, 1989.

21. Sinkjær, T., Nielsen, J.B., and Toft, E., Mechanical and electromyographic analysis of reciprocal inhibition at the human ankle joint, *J. Neurophysiol.*, 74, 849, 1995.

22. Toft, E., Sinkjær, T., and Andreassen, S., Mechanical and electromyographic responses to stretch of the human anterior tibial muscle at different contraction levels, *Exp. Brain Res.*, 74, 213, 1989.

23. Kearney, R.E., Lortie, M., and Stein, R.B., Modulation of stretch reflexes during imposed walking movements of the human ankle, *J. Neurophysiol.*, 81, 2893, 1999.

24. Dietz, V., Human neuronal control of automatic functional movements: interaction between central programs and afferent input, *Physiol. Rev.*, 72(1), 33, 1992.

25. Voigt, M., Komi, P.V., Nicol, C., Andersen, J.B., Ladouceur, M., Haase, J., and Sinkjær, T., Stretch reflex contribution to the human achilles tendon force during sitting and walking, provisionally accepted, *J. Neurophysiol.*, 2001.

26. Komi, P.V., Belli, A., Huttunen, V., Bonnefoy, R., Geyssant, A., and Lacour, J.R., Optic fiber as a transducer of tendomuscular forces, *Eur. J. Appl. Physiol.*, 72, 278, 1996.

27. Andersen, J.B. and Sinkjær, T., An actuator system for investigating electrophysiological and biomechanical features around the human ankle joint during gait, *Trans. Rehab. Eng.*, 3(4), 299, 1995.

28. Komi, P.V., Relevance of *in vivo* force measurements to human biomechanics, *J. Biomech.*, 23(1), 23, 1990.

29. Fellows, S.J., Dömges, F., Töpper, R., Thilmann, A.F., and Noth, J., Changes in the short- and long-latency stretch reflex components of the triceps surae muscle during ischaemia in man, *J. Physiol.*, 472, 737, 1993.

30. Gottlieb, G.L. and Agarwall, G.C., Response to sudden torques about the ankle in man: II. Post-myotatic reactions, *J. Neurophysiol.*, 43, 86, 1980.

31. Gottlieb, G.L., Agarwall, G.C., and Jaeger, R.J., Response to sudden torques about the ankle in man: V. Effect of peripheral ischemia, *J. Neurophysiol.*, 50, 297, 1983.

32. Taylor, J., Stein, R.B., and Murphy, P.R., Impulse rates and sensitivity to stretch of soleus muscle spindle afferent fibers during locomotion in premammillary cats, *J. Neurophysiol.*, 53, 341, 1985.

33. Matthews, P.B.C., The human stretch reflex and the motor cortex, *Trends Neurosci.*, 14, 87, 1991.

34. Berardelli, A., Hallett, M., Kaugman, C., Fome, E., Berenberg, W., and Simon, S.R., Stretch reflexes of triceps surae in normal man, *J. Neurol. Neurosurg. Psych.*, 45, 513, 1982.

35. Thilmann, A.F., Schwarz, M., Töpper, R., Fellows, S.J., and Noth, J., Different mechanisms underlie the long-latency stretch reflex response of active human muscle at different joints, *J. Physiol.*, 444, 631, 1991.

36. Corna, S., Grasso, M., Nardone, A., and Schieppati, M., Selective depression of medium latency leg and foot muscle responses to stretch by an alpha 2-agonist in humans, *J. Physiol. (Lond.)*, 484, 803, 1995.

37. Nardone, A., Grasso, M., Giordano, A., and Schiepatti, M., Different effect of height on latency of leg and foot short- and medium-latency EMG responses to perturbation of stance in humans, *Neurosci. Lett.*, 206, 89, 1996.

38. Dietz, V., Quintern, J., and Berger, W., Afferent control of human stance and gait: evidence for blocking of group I afferents during gait, *Exp. Brain Res.*, 61, 153, 1985.

39. Duysens, J. and Pearson, K.G., Inhibition of flexor burst generation by loading ankle extensor muscles in walking cats, *Brain Res.*, 187, 321, 1980.

40. Pearson, K.G. and Collins, D.F., Reversal of the influence of group Ib afferents from plantaris on activity in medial gastrocnemius muscle during locomotor activity, *J. Neurophysiol.*, 70, 1009, 1993.

41. Dietz, V. and Colombo, G., Effects of body immersion on postural adjustments to voluntary arm movements in humans: role of load receptor input, *J. Physiol.*, 497, 849, 1996.

42. Dietz, V., Evidence for a load receptor contribution to the control of posture and locomotion, *Neurosci. Biobehav. Rev.*, 22, 495, 1998.

43. Stephens, M.J. and Yang, J.F., Loading during the stance phase of walking in humans increases the extensor EMG amplitude but does not change the duration of the step cycle, *Exp. Brain Res.*, 124, 363, 1999.

44. Grey, M.J., Ladouceur, M., Andersen, J.B., Nielsen, J.B., and Sinkjær, T., Group II muscle afferents probably contribute to the medium latency soleus stretch reflex during walking in man, *J. Physiology*, 2001 (in press).

45. Nielsen, J., Sinkjær, T., Baumgarten, J., Andersen, J.B., Toft, E., Christensen, L.O. D., Ladouceur, M., and Morita, H., Modulation of the soleus stretch reflex and H-reflex during human walking after block of peripheral feedback, *Abstract 28th Annual Meeting Society Neuroscience*, Los Angeles, 2103, 837, 16, 1998.

46. Sinkjær, T., Andersen, J.B., Ladouceur, M., Christensen, L.O., and Nielsen, J.B., Major role for sensory feedback in soleus EMG activity in the stance phase of walking in man, *J. Physiol.*, 523, 817, 2000.

47. Petersen, N., Christensen, L.O.D., Sinkjær, T., Morita, H., and Nielsen, J., Evidence suggesting a transcortical pathway from muscle afferents to tibialis anterior moto-neurones in man, *J. Physiol.*, 512(1), 267, 1998.

48. Toft, E., Sinkjær, T., Andreassen, S., and Hansen, H.J., Stretch responses to ankle rotation in multiple sclerosis patients with spasticity, *Electroenceph. Clin. Neurophysiol.*, 89, 311, 1993.

49. Edgley, S.A., Jankowska, E., and Shefchyk, S., Evidence that mid-lumbar neurones in reflex pathways from group II afferents are involved in locomotion in the cat, *J. Physiol.*, 403, 57, 1988.

50. Stein, R.B. and Capaday, C., The modulation of human reflexes during functional motor tasks, *Trends. Neurosci.*, 11, 328, 1988.

51. Faist, M., Dietz, V., and Pierrot-Deseilligny, E., Modulation, probably presynaptic in origin, of monosynaptic Ia excitation during human gait, *Exp. Brain Res.*, 109, 441, 1996.

52. Morita, H., Petersen, N., Christensen, L.O.D., Sinkjær, T., and Nielsen, J., Sensitivity of H-reflexes and stretch reflexes to presynaptic inhibition in humans, *J. Neurophysiol.*, 80, 610, 1998.

53. Grillner, S. and Rossignol, S., On the initiation of the swing phase of locomotion in chronic spinal cats, *Brain Res.*, 146, 269, 1978.

54. Conway, B.A., Hultborn, H., and Kiehn, O., Proprioceptive input resets central loco-motor rhythm in the spinal cat, *Exp. Brain Res.*, 68, 643, 1987.

55. Schomburg, E.D., Petersen, N., Barajon, I., and Hultborn, H., Flexor reflex afferents reset the step cycle during fictive locomotion in cat, *Exp. Brain Res.*, 122, 339, 1998.

56. Merton, P.A., Speculations on the servo-control of movement, in *The Spinal Cord*, Malcolm, J.L., Gray, J.A.B., and Wolstenholme G.E.W., Eds., Little Brown, Boston, 1953, 183.

57. Berkenblit, M.B., Feldman, A.G., and Fukson O.I., Adaptability of innate motor patterns and motor control mechanisms, *Behav. Brain Sci.*, 9, 585, 1986.

10 Canine Motor Neuron Disease: A View from the Motor Unit

Martin J. Pinter, Timothy C. Cope, Linda C. Cork,
Sherril L. Green, and Mark M. Rich

CONTENTS

10.1 INTRODUCTION

The motor neuron diseases are a collection of progressive, neurodegenerative disorders. No effective treatments exist for these disorders primarily because underlying pathological mechanisms are poorly understood. The need for a greater understanding of possible mechanisms has led to the use of several animal models of motor neuron disease. This chapter considers recent work on one of these models called

Hereditary Canine Spinal Muscular Atrophy (HCSMA), first identified by Cork and colleagues.[1,2] General problems and issues associated with human motor neuron disease are considered first, followed by a review of recent work in HCSMA that focuses on the functional properties of motor units and how their function is lost during disease progression.

10.2 HUMAN MOTOR NEURON DISEASE

The most common form of motor neuron disease in humans is amyotrophic lateral sclerosis (ALS), or Lou Gehrig's disease, named after the famous baseball player. Most cases of ALS (85 to 90%) appear without a history of family involvement and are termed *sporadic* while the remainder are inherited and are called *familial* ALS (FALS). Although ALS is viewed by many as the prototypical motor neuron disease, upper motor neuron involvement (corticospinal) is considered to be a cardinal feature of the disease. In general, exclusive involvement of motor neuron degeneration among the motor neuron diseases appears to be rare.[3] Thus, most cases of ALS do not feature exclusive motor neuron degeneration and so are not disorders of a specific neuronal cell type. It is clear, however, that motor neurons are particularly vulnerable, and understanding this vulnerability remains a central focus of research effort.

An intriguing feature of ALS is how the onset of the disorder varies. Approximately 30% of the cases exhibit the first signs of weakness focally among muscles innervated by cranial motor neurons (bulbar onset), 20 to 30% of cases show an onset in distal leg muscles, while about 30% show the first signs in distal hand muscles.[3] Considerable variance is noted in the balance between upper and lower motor neuron signs as well.[3] The basis for this variability is not known, but one possibility is that it is caused by different mechanisms. Other observations, however, indicate that the differing onset versions all tend to regress to a state that features common clinical signs if sufficient time for full disease progression occurs.[3] These observations are more compatible with common underlying mechanisms, while the variability in the onset and character or rate of progression could indicate the existence of modifying factors. Several modifying genes have been identified in one animal version of motor neuron disease.[4] The identification of modifying factors, whether genetic or environmental, could be of particular importance because they could, in principle, be used to control at least the progression of the disorder.

One of the most insidious aspects of ALS is that the actual onset of the disease process occurs well before the victim becomes aware of its existence. Available estimates indicate that as much as 50% of the original innervation in a muscle is lost before weakness is first noted.[5,6] The mechanism underlying this phenomenon is the well-known ability of surviving motor terminals to sprout and reinnervate nearby denervated muscle fibers.[7] Although this mechanism preserves muscle force, it also creates uncertainty in distinguishing clinically between loss of innervation by sprouted motor terminals vs. loss of original innervation. It is thus not surprising that the mechanisms that cause the initial denervation of muscle and loss of motor unit function in ALS are not well understood. An understanding of these mechanisms seems particularly necessary because their operation leads to loss of motor unit function, the single most necessary problem in motor neuron disease.

Classically, the role of motor neuron cell death in the loss of motor unit function has received the most emphasis. In large part, this is due to the relative ease with which motor neuron cell death can be demonstrated with routine histological examination of autopsy material. Human autopsy results, however, are dominated by disease endstage phenomena, and while there is no doubt that cell death explains the permanent loss of motor units and paralysis of ALS, it remains uncertain whether cell death actually accounts for the initial loss of motor unit function. The clinical electrophysiological tests used to diagnose ALS depend on the motor neuron's ability to activate muscle fibers[8,9] and can only detect that denervation has occurred. These methods cannot distinguish between functional denervation that occurs because motor neurons are dysfunctional and denervation that occurs because motor neurons have died.

10.3 UNDERSTANDING THE PROGRESSION OF MOTOR NEURON DISEASE

These considerations underscore the potential importance of understanding events that occur before motor neuron cell death. In the clinical literature, there are reports suggesting that a preliminary phase of motor unit dysfunction occurs in ALS patients. Several investigators have reported abnormal decrement of motor unit potentials during repetitive activation,[8,10–12] and *in vitro* studies indicate that quantal content is decreased at ALS motor terminals.[13] Some of these findings may reflect the functional properties of immature nerve endings belonging to terminal sprouts, but they also raise the possibility that motor unit functional failure precedes motor neuron cell death. Understanding the mechanisms that underlie motor unit failure is particularly important because this failure is the foundation of weakness in motor neuron disease.

Technical issues and other problems limit the ability to obtain from human studies a detailed understanding of how motor units fail in motor neuron disease. Fortunately, a number of animal models of motor neuron disease are available for study. A common concern, however, is that none of these models exactly replicate the human disorder. This concern is partly justified because all these models are in non-primate species which lack the direct (monosynaptic) corticospinal projections to motor neurons that degenerate in human disease. Nevertheless, these animal models provide unique opportunities to test ideas about mechanisms that can cause motor neuron degeneration and dysfunction but cannot be explored at all in human disease. Animal models have been especially instructive regarding certain forms of hereditary motor neuron disease and for expanding our understanding of possible molecular mechanisms. The lack of exact replication of the human disease is perhaps best viewed as an important constraint that must be considered when generalizing results obtained from these models to the human disease.

10.4 HEREDITARY CANINE SPINAL MUSCULAR ATROPHY

In order to examine mechanism issues in motor neuron disease, we have in recent years studied an animal model called Hereditary Canine Spinal Muscular Atrophy

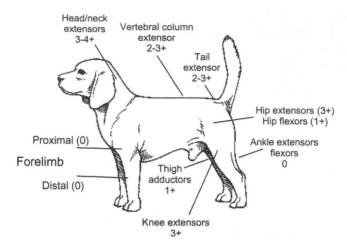

FIGURE 10.1 Muscle locations and grades of spontaneous electromygraphic (EMG) activity in an HCSMA homozygote. Spontaneous EMG activity recorded in resting muscle reflects the presence of denervated muscle fibers. This figure illustrates the extent of spontaneous EMG activity observed in various muscles of an HCSMA homozygote aged about 160 days. EMG activity was recorded with a standard, bipolar, concentric needle electrode with the animal maintained under general anesthesia. Spontaneous activity was graded using a standard clinical rating scale of 0 (no spontaneous activity) to 4 (maximum activity).[57] Denervation appears first in tail muscles at about 10 weeks of age and spreads in rostral and distal directions so that distal hindlimb and forelimb muscles do not exhibit signs of denervation until late in the course of the disease. In the case of ankle extensors, experiments have shown that significant motor unit dysfunction exists by 160 days despite the absence of spontaneous EMG activity.

(HCSMA). HCSMA is an inherited disorder of motor neurons that shares features with human motor neuron disease.[1,14] Genetic studies have shown that HCSMA is an autosomal dominant disorder.[15] Although the defective gene has not yet been identified, a recent study[16] has demonstrated that HCSMA is not caused by the mutations in the survival motor neuron (SMN) gene that are responsible for the human spinal muscular atrophies.[17]

Consistent with its autosomal dominant inheritance, disease in HCSMA manifests as two phenotypes. An accelerated phenotype (presumed homozygous) begins showing weakness about 6 to 8 weeks postnatal with rapid and progressive deterioration that culminates in full tetraparesis by about 6 to 7 months of age. HCSMA homozygotes do not survive to reach sexual maturity. Homozygotes exhibit a stereotyped spatiotemporal pattern of muscle denervation which is first observed in caudal tail muscles. Subsequently, denervation spreads in a rostral and distal direction so that distal hindlimb/forelimb muscles are the last to become involved. An illustration of the spatial distribution and extent of spontaneous electromygraphic (EMG) activity caused by muscle denervation is shown in Fig. 10.1 for an HCSMA homozygote aged 160 days. A more chronic phenotype (presumed heterozygous) begins

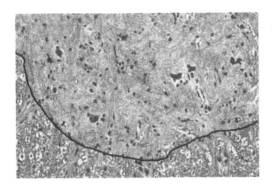

FIGURE 10.2 Motor neuron cell death in an HCSMA heterozygote. Photomicrograph shows a cross-section of lumbar spinal cord from an HCSMA heterozygote aged 5 years. The solid line indicates the border between gray and white matter. Note the absence of large motor neuron cell bodies in the ventral aspect of the spinal gray.

showing weakness at about 8 to 12 months and can survive as long as 7 years. The development of muscle denervation in heterozygotes occurs over a much more protracted time course but exhibits essentially the same spatial pattern as homozygotes.

Histological studies of the brain and spinal cord indicate that pathological involvement in HCSMA is limited to motor neurons.[18] Whether motor neurons are exclusively involved is not known, however, because of uncertainty about whether full disease expression is achieved during the time interval over which these animals can be humanely maintained. More extensive involvement is found, for example, in ALS patients who are maintained for extended periods by artificial ventilation.[19] This illustrates an important point: Limited observations of progressive disorders, perhaps even over the natural disease course, may lead to erroneous conclusions concerning the selectivity of involved neuronal populations.

The pathological features found among motor neurons in HCSMA are similar to those found in other versions of motor neuron disease. These features include abnormal neurofilament accumulations in proximal motor axons, motor neuron chromatolysis, and neuronophagia, all considered evidence of diseased motor neurons.[18] One common feature of motor neuron disease that is not observed in HCSMA homozygotes during the time they can be studied (up to about 6 months) is extensive motor neuron cell death.[18] Since weakness progresses to the point of tetraparesis during this interval, it is apparent that mechanisms other than motor neuron cell death must mediate the progressive weakness in HCSMA homozygotes. As illustrated in Fig. 10.2, however, loss of motor neurons is observed in heterozygotes thus demonstrating that motor neuron cell death is a feature of HCSMA. The relative absence of motor neuron cell death in homozygotes may be related to the accelerated progression rate of weakness in these animals (particularly among neck and proximal limb extensor muscle groups, Fig. 10.1) which renders them moribund before cell death has an opportunity to appear. The much longer time period over which heterozygotes develop symptoms and weakness (years vs. about 2 to 3 months for homozygotes) presumably enables a more complete expression of the disorder.

10.5 MOTOR UNIT FUNCTIONAL PROPERTIES IN HCSMA

A variety of possible mechanisms could lead to loss of motor unit function in HCSMA. To learn how motor units fail in HCSMA, we have investigated the mechanical properties of functionally isolated motor units using intracellular stimulation of motor neuron soma or ventral root motor axons. The studies have focused on motor units in the medial gastrocnemius (MG) muscle which is an ankle extensor muscle that is easily accessible. Because of its distal location, the MG muscle becomes involved later in the disease progression and thus provides an excellent opportunity to investigate the initial stages of motor unit failure. It is important to keep in mind, however, that at all times more proximal muscles, including paraspinous and important neck extensors, are more extensively involved than the MG muscle.

Most of our studies have been performed in HCSMA homozygotes where two types of abnormal motor unit behavior have been observed.

10.5.1 Younger Homozygotes

The first type of abnormal motor unit behavior has been observed only in younger homozygotes, aged about 90 days or less.[20] This is actually not a motor unit behavior per se but rather an absence of motor unit function associated with an otherwise electrophysiologically competent motor neuron. We call these *disconnected* motor neurons because intracellular stimulation of these cells fails to produce detectable motor unit force but recording of single axonal action potentials demonstrates the presence of intact axonal conduction.[20] The basis for this remains uncertain but conduction block between the nerve entry into muscle, loss of conduction within the intramuscular portions of the motor axon, or a complete absence of the motor axon arbor are possibilities. Intracellular stimulation of most of the sampled motor neuron population in these young homozygous animals produced motor unit force, which demonstrates intact motor neuron connections with muscle fibers. Thus, despite the presence of disconnected motor neurons, these muscles probably have a sufficient complement of normally functioning motor units so that no major deficits exist in the ability to extend the ankle joint, and no major weakness is apparent.

10.5.2 Older Homozygotes

We thought initially that older homozygotes (> 90 days) would feature an increased number of disconnected motor neurons and present an extension of the observations made in younger homozgyotes. This did not, however, turn out to be the case; only one disconnected motor neuron has been observed thus far in homozygotes older than 120 days. The fate of disconnected motor neurons remains unknown.

10.5.2.1 Failing Motor Units

In older HCSMA homozygotes, a different type of motor unit failure was encountered. Despite the absence of spontaneous EMG activity indicative of denervation (see Fig. 10.1), motor units were found that did not sustain force output during

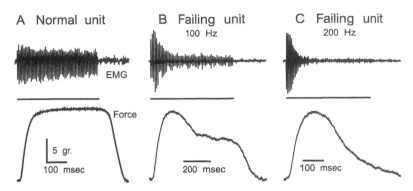

FIGURE 10.3 Motor unit tetanic failure in HCSMA homozygotes. (A) EMG (upper record) and force (lower record) recorded from a medial gastrocnemius (MG) motor unit from symptomless HCSMA animals. A single MG motor axon in the ventral root was stimulated through an intracellular electrode with a train of 60 suprathreshold depolarizing pulses at 200 Hz. Note that force maintains a steady plateau during axon stimulation (duration of axon stimulus train indicated by long horizontal bar). (B) Motor unit force and EMG recorded from the MG muscle of a homozygote aged 165 days. In this case, an MG motor neuron soma was stimulated through an intracellular electrode at 100 Hz (stimulus duration indicated by horizontal bar). Note that both motor unit force and EMG fail after reaching an early peak, and that the EMG signal maintains a reduced level of stimulus-linked activity following the initial failure. This demonstrates that conduction failure in the main trunk of the motor axon does not cause the unit force and EMG failure. (C) Motor unit force and EMG records for 200-Hz stimulation rate. ((B) and (C) from Pinter, M.J. et al., *J. Neurosci.*, 15, 3447, 1995. With permission.)

repetitive activation. Examples of this phenomenon, termed "tetanic failure", are shown in Fig. 10.3. In the typical failing motor unit, both force and motor unit EMG amplitude decline during tetanic stimulation of either the motor neuron soma or motor axon (Fig. 10.3B and C), whereas normal motor units sustain force and EMG amplitude at identical activation frequencies (Fig. 10.3A).

Tetanic failure begins to appear in the MG muscle over a discrete time interval. Before about 90 days, tetanic failure in the MG has not been observed in any HCSMA homozygotes whereas by about 120 days, all but one homozygote studied has shown failing MG motor units. After 120 days, there is considerable variability in the extent of MG motor unit failure among individual animals, thus demonstrating that factors in addition to postnatal age play a role in determining motor unit failure. Based on the fact that proximal muscles are more extensively involved by the time MG motor units first begin exhibiting failure, we assume that motor unit failure begins at an earlier age in these muscles.

During tetanic failure, force and EMG fail in parallel. One possible explanation of this behavior is that conduction failure occurs in the main axon during the repetitive activity. While we cannot exclude this possibility in all cases, conduction failure in the main axon does not appear to be a major cause of tetanic failure in HCSMA. In most cases, motor unit force production does not decrease to zero during tetanic failure as would be expected if conduction failure occurred in the main axon.

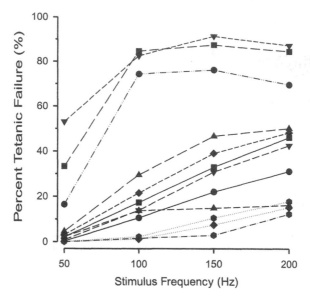

FIGURE 10.4 Motor unit failure increases as activation frequency increases. A plot of unit force failure vs. stimulation rate for 14 motor units recorded from an HCSMA homozygote. Force failure was quantified by measuring the difference between peak unit force and force present at the end of the stimulus train, expressed as a percent of the peak force. Higher values indicate greater force failure. For each motor unit, force failure increases as the motor unit activation frequency increases.

Instead, a small force is very often maintained after the initial fall in force output, thus demonstrating that conduction in the main axon continues (see Fig. 10.3B).

These considerations indicate that the motor terminal is the locus of tetanic failure and illustrate that failure is not uniform within this part of the motor neuron since otherwise it would be complete. Explanations for the simultaneous failure of force output and EMG during tetanic failure include conduction failure in motor terminal arbors and/or failure of transmission at the neuromuscular junction (NMJ). Several additional features of tetanic failure are consistent with the possibility that it arises as a result of neuromuscular transmission failure. As shown in Fig. 10.4, the extent of tetanic failure increases as the frequency of motor unit activation is increased. This is most easily explained in terms of the increased depression of endplate currents that occurs when axon stimulation frequencies are increased (see Fig. 10.6B). Progressively increasing depression during tetanic activation might cause some endplate currents to fall below the threshold of activating muscle fibers thus leading to decreased motor unit force output.

Another property of failing motor units that suggests underlying defects in neuromuscular synaptic transmission involves an increase of motor unit force output following repetitive activity. In many cases, motor unit twitch force is very small when the motor neuron or axon is first stimulated at low (1 Hz) repetition rates (Fig. 10.5A). But following a single, high frequency train of stimuli, however, twitch force of many failing motor units can be dramatically increased (Fig. 10.5B). It is

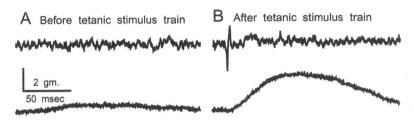

FIGURE 10.5 Motor unit twitch potentiation in failing motor units. Records show force (lower records) and EMG (upper records) for an MG motor unit recorded in HCSMA homozygotes. (A) Records obtained before, (B) records obtained after the motor unit was activated by a single train of 60 axonal action potentials at 150 Hz. The effect of the single train was to potentiate the twitch force and EMG, an effect that has only been observed in failing motor units. (From Pinter, M.J. et al., *J. Neurosci.*, 15, 3447, 1995. With permission.)

unlikely that this reflects potentiation of the force-generating mechanism within muscle fibers since the potentiated twitch is accompanied by a large increase in the amplitude of the motor unit EMG potential (Fig. 10.5B). This indicates that an increased number of muscle fibers become activated following the tetanic stimulation. Maximum tetanic force is also potentiated under these circumstances, but superimposing unpotentiated and potentiated tetanic force records very often shows that the failure occurring during tetanic stimulation is not changed or improved but rather remains proportional to the peak force.[20] This indicates that neurotransmission to those muscle fibers activated as a result of the high-frequency conditioning stimulus train is just as likely to fail during repetitive activation as neurotransmission to those fibers that are active before the conditioning train.

Based on the observation that both motor unit force and EMG increase, we suspect that the post-tetanic increase of motor unit force is caused by post-tetanic potentiation of endplate currents. Prior to the conditioning tetanic stimulus, there are likely to be nerve terminals within these motor units that do not release sufficient transmitter to activate muscle fibers. Following tetanic activation, transmitter output is presumably elevated to enable activation of additional muscle fibers and increased motor unit force output.

10.5.2.2 Effects of 4-Aminopyridine

Additional indirect evidence that motor terminals in failing motor units release low quantities of transmitter has been obtained using the drug 4-aminopyridine (4AP). 4AP blocks voltage-gated potassium channels and has been shown to increase the release of ACh from motor terminals.[21,22] When 4AP is administered systemically while recording force from failing motor units, both motor unit force and EMG increase in parallel whereas no effect is found when recording from a non-failing motor unit. In addition, motor units that exhibit a greater extent of tetanic failure show a larger post-4AP increase of motor unit force and EMG.[23] However, even though unit force can be increased, this is seen at low activation frequencies (1 Hz) whereas tetanic failure seen during activation at higher frequencies is only moderately improved.

At normal motor terminals, 4AP is thought to increase transmitter release by increasing the amount of calcium that enters upon action potential arrival at the motor terminal. By blocking voltage-gated potassium channels, 4AP increases the action potential duration at the motor terminal, which increases the duration of the calcium current that is triggered by the action potential, an effect that increases calcium entry at the terminal. Thus, one possibility in HCSMA is that the amount of entering calcium in motor terminals of failing units is too low to provoke reliable release of transmitter. Defects of motor terminal calcium entry have been suggested to operate in human motor neuron disease, but most often in the context of a postulated autoimmune process directed specifically at calcium channels.[24–26] In HCSMA, it seems unlikely that insufficient calcium entry is the sole explanation of dysfunction because 4AP administration does not eliminate tetanic failure. Other possibilities include increased inactivation of calcium currents during repetitive activity or a deficiency in readily releasable stores of transmitter. While these data provide no definitive insight into the main defect, they support the view that failure is localized to motor terminals and resides in the synaptic release mechanism.

10.5.3 NEUROMUSCULAR TRANSMISSION IN HCSMA

Recently, we began examining the physiological properties of neuromuscular junctions (NMJs) in HCSMA homozygotes to obtain direct evidence that defects in synaptic transmission underlie tetanic failure of motor units. In these studies, we use two-electrode voltage-clamp recording of endplate currents, vital fluorescence microscopy to image muscle fibers and endplates, and the same stimulus patterns to investigate synaptic function as we have used to investigate motor unit properties. We have compared the properties of endplate currents between HCSMA homozygotes and age-matched symptomless members of the HCSMA pedigree or normal, vendor-supplied animals.

This study is not yet complete, but the data we have collected thus far provide a clear indication of how motor unit dysfunction arises in HCSMA. The most important difference we have found is that nerve-evoked endplate quantal content (tested at a nerve stimulation frequency of 1 Hz) is decreased in HCSMA homozygotes relative to normal age-matched dogs by a factor of about 3-fold (HCSMA homozygotes, approximately 6.0 vs. 18.6 for normal MG endplate currents). Consistent with a low probability of transmitter release, we found a large increase in EPC failures at 1-Hz stimulation (15/24 EPCs exhibited failure in one HCSMA homozygote MG muscle vs. 0/26 in one normal control). We have determined that the decrease in EPC quantal content is related specifically to nerve-evoked release of ACh because the amplitudes of spontaneously occurring, miniature endplate currents (mEPCs) are unchanged (HCSMA homozygote, 1.52 nA vs. 1.53 nA for normal dog MG mEPCs). Time-course features such as EPC and mEPC time-to-peak and decay time constant are also unchanged. These data demonstrate that motor nerve terminals in HCSMA release less ACh compared with normal ones. Similar results have been obtained from studies of NMJ function in ALS.[13]

It is conceivable that much of the abnormal motor unit behavior we have seen in HCSMA is related to reduced quantal content at the NMJ. As noted earlier, one remarkable motor unit property observed in HCSMA homozygotes is that force output can be dramatically increased following tetanic activation. This and other evidence suggested that EPCs may potentiate to a greater extent following repetitive nerve activation.[20,23] As summarized in Fig. 10.6, this is exactly the behavior of EPCs observed in HCSMA homozygotes. Repetitive nerve stimulation potentiates EPCs on average by about 38% at normal MG NMJs, but in the homozygote potentiation averages about 130%. Fig. 10.6A shows that the increased EPC potentiation is associated with decreased EPC quantal content at homozygous NMJs.

We have been particularly interested in examining the effects of repetitive activation on EPCs in HCSMA homozygotes because this type of activation leads to tetanic failure.[20] To our surprise, we found that these currents do not depress any more than normal at the same activation frequencies that cause motor unit tetanic failure. This is illustrated in Fig. 10.6C which shows the decrease of EPC amplitude during a 10-pulse, 50-Hz stimulus train (Fig. 10.6B), expressed as a fraction of the EPC amplitude for the first pulse. Values shown are averages of EPCs from 8 MG NMJs from 1 homozygote (aged 170 days) and averages from 14 MG NMJs from 1 normal beagle aged 160 days. These data demonstrate that the relative depression of EPCs during repetitive activation in HCSMA homozygotes is similar to normal.

At present, we suspect that motor unit tetanic failure arises in HCSMA because NMJs in failing motor units feature a low quantal content that is just sufficient to fire muscle fibers when activated at low frequency (1 Hz). When activated at the higher frequencies needed to produce purposeful motor unit force, a normal or even decreased level of depression (Fig. 10.6C) is probably sufficient to lower quantal content so that EPCs drop below the threshold for activating muscle fibers after the first few pulses of the stimulus train. This results in motor unit tetanic failure and weakness.

10.5.4 MECHANISMS RESPONSIBLE FOR TETANIC FAILURE IN HCSMA

In the previous discussion, we considered evidence that defects in neuromuscular synaptic transmission may give rise to motor unit tetanic failure. While this evidence implicates the NMJ as a failure site, it provides little insight into which cellular systems may be involved. Here we consider evidence concerning the structural status of NMJs in muscles that contain failing motor units. Subsequently, we consider evidence concerning the possible role of axonal abnormalities in producing tetanic failure.

10.5.4.1 Neuromuscular Degeneration

A list of specific mechanisms whose failure could account for the appearance of motor unit and neuromuscular transmission failure in HCSMA would be long because it would need to include any process involved in maintaining the normal structure and function of the motor terminal. To gain some insight into possible defective mechanisms that might give rise to tetanic failure, we have attempted to associate the appearance of tetanic failure with other pathological events that occur in HCSMA. Since the pathogenesis of HCSMA includes degeneration of motor nerve terminals and intramuscular nerve branches, we first considered the possibility

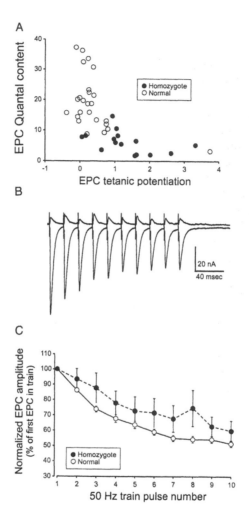

FIGURE 10.6 Properties of neuromuscular synaptic transmission in HCSMA homozygotes. In 1 homozygote aged 160 days and 1 normal, age-matched control dog, endplate currents (EPCs) were studied using voltage clamp recording in crushed fiber biopsy preparations obtained from MG muscles. Muscle fibers were held at –60 mV during current recording. (A) Plot of individual EPC quantal content against maximum EPC amplitude potentiation during repeated trials of alternating train stimuli (150 Hz) and single stimulus. Quantal content was determined directly from averaged records of unpotentiated EPCs and averaged miniature EPCs recorded over 2 to 3 min intervals. The lower quantal contents of EPCs from the homozygote are associated with increased maximum amplitude potentiation. (B) Demonstration of EPC depression during repetitive activity in a control animal. A stimulus train of 10 pulses at 50 Hz was applied to the muscle nerve while recording EPCs. Lower record shows an average of 11 sweeps, while the upper record shows the standard deviation of the mean record. The amplitude of the final ECP was decreased to about half of the initial EPC. (C) Average EPC amplitude depression observed during 10-pulse, 50-Hz stimulus trains for the same animals in (A). In general, depression during repetitive activation was similar between EPCs from normal and homozygote NMJs despite the significantly lower quantal content of EPCs from the homozygote.

that tetanic failure might arise secondarily to these events. To examine this possibility, we studied NMJs in muscles from HCSMA homozygotes that had been investigated physiologically and were known to contain failing motor units.[27] To our surprise, we could find no evidence of degenerative changes at the NMJs in muscles containing up to 60% failing motor units. Immunofluorescence staining and imaging showed that pre- and post-synaptic NMJ components remained perfectly aligned just as in muscles from normal animals (Color Figure 4A*), and that the ultrastructure of NMJs appeared normal. We excluded that these findings were the result of a failure to detect NMJ degeneration by showing that degenerative changes at the NMJs of more involved proximal muscles could be easily demonstrated with immunofluorescent staining and imaging (Color Fig. 4B, C). These results indicate that tetanic failure in HCSMA occurs before degenerative changes appear at the NMJ and suggest that factors involved more directly with the operation or maintenance of neuromuscular transmission are responsible for tetanic failure.

10.5.4.2 Axonal Abnormalities

Other pathological changes that occur in HCSMA involve the properties of the motor axon. We considered that these changes may be relevant for the appearance of motor unit failure because neuromuscular transmission depends critically upon maintenance of normal axonal structural integrity and other functions such as fast axonal transport of synaptic proteins[28,29] and slow axonal transport of structural proteins. In HCSMA, there is a variety of evidence indicating the presence of axonal abnormalities. Motor axon size is decreased relative to normal, age-matched control animals;[30] mRNA for the light neurofilament protein component is decreased.[31] In addition, protein levels and activity of CDK5, a proline-linked kinase known to phosphorylate the heavy neurofilament component, are elevated,[32] and large accumulations of neurofilaments are found in proximal motor axons in HCSMA homozygotes.[18,33] Large accumulations of maloriented neurofilaments in proximal motor axons are also very common in ALS.[34] This and other evidence have led some to propose a central role for neurofilament dysfunction in the pathogenesis of motor neuron disease.[35–37]

The first step in establishing whether the changes described above underlie tetanic failure requires demonstrating temporal links between these phenomena and the appearance of tetanic failure. This is not a straightforward process, however, because the nature of the data is so different. On one hand, tetanic failure is a functional attribute of individually characterized motor units in an identified muscle. In contrast, the pathological findings described above rely on examination of unidentified populations of motor neurons or axons with unknown functional capabilities or the use of tissue homogenates that might include the additional confound of other cell types.

An alternative approach for establishing links to tetanic failure is to use the individual motor axon conduction velocity as an index of axonal functional integrity. The rationale for this is the dependence of conduction velocity on axonal and fiber caliber[38,39] and the dependence of axonal caliber on cytoskeletal properties such as

---

* Color figures follow page 142.

neurofilament number and phosphorylation status.[40–42] We reasoned that if an axonal abnormality is directly or indirectly responsible for motor unit dysfunction in HCSMA, the onset of dysfunction might be associated with changes of axonal conduction velocity or the appearance of proximal swellings in affected motor axons.

To examine these possibilities, we studied the postnatal time course of conduction velocity maturation in HCSMA homozygotes in relation to the onset of motor unit dysfunction. We found that the average conduction velocity of motor axons innervating MG muscles with failing motor units increased linearly and reached adult values by about 180 days, despite the appearance of motor unit failure in the time interval between 90 and 120 days. Furthermore, the rates at which conduction velocity increased did not appear to differ between HCSMA homozygotes and animals that lacked symptoms. We also intracellularly labeled several motor neurons in one homozygote after characterizing motor unit dysfunction for each motor neuron and examined directly for the presence of swellings in proximal motor axons. In two motor neurons that innervated moderately failing motor units, inspection of labeled proximal motor axons revealed no evidence of swellings. In a third motor neuron that innervated a motor unit exhibiting almost complete failure, small swellings were observed in the proximal motor axon, but these swellings were much smaller than those found in nearby spinal cord using immunolabeling for neurofilament proteins.

In terms of the cellular subsystems that might be involved, these results emphasize the selectivity of motor unit tetanic failure in HCSMA. Perhaps the best indication of this is that tetanic failure appears independently of and does not interfere with the postnatal maturation of axonal conduction velocity. The maturation of axonal conduction velocity depends on a variety of mechanisms including the synthesis, transport, and assembly of cytoskeletal and ion channel proteins that mediate axon structure and function as well as interactions between axons and myelinating cells that determine the extent of myelination.[43,44] It is thus tempting to speculate that the appearance of tetanic failure is not due to failure of any of these mechanisms, but more work will be needed to establish this definitively.

Our results make clear that the onset and evolution of motor unit functional failure in HCSMA precede the appearance of other pathological changes such as axonal accumulations of neurofilaments and NMJ degeneration. An analogous situation has recently been reported for transgenic mice expressing an ALS-linked mutation of the SOD1 enzyme where degeneration of NMJs precedes the onset of motor neuron cell death in the spinal cord by a significant amount of time.[45] Thus, in animal models of motor neuron disease where studies of the earliest phase of the disorders can be conducted, dysfunction appears first peripherally. Reports of loss of motor unit function,[8,11,46] deficits in neuromuscular synaptic transmission,[13] and patient complaints of fatigability in involved muscles[47] suggest that an initial phase of neuromuscular dysfunction might also exist in ALS. These findings point to the neuromuscular junction as the site where motor unit function is lost in motor neuron disease. This underscores the importance of understanding the mechanisms that produce this loss, particularly since there is no guarantee that these mechanisms are the same as those that produce the more commonly emphasized pathological changes such as motor neuron cell death or neurofilament dysfunction.

10.6 THE PATHOLOGICAL PROCESS
UNDERLYING HCSMA

The final issue to consider is the general nature of the pathological process in HCSMA. In the broadest sense, this concerns the underlying cause of HCSMA, and while there are some hints, there are no satisfactory answers at present. Central to this issue is the basic genetic defect in HCSMA which, as mentioned above, remains unidentified. Efforts to identify this defective gene continue, but it is important to emphasize that identification of the defective gene might not automatically provide an understanding of the pathogenesis of HCSMA. One reason for this view is that disorders featuring autosomal dominant inheritance patterns (such as HCSMA) can involve novel "gain of function" properties that may not be predictable from an understanding of the affected gene or the function of the normal gene product. While the need for identification of the defective gene in HCSMA (or in any inherited form of MND) is not diminished in any way by this consideration, it does emphasize the potential importance of a detailed understanding of the mechanisms that contribute to the pathogenesis of HCSMA, and more specifically, to the appearance of motor unit failure.

10.6.1 OXIDATIVE STRESS

Recent work has demonstrated that affected HCSMA animals exhibit low serum levels of vitamin E.[48] Additional evidence indicates that this deficiency reflects increased metabolic consumption of vitamin E rather than a dietary insufficiency, and suggests the presence of an unmet demand for vitamin E. Since vitamin E is a potent antioxidant, one interpretation of these data is that oxidative stress is a factor in the pathogenesis of HCSMA. Others have suggested that oxidative stress may play a role in a number of other neurodegenerative disorders as well.[49,50]

10.6.2 THE ROLE OF ACTIVITY

Motor neuron or motor unit activity may play a role in the pathogenesis of HCSMA. This is based on evidence that motor unit tetanic failure appears first in slow or type-S motor units.[20] In individual experiments, tetanic failure tends to be observed in motor units innervated by slowly conducting motor axons, an attribute of slow motor units (Fig. 10.7A). Among data obtained from seven older homozygotes (age > 120 days) in which six or more MG motor units were studied, tetanic failure was observed among only a few motor units with twitch times-to-peak less than 50 to 55 msec while most units with longer contractions times exhibit failure (Fig. 10.7B). Tetanic failure (tested at 100 Hz.) is also significantly greater for units with twitch times-to-peak of 55 msec or greater (51%) than for units with twitch times less than 55 msec (19%). Other analysis shows that there is no change in slow/fast motor unit proportions associated with the appearance of tetanic failure among MG motor units.[20] Additional evidence for the initial involvement of slow motor units has been obtained from MG muscle fiber type analysis which shows that denervation changes appear first among type I muscle fibers which populate slow motor units.[27,51] It is

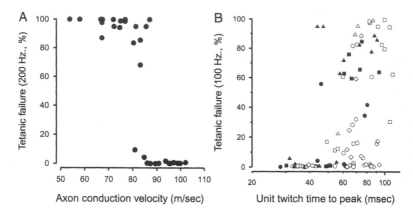

FIGURE 10.7 Motor unit tetanic failure appears first in slow motor units. (A) Plot of MG motor unit tetanic failure at 200 Hz vs. axon conduction velocity for motor units studied in 1 HCSMA homozygote aged 178 days. At this age, evidence of denervation and neuromuscular degeneration has not appeared in the MG muscle.[27] Tetanic failure was quantified as described in Fig. 10.4. Measurement of axonal conduction velocity described in Reference 20. Motor unit failure is present only in motor units innervated by axons with slower conduction velocities. These are slow or type-S motor units. (B) Plot of tetanic failure vs. motor unit twitch contraction time for 7 homozygotes aged 158 to 184 days. Failure occurs primarily among slow motor units possessing twitch contraction times greater than about 50 to 55 msec.

important to emphasize that analysis of more involved, proximal muscles shows that type II muscle fibers (from fast-type motor units) eventually become denervated in HCSMA. Thus, the evidence indicates that slow motor units are initially but not exclusively involved.

The significance of this pattern of motor unit type involvement stems from evidence that shows how motor units are normally used to produce muscle force. Slow motor units are generally recruited first in reflex and voluntary movements,[52] are used to a greater extent in normal movement, and exhibit greater levels of activity than fast units.[53] Our data thus suggest a role for activity in the pathogenesis of HCSMA and indicate that loss of motor unit function and ultimate denervation (caused by motor terminal and intramuscular nerve degeneration) proceed from slow to fast motor units. As slow motor units exhibit greater levels of failure during disease progression, the burden of routine force production must be transferred to fast motor units which are then subjected to greater levels of activity and thus eventually fail as well. It is not known how activity might be injurious to motor neurons, or more specifically, to motor terminals. It is conceivable that normal metabolic byproducts of activity may be processed incorrectly and somehow become toxic. It is of interest that evidence obtained from SOD1 transgenic mice indicates that NMJ degeneration exhibits a different organizational pattern. In these animals, the motor terminals of type-FF motor units appear to degenerate first.[45] Type-FF motor units are generally less active and used under different circumstances than type-S motor units.[53] Thus, motor unit activity may play a different role in the pathogenesis in SOD1 transgenics, and the fundamental mechanisms underlying degeneration may differ between

HCSMA and SOD1 transgenics as well. Further comparisons of neuromuscular structure and function between these models will hopefully yield additional information about the identity of these mechanisms and how they produce similar phenotypes. An important advantage of this approach is that this information can be readily related to human motor neuron disease because of the feasibility of obtaining muscle biopsies.[54]

10.7 SUMMARY

Viewed from the victim's perspective, the central problem in motor neuron disease is weakness. To obtain an effective understanding of the pathogenesis of this disorder, it seems crucial to understand exactly how motor unit function is lost. Our work has shown that in HCSMA loss of motor unit function is due to changes at the NMJ that occur before degeneration or pathological changes such as neurofilament accumulations in axons. In the SOD1 transgenic mouse model of familial ALS, degeneration of NMJs appears well before motor neuron cell death occurs in the spinal cord.[45] These results support the view that loss of motor unit function in motor neuron disease is the result of pathological changes in the periphery that disrupt the function and/or structure of the NMJ. It may be that the mechanisms causing these changes are the same as those underlying subsequent degeneration or motor neuron cell death, so that loss of function can be preempted by inhibiting degeneration or cell death. This view, however, may be too simple since inhibition of motor neuron cell death did not prevent axonal degeneration in the *pmn* model of motor neuron disease.[55,56] Similarly, where loss of motor unit function precedes motor terminal degeneration, as in HCSMA, inhibiting the latter may not be sufficient to prevent loss of function. This situation might be expected if a higher level of cellular differentiation is needed to enable motor unit function than cell survival. These considerations emphasize the need for a better understanding of specific mechanisms that may operate in the motor terminal and axon to cause loss of motor unit function in motor neuron disease.

ACKNOWLEDGMENTS

We thank Drs. R. Balice-Gordon, R. Waldeck and R.E.W. Fyffe for their collaboration on studies of motor unit function and neuromuscular junction and labeled motor neuron morphology, and Ms. Anne Shirley for technical and administrative assistance. The support of the National Institutes of Health is gratefully acknowledged (NS31621, MJP).

REFERENCES

1. Cork, L.C. et al., Hereditary canine spinal muscular atrophy, *J. Neuropath. Exp. Neurol.*, 38, 209, 1979.
2. Lorenz, M.D. et al., Hereditary spinal muscular atrophy in Brittany Spaniels: clinical manifestations. *J. Am. Vet. Med. Assoc.*, 175, 833, 1979.

3. Mitsumoto, H., Chad, D.A., and Pioro, E.P., *Amyotrophic Lateral Sclerosis*, F. A. Davis, Philadelphia, 1998.
4. Cox G.A., Mahaffey, C.L., and Frankel W.N., Identification of the mouse neuromuscular degeneration gene and mapping of a second site suppressor allele, *Neuron*, 21, 1327, 1998.
5. Sharrard, W.J., The distribution of permanent paralysis in the lower limb in poliomyelitis: a clinical and pathological study, *J. Bone Joint Surg.*, 37b, 540, 1955.
6. Dantes, M. and McComas, A., The extent and time course of motoneuron involvement in amyotrophic lateral sclerosis, *Muscle Nerve*, 14, 416, 1991.
7. Brown, M.C., Holland, R.L., and Hopkins, W.G., Motor nerve sprouting, *Ann. Rev. Neurosci.*, 4, 17, 1981.
8. Stalberg, E., Electrophysiological studies of reinnervation in ALS, in *Human Motor Neuron Diseases*, L.P. Rowland, Ed., Raven Press, New York, 1982, 47.
9. Stalberg, E. and Sanders, D.B., Neurophysiological studies in amyotrophic lateral sclerosis, in *Handbook of ALS*, R.A. Smith, Ed., Marcel Dekker, 1992, 209.
10. Mulder, D.W., Lambert, E.H., and Eaton, L.M., Myasthenic syndrome in patients with amyotrophic lateral sclerosis, *Neurology*, 9, 627, 1959.
11. Denys, E.H. and Norris, F.H., Amyotrohic lateral sclerosis: Impairment of neuromuscular transmission, *Arch. Neurol.*, 36, 202, 1979.
12. Bradley, W.G., Recent views on amyotrophic lateral scelerosis with emphasis on electrophysiological studies, *Muscle Nerve*, 10, 490, 1987.
13. Maselli, R.A. et al., Neuromuscular transmission in amyotrophic lateral sclerosis, *Muscle Nerve*, 16, 1193, 1993.
14. Cork, L.C. et al., Hereditary canine spinal muscular atrophy: A canine model of human motor neuron disease, in *Animal Models of Inherited Metabolic Diseases*, Alan Liss, New York, 1982, 449.
15. Sack, G.H. et al., Autosomal dominant inheritance of hereditary canine spinal muscular atrophy, *Ann. Neurol.*, 15, 369, 1984.
16. Blazej, R.G. et al., Hereditary canine spinal muscular atrophy is phenotypically similar but molecularly distinct from human spinal muscular atrophy, *J. Heredity*, 89, 531, 1998.
17. Roy, N. et al., The gene for neuronal apoptosis inhibitory protein is partially deleted in individuals with spinal muscular atrophy, *Cell*, 80, 167, 1995.
18. Cork, L.C. et al., Pathology of motor neurons in accelerated hereditary canine spinal muscular atrophy, *Lab. Invest.*, 46, 89, 1982.
19. Mizutani, T. et al., Development of ophthalmoplegia in amyotrophic lateral sclerosis during long-term use of respirators, *J. Neurol. Sci.*, 99, 311, 1990.
20. Pinter, M.J. et al., Motor unit behavior in canine motor neuron disease, *J. Neurosci.*, 15, 3447, 1995.
21. Molgo, J., Lemeignan, M., and Lechat, P., Effects of 4-aminopyridine at the frog neuromuscular junction, *J. Pharm. Exp. Ther.*, 203, 653, 1977.
22. Argentieri, T.M. et al., Characteristics of synaptic transmission in reinnervating rat skeletal muscle, *Eur. J. Physiol.*, 421, 256, 1992.
23. Pinter, M.J. et al., Effects of 4-aminopyridine on muscle and motor unit force in canine motor neuron disease, *J. Neurosci.*, 17, 4500, 1997.
24. Siklos, L. et al., Ultrastructural evidence for altered calcium in motor nerve terminals in amyotropic lateral sclerosis, *Ann. Neurol.*, 39, 203, 1996.
25. Siklos, L. et al., Calcium-containing endosomes at oculomotor terminals in animal models of ALS, *Neuroreport*, 10, 2539, 1999.

26. Smith, R.G. et al., Altered muscle calcium channel binding kinetics in autoimmune motoneuron disease, *Muscle Nerve*, 18, 620, 1995.

27. Balice-Gordon, R.J. et al., Functional motor unit failure precedes neuromuscular degeneration in canine motor neuron disease, *Ann. Neurol.*, 47, 596, 2000.

28. Dahlstrom, A.B., Czernik, A., and Li, J.-Y., Organelles in fast axonal transport: What molecules do they carry in anterograde vs. retrograde directions, as observed in mammalian systems?, *Mol. Neurobiol.*, 6, 157, 1992.

29. Li, J.-Y. et al., Distribution of Rab3a in rat nervous system: comparison with other synaptic vesicle proteins and neuropeptides, *Brain Res.*, 706, 103, 1996.

30. Cork, L.C. et al., Changes in the size of motor axons in hereditary canine spinal muscular atrophy, *Lab. Invest.*, 61, 333, 1989.

31. Muma, N.A. and Cork, L.C., Alterations in neurofilament mRNA in hereditary canine spinal muscular atrophy, *Lab. Invest.*, 69, 436, 1993.

32. Green, S.L. et al., Alterations in CDK5 protein levels, activity and immunocytochemistry in canine motor neuron disease, *J. Neuropath. Exp. Neurol.*, 57, 1070, 1998.

33. Cork, L.C. et al., Neurofilamentous abnormalities in motor neurons in spontaneously occurring animal disorders, *J. Neuropath. Exp. Neurol.*, 47, 420, 1988.

34. Hirano, A., Cytopathology of amyotrophic lateral sclerosis in *Advances in Neurology, Amyotrophic Lateral Sclerosis and Other Motor Neuron Diseases*, L.P. Rowland, Ed., Raven Press, New York, 1991, 91.

35. Cleveland, D.W., From Charcot to SOD1: mechanisms of selective motor neuron death in ALS, *Neuron*, 24, 515, 1999.

36. Lee, M.K. and Cleveland, D.W., Neurofilament function and dysfunction: involvement in axonal growth and neuronal disease, *Curr. Opin. Cell Biol.*, 6, 34, 1994.

37. Williamson, T.L. et al., Neurofilaments, radial growth of axons and mechanisms of motorneuron disease, *Cold Spring Symp. Quant. Biol.*, 61, 709, 1996.

38. Moore, J.W. et al., Simulations of conduction in uniform myelinated fibers, *Biophys. J.*, 21, 1978.

39. Waxman, S., Determinants of conduction velocity in myelinated nerve fibers, *Muscle Nerve*, 3, 141, 1980.

40. Hoffman, P.N., Griffin, J.W., and Price D.L., Control of axonal caliber by neurofilament transport, *J. Cell. Biol.*, 99, 705, 1984.

41. Hoffman, P.N. et al., Neuorfilament gene expression: A major determinant of axonal caliber, *Proc. Natl. Acad. Sci., USA*, 84, 3472, 1987.

42. Hoffman, P.N. et al., Changes in neurofilament transport coincide temporarily with alterations in the caliber of axons in regenerating motor fibers, *J. Cell Biol.*, 101, 1332, 1985.

43. deWaegh, S.M., Lee, V.M., and Brady S., Local modulation of neurofilament phosphorylation, axonal caliber, and slow axonal transport by myelinating Schwann cells, *Cell*, 68, 451, 1992.

44. Hsieh, S.-T. et al., Regional modulation of neurofilament organization by myelination in normal axons. *J. Neurosci.*, 14, 6392, 1994.

45. Frey, D. et al., Early and selective loss of neuromuscular synapse subtypes with low sprouting competence in motoneuron diseases, *J. Neurosci.*, 20, 2534, 2000.

46. Stalberg, E. and Thiele B., Transmission block in terminal nerve twigs: A single fiber electromyographic finding in man, *J. Neurol. Neurosurg. Psych.*, 35, 52, 1972.

47. Daube, J.R. and Mulder, D.W., Prognostic features in ALS, *Muscle Nerve*, 5, S107, 1982.

48. Green, S.L. et al., Canine motor neuron disease: Clinicopathologic features and selected indicators of oxidative stress, *J. Vet. Int. Med.*, 15, 17, 2001.

49. Tatton, W.G. and Olanow, C.W., Apoptosis in neurodegenerative diseases: the role of mitochondria, *Biochim. Biophys. Acta*, 1410, 195, 1999.

50. Beal M.F., Energetics in the pathogenesis of neurodegenerative diseases, *Trends Neurosci.*, 23, 298, 2000.

51. Burke, R.E., Motor units: anatomy, physiology and functional organization, in *Handbook of Physiology*, V.B. Brooks, Ed., Am. Physiol. Soc., Bethesda, MD, 1981, 345.

52. Cope, T. and Pinter, M.J., The size principle: Still working after all these years?, *News Physiol. Sci.*, 10, 280, 1995.

53. Henning, R. and Lomo, T., Firing patterns of motor units in normal rats, *Nature*, 314, 164, 1985.

54. Maselli, R.A. et al., Anconeus muscle: A human muscle preparation suitable for *in vitro* microelectrode studies, *Muscle Nerve*, 14, 1189, 1991.

55. Sagot, Y. et al., Bcl-2 overexpression prevents motoneuron cell body loss but not axonal degeneration in a mouse model of a neurodegenerative disease, *J. Neurosci.*, 15, 7727, 1995.

56. Sagot, Y. et al., GDNF slows loss of motoneurons but not axonal degeneration or premature death of *pmn/pmn* mice, *J. Neurosci.*, 16, 2335, 1996.

57. Kimura, J., *Electrodiagnosis in Diseases of Nerve and Muscle: Principles and Practice*, F.A. Davis, Philadelphia, 1989.

11 Structural Plasticity of Motoneuron Dendrites Caused by Axotomy

P. Kenneth Rose, Victoria MacDermid, and Monica Neuber-Hess

CONTENTS

11.1 NEURONAL POLARITY

Most neurons have two distinct compartments. As described almost 100 years ago by Ramón Y Cajal,[1] the dendritic domain is composed of relatively short branches that gradually taper and form acute angles between sibling branches. In contrast, processes belonging to the axonal compartment travel for long distances with little tapering and branches usually occur at right angles. Ultrastructurally, the most conspicuous difference is visible at synapses where dendrites are most commonly postsynaptic to presynaptic axonal specializations.[2] These structural differences are matched by an equally distinctive set of molecular characteristics.[3] This morphological and molecular polarity is related to a functional polarity where, with a few notable exceptions, dendrites integrate synaptic signals and axons transmit action potentials that trigger the release of neurotransmitters.[4] Thus, the concept of neuronal polarity as a means of emphasizing the unique features of dendrites and axons, whether at a structural, molecular, or functional level, has become a fundamental principle of cellular neuroscience. The intricately orchestrated steps leading to the formation of axons and dendrites in the developing nervous system[3,5] and the numerous mechanisms that are involved in maintaining neuronal polarity[6,7] have reinforced the importance attached to this integral property of neurons.

Implicit in most descriptions of the polarity of adult neurons is the assumption that it is static. This assumption is questionable. The results of recent experiments suggest that the structural and molecular polarity of adult neurons can be disrupted following long-term axotomy. This plasticity has important consequences for understanding the capacity of the nervous system to recovery from neurotrauma. Much of the evidence in support of a reorganization of neuronal polarity in the adult nervous system is based on studies of permanently axotomized spinal motoneurons. The goal of this chapter is to review and critically evaluate this evidence.

11.2 EARLY STUDIES: STEPS IN THE WRONG DIRECTION?

11.2.1 DENDRITIC TREE SHRINKAGE: THEN

The first descriptions of the effect of axotomy on motoneuron structure provided no evidence for alterations in their polarity. These studies, however, demonstrated that dendritic structure of adult motoneurons was not fixed.

In what would become a landmark paper, Sumner and Watson[8] reported that axotomy leads to a reduction in the size of the dendritic tree of hypoglossal motoneurons. Dendrites of these motoneurons also retracted following intramuscular injection of botulinum toxin, indicating that dendritic loss is partly a consequence of a failure of neuromuscular transmission and not axonal damage alone. The retraction was reversible upon reinnervation or upon regaining functional transmission several weeks after the botulinum toxin injection. The results of the axotomy experiments were subsequently replicated in spinal motoneurons.[9] However, both of these studies suffered from a serious methodological flaw. At the time of these studies, the full extent of the dendritic trees of motoneurons was not fully appreciated. It was standard practice to describe motoneuron dendrites based on Golgistained dendritic branches contained in a single histological section. Based on the results of studies employing serial reconstructions of the dendritic trees of intracellularly stained motoneurons, it is now apparent that this practice will exclude most distal branches due to the complex three-dimensional distribution of the dendritic trees of motoneurons.[10–14] As an example of the seriousness of this problem, Standler and Bernstein[9] reported an average total length of 1.14 mm for dendrites belonging to rat spinal motoneurons that were captured on a single, 200-μm thick section. In contrast, the average total length of intracellularly stained and reconstructed dendritic trees of rat spinal motoneurons is 35.7 mm,[13] a 30-fold difference! Thus, the retraction of dendrites following axotomy, reported by Sumner and Watson,[8] may be an artifact of the techniques used to measure dendritic tree size.

11.2.2 Dendritic Tree Shrinkage: Now

In 1992, Brännström and colleagues[15,16] re-examined the issue of dendritic shrinkage following axotomy of spinal motoneurons. This study avoided the short-comings of the earlier investigations. All motoneurons were identified physiologically and measurements were based on detailed reconstructions of intracellularly stained cells. These measurements provided unequivocal evidence that a permanent axotomy of 12-weeks duration causes shrinkage of the dendritic trees of hindlimb motoneurons in the adult cat. The shrinkage was evident in measurements of total dendritic length, total surface area, and total number of dendritic branches (Fig. 11.1). Cable theory predicts that neuronal input resistance is inversely related to the size of the dendritic trees.[17] Thus, the numerous electrophysiological reports of an increase in the input resistance of motoneurons following axotomy[18–21] were consistent with the morphological results and provided a firm basis for the wide consensus that axotomy of motoneurons leads to a decrease in the size of their dendritic trees.

11.2.3 Axotomy and Loss of Synaptic Integration

Dendritic retraction appears to be part of a larger, well-organized strategy to reduce the integrative capacity of axotomized motoneurons. Other changes that led to the same result include loss of synapses,[18–29] reduction in choline acetyltransferase,[30] and down regulation of neurotransmitter receptors.[31–34] Even the outputs of the motoneuron are not immune to this transformation. Many of the axon collaterals that form the basis for recurrent inhibition are lost following axotomy,[35] leaving the motoneuron deprived of both inputs and outputs. Thus, the prevailing view of axotomy-induced changes in motoneuron dendritic structure emphasizes degenerative events and provides little basis for claims that one of the principal outcomes of axotomy of spinal motoneurons is a change in their polarity. What has happened to change this view?

11.3 STEPS IN A DIFFERENT DIRECTION

11.3.1 Exceptions to the Rule: Dendritic Growth
and Dendraxons

As described above, the remodeling of motoneuron dendritic structure following axotomy is most consistent with a degenerative process. However, some morphological changes appear to contradict this conclusion. As described by Brännström et al.[15] and shown in Fig. 11.2A, a small number (2 of 234) distal dendrites from

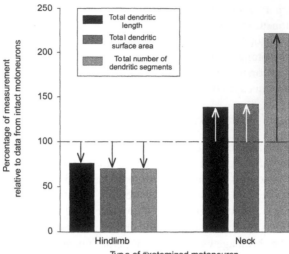

FIGURE 11.1 Comparison of the change in dendritic tree size of hindlimb and neck motoneurons following permanent axotomy. Three indices of dendritic tree size are illustrated: total dendritic length (the sum of the lengths of all dendritic segments for a single motoneuron); total surface area (the sum of the surface areas of all dendritic segments for a single motoneuron); and the total number of dendritic segments per motoneuron. The total number of dendritic segments was not reported. This number was calculated based on their values of the number of stem dendrites per motoneuron and the number of terminal dendrites per stem dendrites, where the number of all dendritic segments per stem dendrite equals the number of terminal dendrites + 1. (Data for axotomized neck motoneurons from Rose and Odlozinski, *J. Comp. Neurol.*, 390, 392, 1998.) As indicated by the direction of the arrows, axotomy caused a decrease in the size of the dendritic trees of hindlimb motoneurons. In contrast, the dendritic trees of neck motoneurons expanded. (Data for total dendritic length and surface area for axotomized hindlimb motoneurons are based on the study of Brännström et al.[15] *J. Comp. Neurol.*, 318, 439, 1992.)

axotomized motoneurons exhibited signs of expansion, instead of retraction. The putative expansion appeared in two forms: a tangle of short preterminal and terminal dendritic segments or a long, meandering, usually thick process that ended simply, with no branches. The meandering trajectory is peculiar because this feature is a hallmark of axons, not dendrites. Moreover, the swelling found at terminations of last-order processes were, as described by Brännström et al.,[15] typical of boutons on axon collaterals. The similarity between these expanding dendrites and axons proved to be only light-microscopically "deep". Electron microscopic observations revealed typical dendritic features, such as synaptic contacts, although contacts were rare on one branch and dense collections of mitochondria were unusually frequent.[15]

In the studies of Brännström et al.,[15] the axon of the motoneuron was transected close to muscle, a distance of approximately 15 to 20 cm from the soma. Cutting motoneuron axons much closer to the soma led to a different result. In a brief report that was subsequently followed by a more detailed description, Lindå, Risling, and Cullheim[36,37] described the structural consequences of a parasaggital incision through

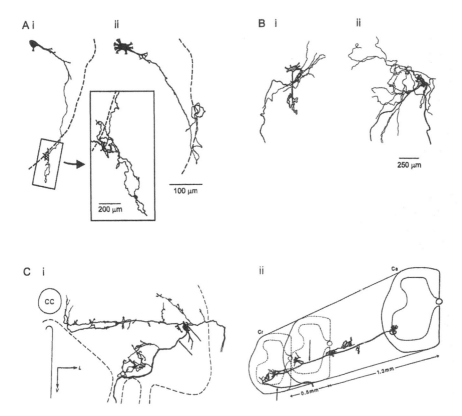

FIGURE 11.2 (A) Unusual distal dendrites of axotomized hindlimb motoneurons. The distal dendrite in (i) gave rise to a complex arbor composed of numerous interwoven and sinuous branches. An expanded view is shown in the inset. The distal dendrite in (ii) did not branch and, unlike dendrites of intact motoneurons, followed a long and meandering path. (From Brännström, T., Havton, L., and Kellereth, J.-O., *J. Comp. Neurol.*, 316, 1, 1992. With permission.) (B) Two examples of dendraxons. These axon-like processes (indicated by thick lines) arose from dendrites of intraspinally axotomized hindlimb motoneurons and projected toward the ventral roots. Only the portion of the dendritic tree that gave rise to the dendraxons is shown. (From Lindå, H., Risling, M., and Cullheim, S., *Brain Res.*, 358, 329, 1985. With permission of Elsevier.) (C) Supernumary axons. The supernumary axon in (i) (double arrow) projected dorsally and medially. Like axon collaterals of the original axon (single arrow), the branches from the supernumary axon, formed numerous *en passant* and terminal boutons. The supernumary axon in (ii) traveled rostrally in the lateral funiculus, for a distance of more than 1 mm. The branches in the gray matter were thick and contorted. (From Havton, L. and Kellerth, J.-O., *Nature*, 325, 711, 1987. With permission.) CC, central canal; L, lateral; V, ventral; Cr, cranial; Ca, caudal.

the lateral and ventral funiculi of L7. This injury transected motoneuron axons 400 to 1400 μm from their somata. Unlike dendrites of distally axotomized motoneurons, where the vast majority of dendrites have a morphology typical of dendrites of motoneurons with intact axons, many distal dendrites of intraspinally axotomized motoneurons were aberrant. The most distinctive feature of these odd dendrites was their unusually large diameter. Typically, the diameter of motoneuron dendrites becomes thinner as they project distally, due to tapering and branching.[13,38–43] The aberrant distal dendrites on proximally axotomized motoneurons either did not taper or they become progressively thicker. Although not examined systematically, some dendrites projected well beyond the usual soma-to-terminal distances of motoneu-rons with intact axons. But the most surprising finding was the presence of myelin surrounding the distal regions of most unusually thick distal dendrites. A small number (n = 3) of these unusual dendrites followed a path that was directed toward the ventral roots (Fig. 11.2B). Since this trajectory mimicked the route taken by axons of intact motoneurons, Lindå, Risling, and Cullheim[36] coined the term "den-draxon" to describe the combination of axon-like and dendritic features of these processes. The trajectory of the dendraxons also suggested that scar tissue caused by the lesion or damage to ventolaterally projecting dendrites might be critical factors in the formation of these processes. However, many unusually thick and distally myelinated dendrites were also found in the gray matter, outside the scar tissue formed by the lesion.[37] Hence, it seems unlikely that scar tissue or damage to the dendritic tree is the primary factor leading to the increase in diameter and myelination.

The aberrant distal dendrites and dendraxons described by Lindå, Risling, and Cullheim[36,37] fulfilled two key criteria for axons. They did not taper and they were myelinated.[2] Thus, the data reported by Lindå, Risling, and Cullheim[36,37] provided the first clues that motoneuron polarity is plastic and can be altered by axotomy. The evidence, however, is not definitive. Distinguishing dendrites from axons based on the presence or absence of tapering may not be warranted if the dendrite is growing. Furthermore, dendrites of some neurons are normally myelinated[43] and, following injury to the dorsal roots, astrocytes are also myelinated.[44] The causal link with axotomy is also questionable. Sectioning the ventral and lateral funiculi will not only axotomize nearby motoneurons, it will also cause a massive deafferention and a persistent disruption of the blood-brain barrier.[45] Either of these events may also contribute to restructuring of the dendritic tree.

11.3.2 SUPERNUMARY AXONS

Although the majority of studies of axotomized motoneurons have been directed to either structural or functional studies of the dendritic tree, changes in axonal structure have not been completely ignored. From the perspective of neuronal polarity and its static or dynamic state, a change in axonal structure that shifts the axon to a phenotype more consistent with dendritic structure would be equal to remodeling in the reverse direction. Observations supporting this type of remodeling have not been reported. However, in 1987, Havton and Kellerth[46] described a transformation of the axonal structure of axotomized motoneurons that has equally important consequences for our understanding of the regulation of neuronal polarity. The form of this reorganization did not alter the polarity of the motoneuron in the strictest sense, but it demonstrated that a generally accepted corollary of polarity, one neu-ron/one axon, is not a rigid feature of the polar organization of motoneurons. Figure 11.2C shows reconstructions of the axonal arborizations of two motoneurons whose axons were sectioned distally. Unlike all motoneurons with intact axons, each of these cells had two axons! One axon from each cell, the original (indicated by single arrows), projected ventrally and gave rise to three or four axon collaterals. The other axon (indicated by double arrows) followed a rostral or caudal trajectory. This second axon gave rise to two types of arborizations. One closely resembled typical axon collaterals: fine diameter branches studded with numerous swellings. The distribution of these swellings was usually outside the zone occupied by boutons of axon collaterals from the original axon. At an ultrastructural level, the swellings contacted neuronal profiles and formed synaptic specialization, but unlike boutons of axon collaterals from motoneurons with intact axons, these boutons only contained dense core vesicles. The other type of arborization had fewer branches, which were thick, formed tangles and had few swellings. Havton and Kellerth[46] used the term "supernumerary" to describe the new axon to emphasize that this axon was *in addition* to the normal complement of one axon/motoneuron.

11.4 WHERE ARE WE?

At this stage in the review, it is useful to retrace our steps and evaluate what progress, if any, has been made toward validation of the claim that axotomy of motoneurons leads to a reorganization of neuronal polarity. To a large extent, support in favor of this claim is dismally weak. The majority of changes that occur in motoneurons post-axotomy have little relationship to neuronal polarity. The few changes that might be associated with a disruption of neuronal polarity are open to other interpretations and may not be causally linked to axotomy. Nevertheless, the morphological studies of Brännström et al.,[15] Lindå et al.[36,37] and Havton and Kellerth[46] proved to be prescient in light of subsequent studies that provided less ambiguous data in favor of the polarity transformation claim.

11.5 A FRESH START: STEPS IN THE RIGHT DIRECTION?

11.5.1 Dendritic Tree Expansion

A principal component of the argument in favor of a link between axotomy and a general regression of motoneuron dendritic function is the consistent demonstration that axotomy causes dendritic shrinkage.[8,9,15,16,37,47] Hence, the results reported by Rose and Odlozinski[48] precipitated a shift in the balance of evidence toward an alternative interpretation of the impact of axotomy on motoneuron dendritic structure and function. Based on detailed reconstructions of the entire dendritic trees of five axotomized motoneurons and eight motoneurons with intact axons, they concluded that axotomy caused an *expansion* of the dendritic tree. Two of the motoneurons that formed the basis for this conclusion are shown in Fig. 11.3. The motoneuron with an intact axon (Fig. 11.3A) had a total dendritic length of 76.3 mm, a total dendritic surface area of 456,000 μm^2, and 231 dendritic branches. These values were similar to the average total dendritic length, 75.2 mm; average total dendritic surface area, 423,000 μm^2 (n = 3); and average number of dendritic branches, 227. In contrast, the axotomized motoneuron shown in Fig. 11.3B had a total dendritic length of 128.6 mm, a total dendritic surface area of 677,200 μm^2, and 721 dendritic

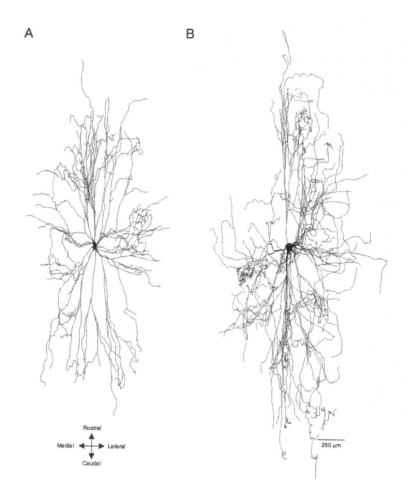

FIGURE 11.3 Drawings of the dendritic trees of intact (A) and axotomized (B) neck motoneurons. Both dendritic trees are shown in the horizontal plane and were drawn, using a computer-assisted reconstruction system, by following each dendrite through serial histological sections. The process ensured that all dendrites were followed to their terminations.

branches. On average, total dendritic length, total dendritic surface, and number of dendritic branches increased 34, 38, and 215%, respectively.

Comparisons of dendritic tree size based on reconstructions of complete dendritic trees suffer from a major drawback. The number of cells studied will inevitably be small because of the time-consuming nature of the reconstruction process. Thus, the representative nature of the sample is questionable. Rose and Odlozinski,[48] therefore, supplemented this analysis with estimates of dendritic tree size based on the correlation between proximal branch diameter and subtree size.[15,38–42,49] This approach was identical to that used by Brännström et al.[15] and provided a means of estimating the total dendritic tree size of a larger number of cells. The results of this

A   B

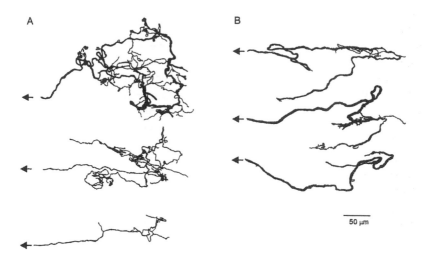

50 μm

FIGURE 11.4 Unusual distal dendrites of axotomized neck motoneurons. These dendrites either formed complex, tangled arborizations (A) or, like axons, did not taper and followed a long tortuous path with few side branches (B). (From Rose, P.K. and Odlozinski, M., *J. Comp. Neurol.*, 390, 392, 1998. With permission.)

analysis are summarized and compared to the data reported by Brännström et al.[15] in Fig. 11.1. Whereas Brännström et al.[15] described a reduction in all measures of dendritic tree size, Rose and Odlozinski[48] found an increase in the same parameters. Moreover, the increases were not trivial; total dendritic length increased 38%, total dendritic surface area increased 42.5%, and the number of dendritic branches rose by 122%. The explanation for these large differences is not immediately apparent. The methods used to measure dendritic tree size and the time frame of the axotomy were identical in each set of experiments. However, some aspects of the experiments were different. The experiments by Rose and Odlozinski[48] were conducted on dorsal neck motoneurons. Brännström et al.[15] examined hindlimb motoneurons. By virtue of the relative proximity of neck muscles to the spinal cord, the selection of neck motoneurons leads to a more proximal axotomy, approximately 15 to 25 mm from the soma, compared to a distance of 150 to 200 mm for the hindlimb motoneurons. Thus, at least two factors, motoneuron type and the proximity of the axotomy to the soma, may have contributed to the different results reported by Brännström et al.[15] and Rose and Odlozinski.[48]

11.5.2 UNUSUAL DISTAL DENDRITES

11.5.2.1 Light Microscopic Characteristics

By itself, expansion of the dendritic tree provides no support for the claim that axotomy of motoneurons leads to a remodeling of their polarity. However, the structural changes leading to the increase in the size of axotomized neck motoneuron dendrites are relevant. The distal dendrites of these cells displayed two unusual features. Some, as shown in Fig. 11.4A, divided to form complex arborizations.

These distal dendritic arborizations had a tangled appearance due to the close proximity and twisting paths followed by the short branches forming the arborization. Web-like expansions and irregular varicosities were common. In contrast, other distal branches did not taper and had unusually large diameters, 3 to 4 μm, instead of 1 to 2 μm.[40] Examples of these branches are shown in Fig. 11.4B. These branches usually followed a meandering path, often reversing directions several times. Some entered the lateral or ventral funiculi where they turned to follow a rostral or caudal trajectory. Branches from these unusually large diameter processes were not common. When present, they were usually short and ended with no obvious specialization or an irregularly shaped appendage. If intracellularly injected with horseradish peroxidase, distal branches with an unusually large diameter were stained in a nonuniform pattern where lengths of darkly stained processes were separated by zones that were either pale or barely visible.

The unusual features of the distal dendrites of axotomized neck motoneurons are reminiscent of distal processes seen on distally and proximally axotomized hindlimb motoneurons. The complex tangled arborizations that are a feature of many distal dendrites of axotomized neck motoneurons are very similar to one of the two unusual distal dendrites described by Brännström et al.[15] in their study of axotomized hindlimb motoneurons. Rose and Odlozinski[48] suggested that these distal dendritic arborizations were indicative of dendritic growth. This conclusion was based on their similarity to some distal dendrites of motoneurons in young cats and rats.[13,50] Moreover, Brännström et al.[15] reported that the tangled distal arborization found on an axotomized limb motoneuron possessed features such as appositions with axon terminals that are consistent with a dendritic phenotype. Hence, this structural alteration provides no support for a change in neuronal polarity following axotomy. In contrast, the unusually thick, highly tortuous, distal branches have three features that are uncharacteristic of dendrites, but are typical of axons: They do not taper; they follow a meandering path; and their non-uniform staining pattern is identical to that seen in myelinated axons after intracellular injections of horseradish peroxidase.[48,51] Presumably, myelin acts to impede the penetration of the reagents used to visualize the intracellularly injected horseradish peroxidase. This interpretation is consistent with the short, darkly stained segments observed in myelinated axons. These likely represent the locations of nodes of Ranvier. Havton and Kellerth[46] also found faintly stained regions along motoneuron axons at the electron microscopic level. These regions were myelinated. Based on these characteristics, Rose and Odlozinski[48] suggested that unusually thick, meandering, and intermittently stained, distal processes from axotomized neck motoneurons were axon-like. This suggestion, however, must be treated cautiously in the absence of ultrastructural confirmation. Nevertheless, the axon-like characteristics of these unusual distal processes may indicate that disruption of the blood-brain barrier and massive deafferentation, features of intraspinally axotomized motoneurons,[36-37] are not prerequisites for the myelination of motoneuron dendrites. Instead, axotomy alone may be sufficient.

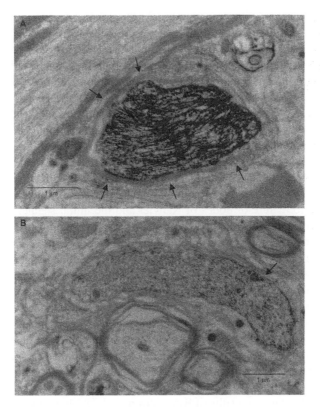

FIGURE 11.5 Electron micrographs of distal processes from the dendritic tree of an axotomized neck motoneuron. This motoneuron was intracellularly stained with horseradish peroxidase to permit visualization of the processes at both the light and electron microscopic
levels. (A) A myelinated process. The myelin (indicated by the arrows) forms a dark band
around most of the circumference of the process. (B) An unmyelinated process. This segment was less intensely stained and permitted a clearer image of the ultrastructure of the
cytoplasm. The reaction product formed by the horseradish peroxidase binds to a dense
network of neurofilaments. In comparison, the neurofilaments in the unstained myelinated axon,
located just below the intracellularly stained process, are faint. In both processes the neurofilaments are uniformly distributed throughout the cytoplasm. At this magnification, microtubules,
the primary cytoskeletal element in dendrites, would appear as thick, tubular structures. The
process from the axotomized motoneuron also contained a dense core vesicle (arrow).

11.5.2.2 Electron Microscopic Characteristics

Confirmation that distal, axon-like processes that emerged from the distal dendrites
of axotomized neck motoneurons are myelinated was provided by Rose and Neuber-
Hess.[52] As shown in Fig. 11.5A, the myelin surrounding the unusually thick and
meandering distal processes was usually thin, 4 to 6 layers, but occasionally reached a
thickness of 20 to 24 layers. As described previously, the presence of myelin, by itself,
is not sufficient to unambiguously distinguish axons from dendrites.[43-44] However, these
processes also contained dense collections of neurofilaments (Fig. 11.5B), which are

the primary cytoskeletal elements of axons.[2] Although the density of neurofilaments appeared to be unusually high, their presence, together with the very low incidence of microtubules, the major cytoskeletal component of dendrites,[2] provides a firm basis for suggesting that axon-like (as defined by their light-microscopic appearance) processes emerging from the distal dendrites of axotomized neck motoneurons are bona fide axons. Two other ultrastructural features of these processes support this suggestion. Small pleomorphic and large, dense core vesicles (Fig. 11.5B) were scattered throughout the cytoplasm and an electron-dense undercoating was occasionally found along the membrane of unmyelinated segments. Small pleomorphic and large, dense core vesicles have only been described in axons and may play a crucial role in the transport of molecules involved in the formation of presynaptic specializations.[53] A dense undercoating along the cytoplasmic side of the membrane is a characteristic feature of nodes of Ranvier and the initial segment of the axon.[2]

The ultrastructural features of axon-like processes arising from distal dendrites of axotomized neck motoneurons provide the best evidence thus far that the polarity of axotomized motoneurons can be rearranged. However, due to the time-consuming nature of correlative light and electron microscopic studies, the axon-like features described above were derived from a study of only two motoneurons. The generality of the observations is, therefore, in doubt. Moreover, a preliminary examination of the ultrastructure of the complex distal arborizations of axotomized neck motoneurons (P.K. Rose, M. Neuber-Hess, and K. Gerrow, unpublished observations) indicates that ultrastructural changes can be complex and not always helpful in addressing questions related to neuronal polarity; for example, the irregular swellings that were a common feature of distal dendritic arborizations did not receive synaptic contacts (in contrast to the results of Brännström et al.[15]). Their cytoplasm contained numerous large, clear, irregularly shaped vesicles and occasional dense-core vesicles. These features are characteristic of regenerating axon terminals in the adult animal.[54] This interpretation is confounded by the presence of dense aggregates of mitochondria. This property is a distinctive feature of dendritic growth cones.[55,56]

11.5.2.3 Molecular Characteristics

Partly as a consequence of the limitations of ultrastructural studies, MacDermid and colleagues[57–59] have re-examined the question of the polarity of axotomized neck motoneurons using a different strategy. This strategy takes advantage of well-known differences in the molecular constituents of axons and dendrites that can be detected at the light microscopic level. Microtubule-associated protein 2a/b (MAP2a/b) is a cytoskeletal protein found only in the somato-dendritic domain of mature neurons.[60] In neck motoneurons with intact axons, immunoreactivity for MAP2a/b extended throughout the dendritic tree and into the most distal dendrites (Color Figure 5B*). In contrast, MAP2a/b immunoreactivity was undetectable in axon-like processes and distal dendritic arborizations (Color Figure 5A). Some distal regions of last-order dendrites with no obvious structural abnormality also lacked MAP2a/b immunoreactivity. The distribution of MAP2a/b in proximal dendrites was not altered by axotomy. These

---

* Color figures follow page 142.

results complement the ultrastructural studies of the axon-like processes. However, the absence of MAP2a/b in complex distal arborizations and the occasional normal last-order process was unexpected, since Rose and Odlozinski[48] had concluded that complex distal arborizations were indicative of dendritic, not axonal, growth. Furthermore, in the studies by Rose and Odlozinski[48] there was little evidence that growth of any kind occurred in dendrites without an obvious abnormality. Once again, there are reasonable grounds to question data used to support claims of a change in the polarity of axotomized motoneurons.

The nature of the MAP2a/b experiments places a strong emphasis on regions that do not contain MAP2a/b. To address concerns related to the interpretation of negative data, MacDermid et al.[57–59] also compared the distribution of growth-associated protein-43 (GAP-43) in intact and axotomized neck motoneurons. In contrast to MAP2a/b, GAP-43 is almost exclusively restricted to the axonal domain of intact neurons in the adult central nervous system.[61] Following axonal injury, GAP-43 expression is upregulated in many neurons and is distributed in axons and somata, but not dendrites.[61] No immunoreactivity for GAP-43 was detected in neck motoneurons with intact axons. This was not true for axotomized neck motoneurons. GAP-43 was found in unusual distal processes that corresponded to axon-like processes (Color Figure 5C) and distal dendritic arborizations. GAP-43 was also located in the somata, the axon, and in some distal processes that appeared structurally normal. Thus, within the dendritic tree, the regions that contain GAP-43, a marker for axons, correspond precisely to the zones that failed to stain using an antibody for MAP2a/b, a marker for dendrites. This distribution provides strong support for the conclusion that axon-like processes, complex distal arborizations, as well as some structurally normal distal processes that arise from the distal dendrites of axotomized neck motoneurons, are indistinguishable from axons.

11.6 HAVE WE ARRIVED AT OUR DESTINATION?

11.6.1 A NEW PERSPECTIVE

At the beginning of this chapter, the concept of neuronal polarity was introduced as one of the cornerstones of cellular neuroscience. From a functional perspective, the separation of input and output by means of dendrites and axons is central to much of our understanding of how the nervous system integrates and relays information in a meaningful fashion. To propose that this fundamental property of neurons is not fixed verges on the absurd. It is for this reason that observations seeming to support this proposal were treated with intense scrutiny. Wherever possible, alternative explanations were found or the data were rejected due to perceived shortcomings. Despite this strategy, the evidence in favor of a reorganization of neuronal polarity following axotomy of adult motoneurons has grown to the point where this claim can no longer be casually dismissed. On its own, each piece of evidence is insufficient to draw a firm conclusion. However, when combined, the evidence indicates that some distal processes emerging from distal dendrites of axotomized motoneurons have the following characteristics: they do not taper; their trajectories are tortuous; they are myelinated; their cytoplasm contains neurofilaments and dense core vesicles; they stain positively to GAP-43, but MAP2a/b is undetectable. All of these characteristics are typical of axons.

11.6.2 FUTURE STEPS

At this stage, the obvious question is whether there are sufficient data to conclude unequivocally that the processes emerging from the distal dendrites of axotomized motoneurons are true axons. The answer to this question must be a qualified "maybe". There are too many outstanding issues to allow a more definitive answer. Foremost among these is whether axon-like processes give rise to functional synapses. Havton and Kellerth[46] demonstrated that supernumary axons formed presynaptic specializations with many of the hallmarks of a functional synapse. Equivalent data for axon-like processes at the distal ends of dendrites are lacking.

It is equally critical to determine if this response to axotomy is generic, especially since much of data marshaled in favor of the claim of a disrupted polarity have been derived from studies of one, perhaps unique, population of motoneurons. On this issue, there are several reasons to suggest that dorsal neck motoneurons are not alone in their ability to generate axon-like processes from distal dendrites following axotomy. Axotomized facial motoneurons develop unusual distal processes identical to those described by Rose and Odlozinski[48] in axotomized dorsal neck motoneurons.[62] Moreover, Havton (personal communication) has found similar distal appendages in lumbosacral motoneurons following a ventral root rhizotomy. There is also evidence that this structural rearrangement is not confined to motoneurons. In a seminal series of experiments, Hall and colleagues[63,64] described several post-axotomy changes in reticulospinal neurons of the giant lamprey, *Petromyzon marinus*. The distal dendrites of these neurons formed sprouts that followed tortuous pathways, formed presynaptic specializations, and contained numerous neurofilaments and few microtubules. In keeping with these morphological characteristics, the sprouts are immunoreactive for phosphorylated neurofilaments, another feature of axons.[65] Thus, the formation of axon-like processes from distal dendrites may be a general response to axotomy.

A key factor in this response appears to be the proximity of the axotomy to the soma, the more proximal the axotomy, the greater the incidence of axon-like processes.[48,63,65] This association has recently been tested directly in axotomized trapezius motoneurons (P. K. Rose, V. MacDermid, J. Mountjoy, C. Ryerson, and M. Neuber-Hess, unpublished observations). Sectioning the spinal accessory nerve at the junction of C1 and the medulla caused a profuse generation of axon-like processes in trapezius motoneurons located within 25 mm of the transection. In contrast, trapezius motoneurons more than 40 mm from the axotomy had few axon-like processes.

This chapter has emphasized the structural and molecular properties of axon-like processes that emerge from the distal dendrites of axotomized motoneurons. This focus reflects the paucity of data describing their functional characteristics; for example, it is not known if these processes initiate and conduct action potentials. Eccles and colleagues[66] described small, all-or-none, transient depolarizations in axotomized motoneurons that were superimposed on EPSPs in response to stimulation of muscle afferents. These observations were confirmed by Kuno and Llinás.[67] At the time of the studies, these partial spike-like responses were attributed to unusually excitable dendrites.[66–69] However, in light of the structural and molecular data described above, the partial spike-like responses may be a consequence of the generation of action potentials in axon-like processes arising from distal dendrites. Action potentials generated at these distal sites would be expected to be greatly attenuated en route to the soma by the intervening, relatively inexcitable, dendritic membrane. Although there is no direct evidence in support of this proposal, it is known that small, spike-like depolarizations in axotomized motoneurons can be eliminated by intracellular injections of QX-314, a blocker of voltage-dependent sodium channels.[70] Furthermore, the proximity of the axotomy to the soma appears to be a critical factor in determining the incidence of partial spikes. In all of the above experiments, the motoneurons were axotomized extradurally at the level of the dorsal root ganglion, in relatively close proximity to the soma. In contrast, partial spikes are absent in distally axotomized motoneurons. [20,21,71,72] Therefore, both partial spikes and axon-like processes are specific consequences of a proximal axotomy. However, this correlation must be tested further by determining the relationship between partial spikes and axon-like processes in the same cell. In addition, it must be shown that the partial spikes originate only from axon-like processes, since dendritic membranes of many neurons possess voltage-dependent sodium channels[73] and dendrites of motoneurons in organotypic spinal cord slice cultures can partially support back propagating action potentials.[74]

There is also a critical need to determine the mechanisms responsible for the formation of axon-like processes following axotomy. These processes have the potential to act as replacements for injured axons and may provide a new means of facilitating functional recovery following traumatic brain injuries. It is equally possible that axon-like processes, if they form synapses, may make inappropriate connections that would be counter-productive to recovery from injury. Based on the temporal sequence of changes in the cytoskeletal contents of proximally axotomized reticulospinal neurons in the lamprey, Hall et al.[65] have proposed that destabilization of microtubules followed by the transport of phosphorylated, high molecular weight neurofilaments is the first step toward the formation of axon-like processes from distal dendrites. This proposal emphasizes the important role that microtubules play in the maintenance of neuronal polarity and is consistent with the models of dendritic differentiation based on the orientation of microtubules.[75,76] However, the study by Hall et al.[65] represents the only attempt thus far to address questions related to mechanism. Further studies will be guided by a growing knowledge of the molecular events responsible for the generation and maintenance of neuronal polarity in general,[5–7,77] and the important roles played by extrinsic factors, such as neurotrophic factors, that promote or impede axonal regeneration.[78–80] Additional insights will be provided by specific features of the axon-like processes that emerge from distal dendrites of axotomized motoneurons; for example, all of the structural and molecular changes associated with the rearrangement of the polarity of axotomized motoneurons occur distally. Thus, whatever the mechanisms that are responsible for their formation, these mechanisms must account for the undisturbed state of the proximal dendritic tree.

11.7 CONCLUDING COMMENTS

Spinal motoneurons have played a pivotal role in our understanding of synaptic integration, the organization of neurons in complex networks, and the response of neurons to injury. The long history associated with these studies often leads to the perception that further examination of motoneurons has little to offer. It is ironic, therefore, that recent studies of this cell provide some of the most compelling evidence for a change in neuronal polarity that challenges rules of neuronal structure and function widely believed to be indisputable.

ACKNOWLEDGMENTS

The preparation of this manuscript was supported by the Canadian Institutes for Health Research and the Ontario Neurotrauma Fund.

REFERENCES

1. Ramón Y Cajal, S., *Histologie du Système Nerveux de L'homme et des Vertébrés,* Maloine, Paris, 1909.
2. Peters, A., Palay, S., and Webster, H. deF., *The Fine Structure of the Nervous System,* W.B. Saunders, Philadelphia, 1976.
3. Craig, A.M. and Banker, G., Neuronal polarity, *Ann. Rev. Neurosci.,* 17, 267, 1994.
4. Kandel, E.R., Schwartz, J.H., and Jessell, T.M., *Principles of Neural Science,* McGraw-Hill, New York, 2000, chap. 2.
5. Baas, P.W., Microtubules and neuronal polarity: lessons from mitosis, *Neuron,* 22, 23, 1999.
6. Winckler, B. and Mellman, I., Neuronal polarity: controlling the sorting and diffusion of membrane components, *Neuron,* 23, 637, 1999.
7. Foletti, D.L., Prekeris, R., and Scheller, R.H., Generation and maintenance of neuronal polarity: mechanisms of transport and targeting, *Neuron,* 23, 641, 1999.
8. Sumner, B.E.H. and Watson, W.E., Retraction and expansion of the dendritic tree of motor neurones of adult rats induced *in vivo, Nature,* 233, 273, 1971.
9. Standler, N.A. and Bernstein, J.J., Degeneration and regeneration of motoneuron dendrites after ventral root crush: computer reconstruction of dendritic fields, *Exp. Neurol.,* 75, 600, 1982.
10. Rose, P.K., Distribution of dendrites from biventer cervicis and complexus motoneurons stained intracellularly with horseradish peroxidase in the adult cat, *J. Comp. Neurol.,* 197, 395, 1981.
11. Brown, A.G. and Fyffe, R.E.W., Direct observations on the contacts made between Ia afferent fibers and α-motoneurons in the cat's lumbosacral spinal cord, *J. Physiol. (Lond.),* 313, 121, 1981.
12. Cameron, W.E., Averill, D.B., and Berger, A.J., Morphology of cat phrenic motoneurons as revealed by intracellular injection of horseradish peroxidase, *J. Comp. Neurol.,* 219, 70, 1983.
13. Chen, X.Y. and Wolpaw, J.R., Triceps surae motoneuron morphology in the rat: A quantitative light microscopic study, *J. Comp. Neurol.,* 343, 143, 1994.

14. Burke, R.E. and Glenn, L.L., Horseradish peroxidase study of the spatial and electrotonic distribution of group Ia synapses on type-identified ankle extensor motoneurons in the cat, *J. Comp. Neurol.,* 372, 465, 1996.

15. Brännström T., Havton, L., and Kellerth, J.-O., Changes in size and dendritic arborization patterns of adult cat spinal α-motoneurons following permanent axotomy, *J.
Comp. Neurol.,* 318, 439, 1992.

16. Brännström, T., Havton, L., and Kellerth, J.-O., Restorative effects of reinnervation
on the size and dendritic arborization patterns of axotomized cat spinal α-motoneurons, *J. Comp. Neurol.,* 318, 452, 1992.

17. Rall, W., Core conductor theory and cable properties of neurons, in *Handbook of
Physiology: The Nervous System. Cellular Biology of Neurons,* Brookhart, J.M. and
Mountcastle, V.B., Eds., American Physiological Society, Bethesda, MD, 1977, 39.

18. Gustafusson, B., Changes in motoneurone electrical properties following axotomy,
J. Physiol. (Lond.), 293, 197, 1979.

19. Gustafusson, B. and Pinter, M., Effects of axotomy on the distribution of passive
electrical properties of motoneurones, *J. Physiol. (Lond.),* 356, 433, 1984.

20. Foehring, C., Sypert, G.W., and Munson, J.B., Properties of self-reinnervated motor
units of medial gastrocnemius of cat. II. Axotomized motoneurons and time course
of recovery, *J. Neurophysiol.,* 55, 947, 1986.

21. Pinter, M. and Vanden Noven, S., Effects of preventing reinnervation on axotomized
spinal motoneurons in the cat. I. Motoneuron electrical properties, *J. Neurophysiol.,*
62, 311, 1989.

22. Blinzinger, K. and Kreutzberg, G., Displacement of synaptic terminals from regenerating motoneurons by microglial cells, *Z. Zellforsch.,* 85, 145, 1968.

23. Kerns, J.M. and Hinsman, E.J., Neuroglial response to sciatic neurectomy. II. Electron
microscopy, *J. Comp. Neurol.,* 151, 255, 1973.

24. Sumner, B.E.H. and Sutherland, F.I., Quantitative electron microscopy on the injured
hypoglossal nucleus in the rat, *J. Neurocytol.,* 2, 315, 1973.

25. Matthews, M.R. and Nelson, V.H. Detachment of structurally intact nerve endings
from chromatolytic neurons of the rat superior cervical ganglion during depression
of synaptic transmission induced by post-ganglionic axotomy, *J. Physiol. (Lond.),*
245, 91, 1975.

26. Chen, D.H., Qualitative and quantitative study of synaptic displacement in chroma-
tolyzed spinal motoneurons of the cat, *J. Comp. Neurol.,* 177, 635, 1978.

27. Delgado-Garcia, J.M., et al., Behaviour of neurons in the abducens nucleus of the
alert cat. III. Axotomized motoneurons, *Neuroscience,* 24, 143, 1988.

28. Johnson, I.P. and Sears, T.A., Ultrastructure of axotomized alpha and gamma motoneurons in the cat thoracic spinal cord, *Neuropathol. Appl. Neurobiol.,* 15, 149, 1989.

29. Brännström, T. and Kellerth, J.-O., Changes in synaptology of adult cat spinal α-motoneurons after axotomy, *Exp. Brain Res.,* 118, 1, 1998.

30. Rende, M., I. et al., Axotomy induces a different modulation of both low-affinity
nerve growth factor receptor and choline acetyltransferase between adult rat spinal
and brainstem motoneurons, *J. Comp. Neurol.,* 363, 249, 1995.

31. Piehl, F., Tabar, G., and Cullheim, S., Expression of NMDA receptor mRNAs in rat
motoneurons is down-regulated after axotomy, *Eur. J. Neurosci.,* 7, 2101, 1995.

32. Popratiloff, A. et al., Glutamate receptors in spinal motoneurons after sciatic nerve
transection, *Neuroscience,* 74, 953, 1996.

33. Alverez, F.J. et al., Downregulation of metabotropic glutamate receptor 1a in motoneurons after axotomy, *Neuroreport,* 8, 1711, 1997.

34. Kennis, J.H. and Holstege, J.C., A differential and time-dependent decrease in AMPA-type glutamate receptor subunits in spinal motoneurons after sciatic nerve injury, *Exp. Neurol.,* 147, 18, 1997.

35. Havton, L. and Kellerth, J.-O., Elimination of intramedullary axon collaterals of cat spinal alpha-motoneurons following peripheral nerve injury, *Exp. Brain Res.,* 79, 65, 1990.

36. Lindå, H., Risling, M., and Cullheim, S., 'Dendraxons' in regenerating motoneurons in the cat: do dendrites generate new axons after central axotomy?, *Brain Res.,* 358, 329, 1985.

37. Lindå, H., Risling, M., and Cullheim, S., A light and electron microscopic study of intracellularly HRP-labeled lumbar motoneurons after intramedullary axotomy in the adult cat, *J. Comp. Neurol.,* 318, 188, 1992.

38. Ulfhake, B. and Kellerth, J.-O., A quantitative light microscopic study of the dendrites of cat α-motoneurons after intracellular staining with horseradish peroxidase, *J. Comp. Neurol.,* 202, 571, 1981.

39. Ulfhake, B. and Kellerth, J.-O., A quantitative morphological study of HRP-labeled cat α-motoneurones supplying different hindlimb muscles, *Brain Res.,* 264, 1, 1983.

40. Rose, P.K., Keirstead, S.A., and Vanner, S., A quantitative analysis of the geometry of cat motoneurons innervating neck and shoulder muscles, *J. Comp. Neurol.,* 239, 89, 1985.

41. Cameron, W.E., Averill, D.B., and Berger, A.J., Quantitative analysis of the dendrites of cat phrenic motoneurons stained intracellularly with horseradish peroxidase, *J. Comp. Neurol.,* 230, 91, 1985.

42. Cullheim, S. et al., Membrane area and dendritic structure in type-identified triceps surae alpha motoneurons, *J. Comp. Neurol.,* 255, 68, 1987.

43. Pinching, A.J., Myelinated dendritic segments in the monkey olfactory bulb, *Brain Res.,* 29, 133, 1971.

44. Bignami, A. and Ralston, H.J., Myelination of fibrillary astroglial processes in long term Wallarian degeneration. The possible relationship to 'status marmoratus', *Brain Res.,* 11, 710, 1968.

45. Risling, M. et al., A persistent defect in the blood-brain barrier after ventral funiculus lesion in adult cats: implications for CNS regeneration?, *Brain Res.,* 494, 13, 1989.

46. Havton, L. and Kellerth, J.-O., Regeneration by supernumerary axons with synaptic terminals in spinal motoneurons of cats, *Nature,* 325, 711, 1987.

47. O'Hanlon, G.M. and Lowrie, M.B., Nerve injury in adult rats causes abnormalities in the motoneuron dendritic field that differ from those seen following neonatal nerve injury, *Exp. Brain Res.,* 103, 243, 1995.

48. Rose, P.K. and Odlozinski, M., Expansion of the dendritic tree of motoneurons innervating neck muscles of the adult cat after permanent axotomy, *J. Comp. Neurol.,* 390, 392, 1998.

49. Kernell, D. and Zwaagstra, B., Size and remoteness: two relatively independent parameters of dendrites, as studied for spinal motoneurones of the cat, *J. Physiol. (Lond.),* 413, 233, 1989.

50. Ulfhake, B. and Cullheim, S., Postnatal development of cat hind limb motoneurons. II. *In vivo* morphology of dendritic growth cones and the maturation of dendritic morphology, *J. Comp. Neurol.,* 278, 88, 1988.

51. Cullheim, S. and Kellerth, J.-O., Combined light and electron microscopic tracing of neurons including axons and synaptic terminals, after intracellular injection of HRP, *Neurosci. Lett.,* 2, 307, 1976.

52. Rose, P.K. and Neuber-Hess, M., Myelinated 'dendrites': a consequence of long-term peripheral axotomy of neck motoneuron in the adult cat, *Soc. Neurosci.,* 23, 608, 1997.

53. Ahmari, S.E., Buchanan, J., and Smith, S, J., Assembly of presynaptic active zones from cytoplasmic transport packets, *Nature Neurosci.,* 3, 445, 2000.

54. Keirstead, H.S., Hughes, H.C., and Blakemore, W.F., A quantifiable model of axonal regeneration in the demyelinated adult rat spinal cord, *Exp. Neurol.,* 151, 303, 1998.

55. Sotello, C. and Palay, S.L., The fine structure of the lateral vestibular nucleus in the rat, *J. Cell Biol.,* 36, 151, 1968.

56. Ramirez, V. and Ulfhake, B., Anatomy of dendrites of motoneurons supplying the intrinsic muscles of the foot sole in the aged cat: evidence for dendritic growth and neo-synaptogenesis, *J. Comp. Neurol.,* 316, 1, 1992.

57. MacDermid, V. et al., Distribution of immunoreactivity for MAP2 and GAP-43 in distal dendrites of permanently axotomized motoneurons in the adult cat: evidence of neuronal polarity alteration, *Soc. Neurosci.,* 24, 1034, 1998.

58. MacDermid, V., Neuber-Hess, M., and Rose, P.K., Multiple axonal growth within the distal dendritic tree of permanently axotomized motoneurons in the adult cat, *Soc. Neurosci.,* 25, 2287, 1999.

59. MacDermid, V., Neuber-Hess, M., and Rose, P.K., On a quest for a new axon: the molecular and morphological evolution of distal dendrites to axons in permanently axotomized motoneurons in the adult cat, *Soc. Neurosci.,* 26, 861, 2000.

60. Tucker, R.P., The roles of microtubule-associated proteins in brain morphogenesis: a review, *Brain Res. Rev.,* 15, 101, 1990.

61. Benowitz, L.I. and Routtenberg, A., GAP-43: an intrinsic determinant of neuronal development and plasticity, *Trends Neurosci.,* 20, 84, 1997.

62. Nagase, Y. et al., Changes in size and dendritic structure of cat facial motoneurons after permanent axotomy, *Soc. Neurosci.,* 25, 653, 1999.

63. Hall, G.F. and Cohen, M.J., The pattern of dendritic sprouting and retraction induced by axotomy of lamprey central neurons, *J. Neurosci.,* 8, 3584, 1988.

64. Hall, G.F., Poulos, A., and Cohen, M.J., Sprouts emerging from the dendrites of axotomized lamprey central neurons have axonlike ultrastructure, *J. Neurosci.,* 9, 588, 1989.

65. Hall, G.F. et al., Cytoskeletal changes correlated with the loss of neuronal polarity in axotomized lamprey central neurons, *J. Neurocytol.,* 26, 733, 1997.

66. Eccles, J.C., Libet, B., and Young, R.R., The behavior of chromatolysed motoneurones studied by intracellular recording, *J. Physiol. (Lond.),* 143, 11, 1958.

67. Kuno, M., and Llinás, R., Enhancement of synaptic transmission by dendritic potentials in chromatolysed motoneurones of the cat, *J. Physiol. (Lond.),* 210, 807, 1970.

68. Dodge, F.A., The nonuniform excitability of central neurons as exemplified by a model of the spinal motoneuron, in *The Neurosciences, Fourth Study Program,* Schmitt, F.O. and Worden, F.G., Eds., MIT Press, Cambridge, 1979, chap. 25.

69. Traub, R.D. and Llinás, R., The spatial distribution of ionic conductances in normal and axotomized motorneurons, *Neuroscience,* 2, 829, 1977.

70. Sernagor, E., Yarom, Y., and Werman, R., Sodium-dependent regenerative responses in dendrites of axotomized motoneurons in the cat, *Proc. Natl. Acad. Sci. U.S.A.,* 83, 7966, 1986.

71. Mendell, L.M., Munson, J.B., and Scott, J.G., Connectivity changes of Ia afferents on axotomized motoneurones, *Brain Res.,* 73, 338, 1974.

72. Mendell, L.M., Munson, J.B., and Scott, J.G., Alterations of synapses on axotomized motoneurones, *J. Physiol. (Lond.),* 255, 67, 1976.

73. Magee, J.C., Voltage-gated ion channels in dendrites, in *Dendrites,* Stuart, G., Spruston, N., and Häusser, M., Eds., Oxford, New York, 1999, chap. 6.
74. Larkum, M.E., Rioult, M.G., and Lüscher, H.-R., Propagation of action potentials in the dendrites of neurons from rat spinal cord slice cultures, *J. Neurophysiol.,* 75, 154, 1996.
75. Black, M.M. and Baas, P.W., The basis of polarity in the neuron, *Trends Neurosci.,* 12, 211, 1989.
76. Yu, W. et al., Depletion of a microtubule-associated motor protein induces the loss of dendritic identity, *J. Neurosci.,* 20, 5782, 2000.
77. Mattson, M.P., Establishment and plasticity of neuronal polarity, *J. Neurosci. Res.,* 57, 577, 1999.
78. Bregmann, B.S., Regeneration in the spinal cord, *Curr. Opin. Neurobiol.,* 8, 800, 1998.
79. Tetzlaff, W. and Steeves, J.D., Intrinsic neuronal and extrinsic glial determinants of axonal regeneration in the injured spinal cord, in *Degeneration and Regeneration in the Nervous System,* Saunders, N.R. and Dziegielewska, K.M., Eds., Harwood Academic, Amsterdam, 2000, chap. 5.
80. Bandtlow, C.E. and Schwab, M.E., NI-35/250/nogo-a: a neurite inhibitor restricting structural plasticity and regeneration of nerve fibers, *Glia,* 29, 175, 2000.

12 How Does Nerve Injury Strengthen Ia-Motoneuron Synapses?

Timothy C. Cope, Kevin Seburn, and Charles R. Buck

CONTENTS

12.1 INTRODUCTION

Synapses made in the spinal cord by neurons whose axons are severed several centimeters distant in the periphery can express substantial changes within hours of the injury. At the synapses made between group Ia muscle stretch afferents and alpha motoneurons (Ia-MN synapses), the excitatory postsynaptic potentials (EPSPs) are significantly enlarged soon after and for several days following nerve section in adult rats.[1-3] This observation has captured our attention for a variety of reasons. First, the *direction of change* may represent a unique form of synaptic plasticity, whereby presynaptic inactivity enhances synaptic strength. Second, the *speed of change* demonstrates that steady-state synaptic strength can be adjusted on a time scale of hours, suggesting close and continuous regulation of mature central synapses. Third, the *potential role of neurotrophins* in the regulating function of mature synapses might be significantly advanced in light of recent findings on neurotrophin expression by primary afferents, motoneurons, and muscle, and changes in this expression following nerve section. Fourth, the *environment of change* is uniquely relevant to whole-animal behavior because the changes are observed *in vivo*.

12.2 THE Ia-MN SYNAPSE: A PERSPECTIVE ON CONTINUED STUDY

The first intracellular records of postsynaptic potentials in the mammalian central nervous system were obtained at Ia-MN synapses in studies reported by Eccles and colleagues in 1952.[4] The unique experimental accessibility to function at these synapses motivated hundreds of subsequent studies and elevated the Ia-MN synapse to the status of the prototype synapse in the mammalian central nervous system. Over the past 50 years, the Ia-MN synapse has provided crucial and novel insights into central synaptic function. The following topics were significantly advanced at the Ia-MN synapse: electrotonic decay of synaptic current in passive dendrites; nonlinear summation of synaptic currents; frequency dependent modulation of synaptic potentials; quantal nature of transmitter release; specificity of synaptic connections; and presynaptic inhibition. The reader can find discussion of these and numerous other examples in References 5–12.

While these historical considerations establish the early value of information about the Ia-MN synapse, for some readers they may also raise the question, "Does further examination of the long-studied Ia-MN synapse have a place in a book dedicated to frontiers in neuroscience?" The answer in our opinion is undeniably "yes." First, our understanding of the normal operation and regulation of function at this synapse remains incomplete. In the course of discussion of selected candidate factors that establish and adjust steady-state synaptic strength, this chapter identifies important areas of uncertainty; for example, the fundamental relation between efficacy and activity at Ia-MN synapses is not yet settled. Making this determination is not only key to understanding the basic cellular mechanisms of synaptic function at this and, perhaps, at other synapses, but also it has important implications for abnormal motor behaviors such as hyperactive tendon-jerk reflexes that follow spinal injury and stroke. A second reason for our positive answer is that study of Ia-MN synapses continues to provide exciting new information. For example, a recent study of developing Ia afferents and motoneurons shows that these neurons have a matched expression of particular genes when they come to innervate the same muscle.[13] This observation suggests a mechanism by which synaptic connections might be specified between Ia afferents and motoneurons, and perhaps between other neuron types in the CNS. A third rationale for continuing study of the Ia-MN synapse is that this synapse is uniquely suited to examination in the intact central nervous system of living mammals. The Ia-MN synapse can be exploited to test the physiological relevance of findings made in more reduced preparations, e.g., spinal or brain slices.

12.3   Ia-MN SYNAPTIC FUNCTION

In this chapter we attempt to advance understanding of the function and regulation of central synapses by examining the injury-induced enlargement of EPSPs at the Ia-MN synapse. We begin in this section by defining the composite Ia EPSP and by assessing its usefulness as a measure of Ia-MN synaptic function. This section is necessarily brief and not intended to provide the thorough discussion of details that can be found in several earlier reviews.[5–12]

It is important to keep in mind that while the EPSP enlargement under consideration here was observed in rat, some of the relevant observations used to evaluate this enlargement were made in cat. Although there are no clear indications of species differences in Ia-MN synaptic function, greater assurance will require more data. Indeed, it is not known whether Ia EPSPs are actually enlarged in the cat 1 week after muscle nerve section as they are in the rat.

12.3.1   SYNAPTIC PATHWAYS INFLUENCING THE Ia* EPSP

Included among the large number of sensory afferents innervating a single skeletal muscle are the afferents supplying muscle spindles. Each spindle-bearing muscle sends multiple spindle afferents, groups Ia and II, into the spinal cord, where the afferents synapse with a variety of neurons including αMNs.[14] Further detail about spindle-afferent synapses with MNs derives from studies of anesthetized adult cats, wherein EPSPs produced by individual afferents are measured in MNs using the spike-triggered averaging (STA) technique.[15] Physiologically identified group Ia afferents generate EPSPs with monosynaptic latency at synapses made with MNs supplying the same muscle as the afferent (homonymous synapses) and with MNs innervating synergist muscles (heteronymous synapses). For example, each one of

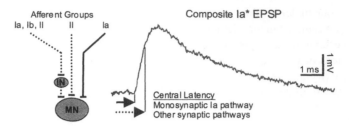

FIGURE 12.1 The composite Ia* EPSP and its contributing afferent pathways. The voltage trace to the right was recorded intracellularly from a medial gastrocnemius motoneuron (conduction velocity 50 m/s) upon stimulation (0.5 hz) of the lateral gastrocnemius soleus nerve in an anesthetized adult rat. The trace is an average of 10 sweeps. Neither pre- nor postsynaptic neurons were axotomized. Arrows estimate central latency of action potentials conducted in afferent pathways from the time of their arrival at the spinal cord (onset of each arrow) to the initiation of postsynaptic potentials (to the tip of each arrow). Solid arrow identifies central latency for the monosynaptic Ia afferent pathway; broken arrow shows central latency for other pathways (involving group Ia, Ib, and II primary afferents) and indicates the potential for these pathways to contribute to the EPSP before it reaches its peak amplitude. All pathways are represented in the diagram to the left, where the solid and broken lines depict, respectively, the pathways that yield the central latencies shown as solid and broken arrows superimposed on the EPSP. The asterisk in Ia* EPSP designates the potential contribution from sources other than the monosyanptic Ia pathway.

60 Ia afferents from the cat medial gastrocnemius (MG) muscle makes homonymous synapses with virtually all 300 MG MNs and heteronymous synapses with about 2/3 of approximately 450 lateral gastrocnemius-soleus (LG-S) MNs.[16] Amplitudes of EPSPs produced by single Ia afferents range from ca. 1 to 600 μV.[17–20]

Electrical stimulation of selected muscle nerves produces composite EPSPs at short latency that range in peak amplitude from less than 1 to 12 mV in cat lumbosacral MNs[21,22] and from less than 1 to around 5 mV in rat.[2,3,23] The functional anatomy described above for single Ia afferents leads to the supposition that this short-latency EPSP is the composite synaptic event[24] produced by groups of Ia afferents that are activated by electrical activation of the nerve. This composite EPSP is the event shown to enlarge after muscle nerve section, and the extent to which it represents Ia-MN synaptic function requires careful consideration.

The strength of electrical stimulation required to activate all Ia afferents in a muscle nerve will also activate group Ib and some group II afferents. In the rat, there is no obvious demarcation in the distribution in conduction velocity for afferent groups Ia and II,[25] making it likely that there is considerable overlap in the electrical thresholds of these afferents. It is important then to consider the contribution from these other afferents to the putative composite Ia EPSP (Fig. 12.1). We begin by estimating that monosynaptic EPSPs produced by single Ia afferents reach their peak amplitudes typically 1.5 msec after Ia action potentials arrive at the dorsum of the spinal cord. This latency includes conduction time through the spinal cord up to initiation of the EPSP in a MN, i.e., the central latency, which for single Ia afferents is commonly 0.7 to 0.8 msec and ranges from 0.4 to 1.1 msec.[26,27] Added to this is the rise time of the EPSP, which from 10 to 90% of the peak EPSP averages between

0.6 and 0.9 msec and ranges between 0.2 and 3.0 msec.[15,18,20,26] In comparison, the central latency for synaptic potentials produced either monosynaptically for some group II afferents,[28,29] or disynaptically for other group II afferents and for group Ib and Ia afferents, ranges between 1.2 and 2.8 msec.[26,29] This means that synaptic potentials, both inhibitory and excitatory, evoked electrically through pathways other than the monosynaptic group Ia pathway, can be initiated before the group Ia EPSP reaches peak amplitude (Fig. 12.1).[30–32] These considerations make it plain that multiple afferent pathways have the capacity to contribute to the rising phase and peak amplitude of short-latency EPSP.

In addition to the extrinsic synaptic influences that act postsynaptically to modify the short-latency EPSP, other effects may be introduced presynaptically as a result of afferents that synapse with Ia afferents and produce presynaptic inhibition.[10] The influence of tonic presynaptic inhibition on short-latency EPSPs is suggested by the large increase (up to 60%) that is observed in these potentials soon after treatment with a $GABA_B$ antagonist.[23,33]

As for the contribution of the Ia-MN synapse to the short-latency EPSP, the following indirect evidence suggests an important if not predominant contribution. First, the mean amplitude of the composite EPSP produced by electrical stimulation approximates that calculated as the product of the number of activated Ia afferents and the average EPSP produced by each.[17,18] Second, the amplitude of the steady-state EPSP evoked by muscle vibration, a stimulus that selectively activates Ia afferents in cats, covaries with the short-latency composite EPSP produced by electrical stimulation of the nerve.[34] Third, the strength of reflex contractions initiated by muscle stretch varies among triceps surae muscles in a pattern that matches the pattern of short-latency EPSP amplitudes distributed in this system.[35]

Considering all of the above, we arrive at the perspective that the short-latency composite EPSP is generated predominantly at Ia-MN synapses but modified by transmission through other afferent pathways. In order to acknowledge potential contributions from these other pathways we use an asterisk when referring to the composite Ia* EPSP. Strong support for the assertion that the Ia-MN synapse itself contributes to the axotomy-induced enlargement of the Ia* EPSP is given below (12.4.1).

12.3.2 OTHER INFLUENCES ON Ia* EPSP AMPLITUDE

Theoretical considerations identify several anatomical and biophysical properties of both pre- and postsynaptic elements of the Ia-MN synapse that are expected to influence Ia* EPSP size. These properties, e.g., MN cable properties and synaptic density of Ia afferent terminations on MNs, have been the subject of extensive discussion and study.[5,6,8,11,24] We expect that the explanation for Ia* EPSP enlargement resides in the changes induced by axotomy in one or several of these cellular properties of the Ia-MN synapse, and some possibilities are discussed below (12.4.3). Limited space precludes further discussion. Before continuing, however, we point out that because of its dependence on multiple features of the Ia-MN synapse, the amplitude of the Ia* EPSP is sensitive to a broad range of changes at the synapse. This sensitivity has great value in enabling detection of synaptic plasticity. Knowledge of the pre- and postsynaptic factors that covary with Ia* EPSP amplitude also assists with data analysis and interpretation, because these factors enable assessment of the comparability of pooled samples of data taken from different treatment groups, e.g., nerves intact vs. cut.

It is important to realize that description of the Ia* EPSP derives predominantly from studies of animals anesthetized by barbiturate or ketamine-xylazine. The EPSP enlargement that we evaluate in this chapter was obtained from anesthetized rats. One advantage of this condition is that it suppresses voltage-gated channels that are activated in MNs by synaptic potentials in cats that are decerebrated and untreated by anesthetic drugs.[36] Thus, although it will be of interest to determine whether these channels might otherwise contribute to synaptic plasticity, the use of anesthetic drugs simplifies interpretation of EPSP amplitude and its changes. Nonetheless, anesthetics themselves can introduce confounding effects and are known to influence Ia* EPSP amplitude.[37]

12.3.3 STEADY-STATE SYNAPTIC STRENGTH

Throughout this chapter, *synaptic strength* is equated to the peak amplitude of Ia* EPSPs measured in units of millivolts. The term strength has meaning with regard to the input–output relation of the Ia-MN circuit, because motoneuron firing probability increases in direct proportion to the size of an EPSP.[38–41]

We define *steady-state synaptic strength* at Ia-MN synapses as the maximum amplitude of the Ia* EPSP produced when a muscle nerve is stimulated at low frequency (≤ 1 pps). At low stimulation frequency, EPSP amplitude remains steady over repeated stimuli.[3,42,43] At higher stimulation frequencies, especially rates exceeding ca. 10 to 20 pps, EPSP amplitude increases at some Ia-MN synapses and decreases at others (see 12.4.3.1). Relationships between the direction and amplitude of this dynamic behavior with the size of the steady-state Ia* EPSP and with MN membrane resistance[3,23,44–46] provide important insights into Ia-MN function. These relationships may represent systematic differences in the transmitter release properties of Ia afferents, incomplete invasion of all of the terminal boutons of Ia afferents, or the nonlinear nature of the relation between voltage and conductance at chemical synapses.[44] Most pertinent to the present discussion, steady-state Ia* EPSP amplitude represents a broad range of synaptic functions and properties of Ia-MN synapses.

12.4 PERIPHERAL NERVE SECTION STRENGTHENS Ia-MN SYNAPSES

12.4.1 THE PHENOMENON OF Ia* EPSP ENLARGEMENT

Enhanced transmission strength at Ia-MN synapses in response to nerve section is documented in three reports: Miyata and Yasuda;[1] Manabe et al.;[2] Seburn and Cope.[3] In all three studies, Ia* EPSPs were sampled *in vivo* by intracellular recording from spinal MNs in anesthetized rats. Fig. 12.2 is reproduced from the study of Miyata and Yasuda[1] for composite EPSPs recorded from homonymous MG Ia-MN synapses. The mean amplitude of Ia* EPSPs sampled from control rats without nerve cut is plotted at time zero and represented by the horizontal dotted line. Mean amplitudes are plotted also for Ia* EPSPs sampled from rats grouped by the time interval

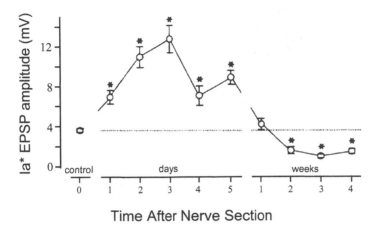

Time After Nerve Section

FIGURE 12.2 Ia* EPSP amplitude increases substantially before decreasing after nerve section. Mean values (open circles) and standard errors of the means (bars) for pooled samples of homonymous EPSPs evoked by electrical stimulation of the medial gastrocnemius (MG) nerve and recorded in MG motoneurons. Samples were taken from rats grouped at different times following section of the MG nerve and from rats with no nerve section (average amplitude for control data is plotted at time 0 and extended as dotted line). Asterisks indicate significant difference from control. Modified from Y. Miyata and H. Yasuda, *Neurosci. Res.*, 5, 338, 1988. With permission.

following section of the MG nerve in the periphery (1 day to 4 weeks). Fig. 12.2 shows that at these synapses, for which both pre- and postsynaptic axons were severed, Ia* EPSPs undergo a biphasic change. At intervals longer than 1 week, the mean size of Ia* EPSPs is smaller than normal. This reduction in synaptic strength following long periods of nerve section is amply established, particularly for Ia-MN synapses in the cat.[47] At shorter intervals, EPSPs are significantly larger than normal: 3.4 times larger after 3 days (see Fig. 12.3) and nearly 2 times larger after 1 day (between 19 and 25 hours). The study of Manabe, Kaneko, and Kuno[2] places a lower limit on the time required for this effect by showing no significant change in amplitude earlier than 12 hours after nerve section.

A similar change in EPSP size occurs following section of the afferent limb of the Ia-MN synapse.[1,3] Thus, electrical stimulation of group I afferents in the severed MG nerve evoked composite Ia* EPSPs in uncut LG-S MNs that were significantly larger than normal beginning 1 day after nerve cut. At the 3-day mark, Miyata and Yasuda[1] showed that EPSPs were on average 2.6 times larger than the normal amplitude (Fig. 12.3). Seburn and Cope[3] confirmed this increase under similar experimental conditions, although the increase in Ia* EPSP size was smaller, amounting to 1.7 times normal. The quantitative difference may be attributable to differences between studies in the rat species (Wistar vs. Sprague Dawley), anesthetics (pentobarbital vs. ketamine-xylazine), or the nerve selected for cut (MG vs. LG-S) (Miyata and Yasuda[1] vs. Seburn and Cope,[3] respectively). Despite these different conditions, presynaptic axotomy significantly elevated transmission strength at the Ia-MN synapse.

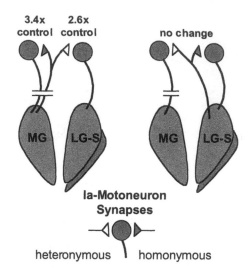

FIGURE 12.3 Schematic diagram of divergent monosynaptic pathways from Ia afferents onto motoneurons supplying medial gastrocnemius (MG) and lateral gastrocnemius-soleus (LG-S) muscles. Legend at bottom shows synaptic terminals made with motoneurons by homonymous Ia afferents (shaded terminals from afferents supplying the same muscle as the motoneuron) and by heteronymous Ia afferents (open terminals from afferents supplying a different muscle than the contacted motoneuron). Both MG and LG-S Ia afferents make homonymous and heteronymous synapses in the rat, but are separated for clarity (left and right). Changes relative to control in mean Ia* EPSP amplitude after 3 days of MG nerve section (indicated by interrupted lines) are given as reported by Miyata and Yasuda.[1]

In an attempt to discriminate the effects of afferent axotomy on transmission specifically at the Ia-MN synapse, we re-examined our published data.[3] This analysis rests on the argument that the earliest portion of the rising phase of the short latency EPSP is generated exclusively by current at Ia-MN synapses (Fig. 12.1). In addition, we expect that if these synapses are strengthened by axotomy, then the rate of rise in voltage during this early portion of the Ia* EPSP should be increased. The results of reanalyzing our data met this expectation: the mean rate of rise over first 0.25 ms of the rising phase of the EPSPs from the 3-day axotomy rats (288.4 V/s ± 244.7 SD; n = 38) was significantly larger (p = 0.0008; independent t test) than that obtained from untreated rats (144.2 V/s ± 85.3 SD; n = 40). These findings provide strong evidence that the Ia-MN synapse is strengthened 3 days after axotomy.

By contrast, EPSPs elicited by electrically stimulating uncut afferents were unchanged up to 2 weeks following MN axotomy. MN axotomy is not without effect, however, since it yields a greater Ia* EPSP increase when combined with afferent axotomy than does afferent axotomy alone (3.4× vs. 2.6× normal, respectively). Fig. 12.3 also indicates that homonymous synapses made by uncut afferents with uncut LG-S MNs express no change following section of the nerve supplying a close synergist muscle, i.e., MG.

In sum, these studies show that the steady-state synaptic strength *increases* at synapses made within the spinal cord between sensory and motor neurons whose axons are cut in the periphery. The increase occurs not immediately, but within several hours following axotomy. Section of the afferent axon is necessary, and section of the motor axon can amplify this effect, but is insufficient itself to increase EPSP amplitude. The remaining discussion focuses on the signals that might initiate and the mechanisms that might underlie this early increase in steady-state synaptic strength.

12.4.2 POTENTIAL INITIATING SIGNALS FOR Ia* EPSP ENLARGEMENT

The enhancement of synaptic strength might be initiated by any of several different changes set off by cutting the muscle nerve. The possibility of a generalized systemic effect is excluded by the selective nature of the synaptic enhancement, occurring at some but not other Ia synapses even on the same MNs (Fig. 12.3). The group Ib, II, III, and IV primary afferents that are axotomized together with Ia afferents when the muscle nerve is cut represent another potential means of initiating enhanced strength at Ia-MN synapses. These primary afferents diverge widely to contact both segmental and ascending neurons,[48] and their axotomy would affect myriad circuits extrinsic to the Ia-MN synapse. Although some influence of extrinsic circuits cannot be ruled out, the narrow distribution of the Ia* EPSP enhancement by nerve section contrasts with the broad distribution of group II–IV afferents. Group III and IV afferents supplying the MG muscle, for example, have strong reflex actions on the soleus muscle.[49-51] Thus, if these afferents are somehow involved in altering homonymous MG Ia-MN synapses, they should also produce some change at homonymous soleus Ia-MN synapses. The failure to observe such widespread changes in synaptic strength diminishes the likelihood that damage to afferents other than the Ia initiates synaptic enhancement at the Ia-MN synapse.

The most direct induction of synaptic change would derive from the responses initiated by cutting the pre- and/or postsynaptic elements of the synapse expressing the change. Support for this possibility is given in Fig. 12.3 where it is seen that synaptic strength is enhanced at all Ia-MN synapses in which the cut Ia afferent participates. The MN may also participate in initiating synaptic change; although cutting the MN axon is not a sufficient condition, it does amplify enhancement. For these reasons, we focus further discussion on the changes induced by axotomy in both Ia afferents and MNs. Two changes are examined in detail. One is the change in firing behavior and synaptic activity of axotomized Ia afferents and MNs. The other is the alteration of trophic factors that occurs when axotomy separates the somata and central synapses of Ia afferents and MNs from their muscle. Peripheral nerve section alters both synaptic activity and trophic support and both have the capacity to modify synaptic strength.

12.4.2.1 Synaptic Activity

12.4.2.1.1 Axotomy

It is proposed that the increase in Ia-MN synaptic strength is attributable to disuse or inactivation of the synapse that results when Ia afferents are axotomized.[1,2] In support of this possibility, it is typically found that a substantial fraction of primary afferents falls silent when axotomy separates the sensory axon from its receptor ending in the muscle.[52] For example, Seburn et al.[53] found that only 13% (29/228) of cut Aα/Aβ afferents generated spontaneous action potentials in anesthetized rats studied 3 days after sciatic nerve section. This fraction was down from the 22% of active cut afferents observed over the first 7 hours following nerve section. These findings suggest that many of the cut group Ia afferents are inactive over the period that synaptic enhancement is observed at the Ia-MN synapse. This is not to say, however, that a contribution of a few active group Ia afferents can be overlooked. The synaptic enhancement that we explore in this chapter is assessed from the amplitude of composite Ia* EPSPs that are evoked by the electrical stimulation of all group Ia afferents, including ones that are either active or silent prior to the recording session. For this reason it is of interest to look more closely at the behavior of the spontaneously active afferents.

Fig. 12.4A illustrates data obtained in one decerebrate cat from physiologically classified group Ia afferents before, during, and after cutting the MG nerve.[54] Action potentials were recorded from two afferents that were simultaneously penetrated by independent microelectrodes in a dorsal root. Both afferents responded with high-frequency injury discharge immediately after and for several seconds after nerve cut. Afferent #1 fired only infrequently after about 30 sec following nerve cut. The other afferent continued firing at impressively high rates in a bursting pattern for as long as it was monitored (67 min). In the study of Seburn et al.,[53] the 13% that fired did so sporadically or at steady rates averaging 28 pps after 3 days of sciatic nerve cut. Examples are shown in Fig. 12.4B for sporadic or steady firing recorded in rat from 2 Aα/Aβ afferents axotomized for 3 days. Because the spontaneously firing afferents in the rat are probably muscle and not cutaneous afferents,[55] some of the active ones are likely to be group Ia. It is unknown whether cut afferents maintain their activity or silence, as opposed to switching on and off following injury.

The effect of spontaneous afferent activity on EPSPs at the Ia-MN synapse is difficult to assess. The early injury discharge is unlikely to have long-term effects on EPSP amplitude, because brief periods (10s to 100s ms) of high-frequency (ca. 200 to 500 Hz) stimulation produce post-tetanic potentiation and/or depression that last no longer than a couple of minutes.[42,44] To date, there is no evidence for long-term potentiation at Ia-MN synapses in anesthetized adult rats. As for the effects of the prolonged and unusual discharge rates and patterns of the sort exhibited by one cut Ia afferent in Fig. 12.4A, there are no data that address how synapses might respond. It is as plausible that the active afferents cause the EPSP enlargement as it is that they retard its full development. Distinguishing between these possibilities will require direct comparison of the EPSPs produced by individual Ia afferents that are either inactive or spontaneously active.

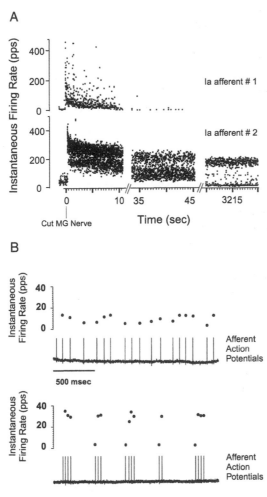

FIGURE 12.4 Instantaneous firing by afferents following axotomy. (A) Data recorded intra-axonally from two group Ia afferents supplying the medial gastrocnemius (MG) muscle in cat before and for many minutes after MG nerve section.[54] Total duration of recording from afferent #1 was about 44 secs and for afferent #2 about 67 min (last 12 min not shown). (B) Samples of data recorded intra-axonally from two group Aα/Aβ afferents that were cut 3 days earlier in a rat. Instantaneous firing rates are plotted in upper traces for the recorded action potentials shown in lower traces.

Motoneurons continue to receive excitatory synaptic drive following axotomy and continue to fire in response to that drive. In decerebrate cats, MG MNs that are recruited in cutaneous reflexes before MG nerve cut are recruited in the same reflex immediately and for several hours after the cut.[54] Moreover, cut muscle nerves continue for many months to fire in relation to other nerves as they do normally, although the activity level of axotomized MNs declines progressively, beginning very soon after injury.[56] To compensate for this loss, synergistic muscles quickly become much more active than they are normally.[57] This difference in activity levels of axotomized vs. uncut MNs is interesting in light of the difference in EPSPs produced in these two classes of MNs by cut Ia afferents (Fig. 12.3). Taken together, these observations lead us to speculate that the enlargement of Ia* EPSPs induced by cutting afferents is enabled or amplified by the reduced activity of the homonymous MN, and suppressed or not promoted by the increased activity of the heteronymous MN.

12.4.2.1.2   TTX Treatment

Distinguishing the effects of altered activity on synaptic strength requires isolation of the confounding factors introduced by nerve section. Nerve section alters the activity of the Ia afferents in the uncontrolled manner described above and introduces metabolic, anatomic, and functional changes in response to axonal injury, changes that are referred to collectively as the axon or retrograde reaction.[58,59] Some of these cellular changes can occur soon enough after injury to account for the early changes in synaptic strength under discussion here. These confounding variables are eliminated or constrained by an experimental approach in which the voltage-gated sodium channel blocker tetrodotoxin (TTX) is continuously applied to a small section of a peripheral nerve.[60] TTX prevents the central propagation of action potentials in primary sensory axons, although conduction may not be blocked in the small diameter afferents due to the presence of TTX-insensitive sodium channels.[61,62] With regard to the large Aα/Aβ afferents, intra-axonal recording from dorsal roots in anesthetized rats shows a complete absence of action potentials in all axons sampled (25/25) after 7 days of TTX treatment (Seburn and Cope, unpublished observations). Because the recording configuration would have detected action potentials generated at any location central to the TTX treatment site, we can rule out the possibility of action potential generation at ectopic sites, e.g., dorsal root ganglion. TTX treatment also has the advantage of minimizing damage to the axons[63] and interference with axoplasmic transport.[64,65]

Action potentials blocked from entering the central projections of primary sensory axons fail to invade and evoke transmitter release from synaptic terminals. This condition makes it possible to assess how synaptic strength might be influenced by some period of synaptic inactivity. It is important to note, however, that this experimental procedure introduces additional factors whose contributions to changes in synaptic function must be considered. Even though impulse invasion of the synaptic terminal is prevented, spontaneous release of transmitter may continue as it does at the neuromuscular junctions of TTX-treated motor axons.[66,67] In addition, TTX treatment of a muscle nerve affects transmitter release from more than just Ia afferents. One of these effects is blockade of action potential propagation in primary afferents other than group Ia in the treated nerve, and the ensuing alteration of activity in diverse spinal circuits. Another effect of TTX treatment of muscle nerves is the blockade of impulses arriving at the neuromuscular junction and the resultant muscle paralysis.

The response of Ia-MN synapses to the effects of impulse blockade by TTX treatment was first examined by Gallego et al.[60] in anesthetized cats. Ia* EPSPs were evoked in triceps surae MNs by electrical stimulation of the MG nerve central to the site of continuous TTX treatment. Two weeks of TTX blockade produced a 1.5-fold increase in amplitude of the Ia* EPSPs produced by TTX-treated Ia afferents in MNs that were or were not treated. Webb and Cope[68] corroborated this effect under experimental conditions that were similar, but that eliminated the widespread limb denervation that was part of the experimental design applied by Gallego et al.[60] Shorter durations of TTX treatment were not examined in the cat studies. Manabe, Kaneko, and Kuno[2] reproduced the increase in Ia* EPSP amplitude in rats following TTX application to the sciatic nerve. Synaptic modification in the rat was detectable within 1 day, and achieved a maximum increase of 1.5 times the normal EPSP amplitude after 2 days of TTX treatment. These findings give suggestive evidence that *prolonged inactivity at Ia-MN synapses can enhance synaptic strength.*

At the neuromuscular junction, blockade of action potential invasion of the motor terminal by TTX treatment of the motor axon is presumed to inactivate the postsynaptic cell, i.e., the muscle fiber. Although some caution in interpretation is required because spontaneous myogenic action potential activity may occur, the presumed postsynaptic inactivation coupled with presynaptic inactivity is associated with an enhancement of synaptic transmission at the neuromuscular junction.[66,67] These observations contrast strongly with the findings described above for Ia-MN synapses, where synaptic strength increases when continued postsynaptic activity, albeit reduced, is coupled with prolonged presynaptic inactivation that is achieved by TTX treatment and, at least partially, by axotomy. Serious caution is required in interpreting these findings, because the experimental procedures introduce confounding factors mentioned above that have yet to be critically examined. Still, one reasonable interpretation is that dissonant firing between pre- vs. postsynaptic neurons may actually enhance synaptic strength at the Ia-MN synapse, and possibly at other synapses. This form of plasticity contradicts existing predictions emerging from Hebbian theory and to our knowledge represents a form of synaptic plasticity that has not been documented at any other synapse. For example, using a cell culture system, Fields, Yu, and Nelson[69] compared synaptic strength at synapses made by stimulated vs. unstimulated afferents with mouse spinal cord neurons. Because the postsynaptic cells fired spontaneously, synapses made with the unstimulated afferents experienced dissonant firing that has been postulated to weaken the synapse.[70] Indeed, EPSP amplitude was significantly smaller when produced by afferents that were unstimulated compared to ones that were stimulated in a phasic pattern for 3 to 5 days. Thus, findings at the Ia-MN synapse may extend our understanding of the full set of rules by which synaptic function is regulated in the adult central nervous system, that is, if synaptic enhancement by presynaptic disuse can be authenticated.

12.4.2.1.3 Conclusion

Manabe, Kaneko, and Kuno[2] conclude that "… the early synaptic enhancement produced by section of the peripheral nerve could be accounted for entirely by the deprivation of sensory impulse activity." Data presented above together with other details carefully considered by them[2] are consistent with this proposal. However, the data do not prove and we are not yet convinced of an exclusive role for synaptic disuse in accounting for synaptic enhancement. One cause for skepticism is the finding that the enhancement seen after nerve section is about 2× greater than that observed after TTX treatment. This quantitative difference is the opposite of what one would predict based upon synaptic disuse, which is complete at the Ia-MN synapse following nerve treatment with TTX but not after nerve section. Another reason for doubting an exclusive role for disuse is the observation that the increase in EPSP amplitude produced by TTX is increased even further by the addition of a distal nerve cut. One would have predicted instead no further increase in EPSP size, because nerve cut adds no additional synaptic inactivity (but see Manabe, Kaneko, and Kuno[2] for an alternate interpretation). These discrepancies between observation and prediction draw attention to other factors that may contribute to synaptic enhancement.

12.4.2.2 Neurotrophins

Our attention has recently turned toward neurotrophins because of a growing number of reports that these molecules modify synaptic transmission.[71–74] For example, Kang and Schuman[75] showed that neurotrophin-3 (NT-3) and brain-derived neurotrophic factor (BDNF) increased synaptic strength at synapses made between Schaffer collaterals and CA1 neurons in slices of rat hippocampus. Within minutes of bath application of these neurotrophins and lasting for tens of minutes thereafter, EPSPs increased in size by 2.5 to 3 times normal. Most pertinent to our interests, these observations were made in mature rats (average age about 46 days). This means that in addition to well-established actions in developing animals,[76] neurotrophins have the capacity to modify synaptic function in adult animals. Taken together with the presence of neurotrophins in muscle, MNs, and primary sensory afferents and the changes induced in neurotrophin expression by those cells following muscle nerve section, a role for neurotrophins in producing the early enhancement of Ia-MN synaptic strength seemed important to explore.

12.4.2.2.1 Trophic Dependence of Ia-MN Synaptic Function in Adult Animals

The possibility that factors in addition to activity regulate Ia-MN synapses in adult animals is promoted by studies performed *in vivo* on anesthetized cats. Goldring et al.[77] demonstrated that the significant decline in Ia* EPSP size months after cutting a muscle nerve is at least partially reversed when the nerve is allowed to reinnervate muscle. Of particular interest was the finding that Ia* EPSPs were restored to their normal size even when long delays in the reinnervation process (2 to 8 months) prevented recovery of group I afferent stretch sensitivity. These findings suggest that something about reconnection of cut afferents with muscle, something that does not depend upon recovery of afferent activity, is sufficient to restore synaptic strength. This suggestion has more recent support in the work of Mendell et al.[78] who found partial recovery of Ia* EPSP amplitude when cut group I afferents were forced to reinnervate skin. These investigators speculated that certain neurotrophins known to reside in both skin and muscle might act to "rescue" muscle afferents, and perhaps the functional properties of synapses. Consistent with this notion, Munson et al.[79] and Mendell et al.[80] demonstrated that prolonged treatment of cut muscle nerves with exogenous neurotrophin not only reversed the decline in Ia* EPSP amplitude, but increased EPSP size to values significantly greater than normal. Although these observations are made more than 1 week following nerve section and, therefore, have unknown relevance to the early changes under consideration in this chapter, they demonstrate that adult Ia-MN synapses are sensitive to the status of their connections in the periphery, possibly as signaled by neurotrophins.

12.4.2.2.2 Expression and Cellular Localization of Neurotrophins in Relation to the Ia-MN Synapse

A first step toward understanding the functional role of neurotrophins at the Ia-MN synapse, or in any other system, is to obtain a complete and accurate picture of the synapse's access to neurotrophin. This brings us to consider expression of both the neurotrophins and their receptors by Ia afferents and MNs and their associated tissues and cells, including muscle and glia. The source of neurotrophin that is most relevant to Ia-MN function is unknown, and accumulating evidence is not resolving this issue. The classic "neurotrophic hypothesis" proposing that target tissue provides a limited supply of factor(s) to the neuron[81] is challenged by numerous studies in both developing and mature systems.[82–84] For neurons in the adult spinal cord, this hypothesis seems, at best, an oversimplification.

NT-3, neurotrophin-4 (NT-4), and BDNF mRNAs have been detected by RNA blot and RNase protection analyses of whole spinal cord,[85,86] sensory ganglia,[87–90] and muscle.[85,86,88,90–93] More recently, reverse transcriptase polymerase chain reaction (RT-PCR)[94] and sensitive *in situ* hybridization (ISH) analyses[89,95–100] have localized expression of these mRNAs to MNs and to both neurons and support cells in the sensory ganglia. Additionally, a significant proportion of adult MNs express more than one neurotrophin,[97,98] and adult rat DRG cells may also express multiple neurotrophins.[101]

Increasingly sensitive antibody reagents have now enabled detection of neurotrophin protein expression by immunohistochemistry (IHC) and provide further support for multiple neurotrophin sources and for local production of NT-3, BDNF, and NT-4 in MNs and DRG neurons.[94,97,102–104] In addition to MNs, these factors have been localized to astroglial cells in the ventral horn and white matter[104] and to CNS microglial cells in culture.[105] We have also localized expression of both mRNA and protein for NT-3, NT-4, and BDNF to spinal cord interneurons, astroglia and microglia *in vivo*. Some of these results are illustrated in Color Figure 6.*

There is no shortage, therefore, of expression data for neurotrophin mRNA and protein in the Ia-MN circuit. Quantifying expression of these molecules *in vivo*, however, has been notoriously problematic. Enzyme-linked immunosorbent assays (ELISA) have been extremely difficult to establish with reliability and reproducibility for neurotrophins. A sensitive two-site ELISA for NGF was reported nearly 30 years ago,[106] thanks largely to a rich source of endogenous NGF in the rodent submandibular gland, which provided an invaluable control for detection of this neurotrophin in tissues. Similar assays for the other neurotrophins have proven problematic for many reasons, including the lack (until quite recently) of specific and sensitive antibody reagents to detect the neurotrophins; frequent false-positive results; inefficient extraction of neurotrophins from tissue sources; and the extremely low levels of

---

* Color figures follow page 142.

endogenous expression of these molecules.[107] Some of these difficulties continue to plague attempts at quantitative detection of neurotrophins *in vivo*, including NGF, so that much caution should be exercised in interpreting reported neurotrophin levels obtained from ELISA. More reliable assays are slowly becoming available, however, and limited information on precise levels of neurotrophins is emerging.[108,109]

Determination of neurotrophin protein levels aside, biological activity of endogenous neurotrophins expressed in the CNS has not been demonstrated. This is surprising since the initial characterization of NGF was based on a simple but sensitive neurite outgrowth bioassay.[110] We have recently employed the embryonic chick DRG neurite outgrowth assay to demonstrate robust neurotrophin activity in extracts of adult rat spinal cord, presumably resulting from the neurotrophins we have detected in this tissue by *in situ* hybridization and immunohistochemistry.[97] We are presently developing immunological and biochemical assays to distinguish the various neurotrophins and to quantify the neurite outgrowth activity with the bioassay as a measure of biologically relevant neurotrophin expression.

Neurotrophins act through high-affinity Trk receptors and the widely expressed lower-affinity p75 receptor.[111] Thus, receptor expression represents an additional means of regulating function. The profile of expression of these receptors is also complex, but the reagents available to detect these molecules have been more reliable. Most MN somata express TrkB and TrkC receptors,[98,112,113] and the majority of lumbar DRG cells, including those falling in the size range of the Ia afferents, express more than one Trk receptor.[99,114]

The preceding summary of expression data demonstrates that the neurotrophic environment of the Ia-MN synapse is complex. These synapses have multiple potential sources of neurotrophin within the spinal cord and dorsal root ganglion, seemingly independent of the target muscle. Evidence for the possibility that neurons can utilize local neurotrophic support in an autocrine or paracrine manner has also been reported,[115-119] and this may apply to the MN or its synaptic inputs. The complex combinations of neurotrophin and Trk receptor expression within and across adult motor and sensory neuron populations, as well as expression in local supporting cells and in peripheral nerve and target muscles, render difficult the task of determining their relative physiological roles *in vivo*. Achieving such understanding requires a means of manipulating and quantifying changes in neurotrophin expression in order to test their effect on Ia-MN synaptic properties.

Conditional deletion of genes encoding neurotrophins and/or receptors for these molecules will allow for relatively localized manipulation of neurotrophin signaling in mature animals. A recent illustration of this type of approach delineates the role of TrkB in the production of LTP (long-term potentiation) in the adult hippocampus. Xu et al.[120] performed experiments in which they selectively flanked the TrkB gene with loxP sequences by homologous recombination. Transgenic animals carrying the modified TrkB gene were mated with transgenic mice expressing the *Cre* recombinase selectively in frontal cortex and CA1 hippocampal fields. This enzyme recognizes the lox sites flanking TrkB sequences and removes DNA between these sites, thereby deleting the TrkB gene in cortical and CA1 pyramidal neurons. Examination of LTP in hippocampal slice preparations obtained from these mice allowed the authors[120] to conclude that BDNF acts through TrkB presynaptically, but not postsynaptically, to modulate LTP. The general characteristics of this approach, postnatal manipulation of a single receptor in a cell-specific manner, could be very useful for dissecting the role of neurotrophins in axotomy-induced strengthening of the Ia-MN synapse.

New information about neurotrophin signaling reveals novel mechanisms that might participate in the axotomy-induced enhancement of Ia-MN synaptic strength. For instance, cells that express more than one receptor may produce different outcomes depending upon whether one or both ligands are bound[121] and/or the binding of one neurotrophin may alter the response of binding by a second.[99] Thus, the reduction of one neurotrophin following axotomy might have synaptic effects as a result of changing the effectiveness of the remaining neurotrophins. Moreover, recent studies demonstrate that the neurotrophin receptor response at the cell surface can be distinguished from responses mediated by internalized, retrogradely transported neurotrophin/receptor complexes. Neurotrophin-mediated cell survival does not require internalization of the neurotrophin/Trk receptor complex, whereas neurotrophin-induced differentiation does.[122] Second-messenger systems activated in response to neurotrophins that lead to survival or differentiation may also be distinct.[123] Distinct functions of cell surface-activated Trk receptors may lead to distinct MN responses to neurotrophins (or absence thereof) retrogradely transported from target muscle compared with those available in an autocrine or paracrine manner within the spinal cord. These and anticipated new complexities of neurotrophin actions are likely to provide fertile grounds for generating hypotheses about neurotrophin influences on synaptic function.

12.4.2.2.3 Axotomy-Induced Changes in Neurotrophins

Following sciatic nerve transection in adult rats, mRNA levels for BDNF, and NT-4 and the TrkB receptor for these molecules as well as NT-3 and its receptor TrkC are differentially modified in the target muscle, sciatic nerve, and spinal cord.[85,86] Table 12.1 shows that many of the tissue-specific and heterogeneous changes in neurotrophins and their cognate receptors occur as early as 6 to 12 hours following axotomy. These early changes *precede* the axotomy-induced increase in Ia-MN synaptic strength that is first detected at 12 hours and are, therefore, eligible candidates for inducing the increase in synaptic strength. Table 12.1 further indicates that the direction of change may reverse with time. To determine direction of change in the expression of the neurotrophins at the peak of the increase in synaptic efficacy (see Fig. 12.2) we performed non-radioactive *in situ* hybridization (ISH) experiments to measure cell-specific expression of BDNF, NT-3, and NT-4 in rat lumbar MNs 3 days after sciatic nerve section. To our surprise, the results pooled from 3 rats revealed no significant difference ($p > 0.1$; independent t-test) in the percentages of intact vs. axotomized MNs expressing mRNA for any of the three neurotrophins: intact vs. axotomized MNs for NT3 = 87% ± 5.3% (SD) vs. 84% ± 3.1%, for BDNF = 81% ± 6.6% vs. 78% ± 2.7%, and for NT4 = 77% ± 3.1% vs. 73% ± 9.0%. From these findings we conclude either that the reported reduction of BDNF and

TABLE 12.1

Tissue	Post-Axotomy Period	NT-3	TrkC	NT-4	BDNF	TrkB
Muscle	Early[a]	n.c.[c]	n.d.[d]	⇑	⇓	n.d.[d]
	Late[b]	n.c.[c]	n.d.[d]	⇓⇓	⇑	n.d.[d]
Sciatic nerve	Early[a]	⇓⇓	⇓	⇓	undetected	⇑
	Late[b]	n.c.[c]	⇑⇑⇑	⇑⇑	⇑⇑	n.c.[c]
Spinal cord	Early[a]	⇓	n.c.[c]	n.c.[c]	⇓	n.c.[c]
	Late[b]	⇓	⇑	n.c.[c]	⇓	⇓⇓

[a] 6 to 12 hours post-axotomy

[b] 7 to 14 days after axotomy

[c] no change

[d] not determined

Table data taken from Funakoshi et al., *J. Cell Biol.*, 123, 455, 1993 and Griesbeck et al. *J. Neurosci.*, 42, 21, 1995. With permission.

NT-3 neurotrophin mRNA in the spinal cord following axotomy (Table 12.1) is due to a reduced expression by cells other than MNs, or that changes in MN expression fall below the sensitivity threshold for ISH.

The common p75 receptor is dramatically increased in MNs following nerve injury.[124] The injury response of hypoglossal MNs again suggests complexity in trophic support for injured MNs. Axotomy alone, in the absence of proximal crush injury, results in decreased choline acetyl transferase (ChAT), a marker for MN function, but not the dramatic increase in p75. A crush injury proximal to the pure axotomy site was required to elicit the increase in MN p75 expression. These data suggested independent trophic support mechanisms for the maintenance of ChAT expression (target-derived), and for the p75 neurotrophic factor increase (local signals at the site of regeneration).[125]

12.4.2.2.4 Effects of Manipulating Neurotrophins on MNs, Afferents, and Their Synapses

About 1 week and longer after a muscle nerve is cut and before it reinnervates its target, axonal conduction velocity (CV) of the cut MNs and afferents and the amplitude of the associated Ia* EPSPs fall significantly below normal values (e.g., Fig. 12.2). Although not the focus of this chapter, these physiological changes are worthy of brief discussion because they are the only ones for which the effects of neurotrophin manipulations have been examined in adult animals *in vivo*. The continuous application of exogenous NT-3 or NT-4 to the central cut ends of muscle nerves in rats[126] and cats[79,80] reversed the fall in MN and/or afferent CV and/or in Ia* EPSP amplitude. Conversely, sequestration of endogenous neurotrophin by continuous infusion of Trk-IgG receptor body molecules onto muscles with intact nerves acted in some cases to slow CV of uninjured MNs and/or afferents.[126]

Outwardly, these findings suggest that selected functional properties of MNs, afferents, and their synapses are differentially regulated by target-derived neurotrophins. The physiological relevance of these findings is questionable, however, because of the extremely large amounts of exogenous neurotrophin applied over 1 to 5 weeks directly to the cut nerve. If the daily regimen of neurotrophin (60 µg/day) were delivered in the relatively large volume of 1 ml, the concentration of NT-3 in this paradigm would be 2.2 µM, approximately 200,000 times higher than the dissociation constant of the TrkC receptor (1×10^{-11} M) and 2000 times higher than that for the low affinity p75 receptor for NT-3! Similar concerns should be sounded about the very high concentrations of Trk-IgG receptor bodies. Pertinent to this concern is the demonstration in visual cortical cultures from developing rats, for example, of a dose–response relation in which synaptic current amplitude changes substantially between 0.5 and 25 ng/ml BDNF[127] (approximately 1×10^{-9} M). In addition, it is somewhat unsettling that the effects of neurotrophins differ so dramatically between rats and cats. Both NT-3 and NT-4 are effective in partially restoring CV in cut MNs in rat,[126] but neither are effective in cat;[80] both NT-3 and NT-4 raise the CV of cut afferents in cat,[80] but only NT-3 has this effect in rat.[126] Inconsistency is also found in the effect of exogenous NT-3 applied to cut nerves, in that Ia* EPSPs sampled from different treated animals range from 5 times normal to not significantly different than normal.[79,80] These considerations raise caution about the use of exogenous neurotrophin administration for purposes of identifying possible roles for these molecules *in vivo*.[128–131] Investigations employing these strategies must demonstrate that the neurons in question have access to exogenously added neurotrophins or blocking agents and, most importantly, the concentration of these molecules at that site must be determined.

12.4.2.2.5 Relationship between Activity and Neurotrophins

In this chapter we identify two changes that are caused by cutting the peripheral nerve and that may induce an increase in Ia* EPSP size: alterations in nerve impulse activity and in trophic support. These two changes cannot be considered independently when investigating the potential role of neurotrophins in altering synaptic function, because expression of both the neurotrophins and their receptors has been shown to be modulated by neuronal activity. In fact, evidence from neocortical cultures suggests that neural activity regulates synaptic current through its influence on BDNF expression.[127] Thus, future studies may show that neurotrophins carry the signal for activity-dependent synaptic plasticity, perhaps at the Ia-MN synapse.

Funakoshi and colleagues[91] first suggested the possibility that neurotrophins may provide activity-dependent, muscle-derived trophic support for adult MNs. Following direct electrical stimulation of muscle, these investigators found a dramatic but transient increase in the muscle mRNA levels for NT-4, but not NT-3 or BDNF. These results remain controversial,[104] however, and to our knowledge have not been replicated.

Changes in expression of neurotrophins in postsynaptic cells induced by afferent activity have been reported in the CNS, e.g., hippocampus, reviewed by Thoenen.[132] Some support for activity-related regulation of neurotrophins in the spinal cord is provided by a recent report that exercised rats show a 50% increase in the number of small diameter non-neuronal cells showing TrkB immunoreactivity.[133] This is remarkable given the relatively low intensity (walking) and short duration (5 days/wk for 4 wk) of the exercise and suggests that changes in activity at the level of the whole organism may produce more dramatic alterations than more localized changes affecting only a subpopulation of cells. It remains to be determined whether spinal synapses respond to these kinds of changes in neurotrophin signaling.

12.4.2.2.6   Summation and Evaluation

Observations of the sort briefly discussed above give support to the possibility of neurotrophin involvement in the axotomy-induced enhancement of steady-state synaptic strength at the Ia-MN synapse. These observations include demonstrations of neurotrophin effects on mature synapses; neurotrophin availability to Ia afferents, MNs, and their synapses; neurotrophin changes in response to axotomy and preceding Ia* EPSP enlargement; and neurotrophin dependence on neuromuscular activity. Still, the case for neurotrophin participation is based strictly on circumstantial and correlative evidence and requires more direct substantiation.

12.4.3   POTENTIAL MECHANISMS FOR Ia* EPSP ENLARGEMENT

The cellular changes responsible for the EPSP enlargement that follows soon after axotomy are not known. Any one or more of the several pre- and/or postsynaptic factors that determine Ia* EPSP amplitude may participate (see 12.3). The participation of certain factors can be downplayed by the observation that, for example, Ia* EPSP enlargement requires neither axotomy of the MN (see Fig. 12.3) nor any measurable change in whole-cell electrical properties of the MN, including input resistance.[1,3] We turn attention instead to our studies of two factors, one ostensibly presynaptic (transmitter release) and one postsynaptic (glutamate receptor composition).

12.4.3.1   Alteration in High-Frequency Modulation of Ia* EPSP Amplitude

When muscle nerves are electrically stimulated at rates exceeding 10 to 20 pps, the evoked composite Ia* EPSPs display a progressive change in amplitude during the stimulus train. Fig. 12.5 adapted from Seburn and Cope[3] illustrates the progressive decline in Ia* EPSP amplitude during stimulation at 18 Hz and at a conventional standard frequency of 167 Hz. Repetitive, high-frequency stimulation of single Ia afferents yields similar amplitude modulation of the evoked EPSP,[41,43,134] thereby verifying this behavior for Ia-MN synapses. The change in Ia* EPSP amplitude varies in magnitude and direction from one MN to the next. In our studies of the rat, amplitude changes predominantly in the direction of a progressive decline, defined here as synaptic depression and called negative modulation in earlier reports.[135]

The mechanism of depression observed at normal Ia-MN* synapses has been inferred solely from observations on the relationship found between the size of the steady-state Ia* EPSP and the magnitude of depression.[134] In our study,[3] for example, we found that the largest steady-state Ia* EPSPs exhibited substantial depression during the course of stimulation at 167 pps, while smaller Ia* EPSPs typically decreased by lesser amounts or even increased in size. This observation draws attention to findings made at other synapses where the magnitude of depression during repetitive stimulation is directly proportional to the amplitude of the unconditioned or steady-state synaptic potential or current.[136,137] It is hypothesized that this relationship results because

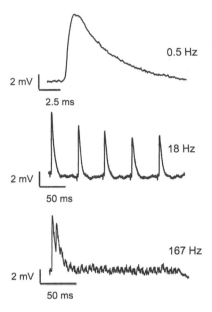

FIGURE 12.5 Ia* EPSPs demonstrate amplitude depression at high stimulation frequency. Records obtained in rat from medial gastrocnemius motoneuron taken at 3 different frequencies of stimulation of a lateral gastrocnemius-soleus nerve cut 3 days earlier. In contrast with Ia* EPSPs that exhibit no systematic variation in amplitude when evoked at 0.5 Hz, Ia* EPSPs fall progressively in amplitude during stimulation at 18 and 167 Hz. (Modified from Seburn, K. and Cope, T., *J. Neurosci.*, 18(3) 1142, 1998. With permission.)

synapses with a higher probability of transmitter release experience greater depletion of the available pool of releasable transmitter during repetitive stimulation than do synapses with a lower probability of release. This hypothesis guided our thinking about the cellular mechanism(s) by which axotomy might enhance synaptic strength at the Ia-MN* synapse; we reasoned that if Ia* EPSP enlargement results from an increase in the probability of transmitter release, then Ia* EPSP depression should also increase. Consistent with this notion, our study showed that Ia* EPSPs sampled 3 days after nerve section were not only enlarged but also significantly shifted toward a larger than normal magnitude of depression (Fig. 12.6). This meant that axotomy might increase the probability of transmitter release, but other mechanisms are not ruled out.

Returning to considerations of the mechanism(s) of depression at normal synapses, a number of possibilities other than transmitter depletion need to be appreciated. With respect to presynaptic mechanisms, Hsu, Augustine, and Jackson[138] demonstrate Ca^{++}-dependent adaptation in the rate of synaptic vesicle fusion at squid synapses, and Bellingham and Walmsley[139] speculate that Ca^{++} can act to transiently inhibit transmitter release at synapses in slices of cochlear nucleus in developing rats. On the postsynaptic side of the synapse, Otis, Zhang, and Trussell[140] give direct evidence for desensitization of glutamate receptors of neurons studied in slices of embryonic chick cochlear nucleus.

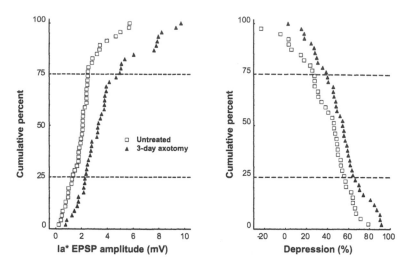

FIGURE 12.6 Presynaptic axotomy increases both high frequency depression and amplitude of Ia* EPSPs. Ia* EPSPs were recorded from intact medial gastrocnemius (MG) motoneurons upon electrical stimulation of lateral gastrocnemius-soleus nerves that were either untreated or cut for 3 days in rats. Cumulative histograms for pooled samples show shifts toward greater than normal values that were significant ($p < 0.05$; nested ANOVA) for both the amplitude of Ia* EPSPs measured at low stimulation frequency (0.5 Hz; left panel) and for the decline in amplitude of Ia* EPSPs measured over the course of high stimulation frequency (167 Hz; right panel). Note that the negative depression indicated for one point represents an increase in Ia* EPSP amplitude during high frequency stimulation. (Modified from Seburn, K. and Cope, T., *J. Neurosci.*, 18(3) 1142, 1998. With permission.)

Any of these mechanisms might be important to the process of synaptic depression normally and after axotomy at the Ia-MN synapse. Moreover, closer inspection raises some doubt about the contribution of transmitter depletion to depression at Ia-MN synapses. The relationship between steady-state Ia* EPSP size and high-frequency amplitude modulation is not strong; variation in Ia* EPSP amplitude accounts for no more than 25% of variation in modulation across Ia-MN* synapses in the rat.[3,23] In addition, the expected serial dependence between Ia* EPSP pairs obtained through paired-pulse testing is not found among pre-tetanic control Ia* EPSPs.[44] These observations, together with recognition of multiple potential mechanisms for synaptic depression, raise considerable uncertainty about the extent to which synaptic depression at the Ia-MN synapse is due purely or even partially to transmitter depletion. The only supportable conclusion at this time is that our data do not rule out the possibility that axotomy alters release probability.

Our observations on the high frequency behavior of Ia* EPSPs indirectly address the possibility that they enlarge because axotomy increases the number of active Ia synaptic terminals, either by activating silent Ia synapses or generating new ones. The prospect of new functioning synapses is supported by observations that single Ia afferents make functional synaptic connections with greater than normal numbers of motoneurons soon after spinal cord injury in cats.[141] Axotomy might have the same effect; however, we would not have expected to see increased depression with the simple addition of Ia synapses that express the same transmitter release properties as the extant Ia terminals. By this reasoning, it seems likely that if new Ia synapses are added, then they must have release properties that differ from the original Ia synapses.

12.4.3.2 Alteration of Glutamate Receptor Composition

The weight of evidence suggests that the Ia-MN synapse is glutamatergic, although some lingering uncertainty merits attention.[8] All reports are consistent in showing that transmission occurs at least in part through the AMPA/KA (α-amino-3-hydroxy-5-methyl-4-isoxazole proprionate/kainate) subtype of glutamate receptor.[142–147] By contrast, reports are inconsistent on whether NMDA receptors participate in mediating Ia-MN transmission, possibly because of differences in the ages of animals studied and the potential for NMDA participation to change over the course of development (for discussion and citations, see Pinco and Lev-Tov[144]). Uncertainty about NMDA receptor actions and the lack of evidence for the phenomenon of long-term potentiation at mature Ia-MN synapses, cause us to turn our attention in this chapter toward non-NMDA mechanisms in explaining short-term enhancement following axotomy. In addition, space limitations and the paucity of information about the effects of metabotropic glutamate receptors on Ia-MN transmission explain their omission from this discussion, although we have recently presented evidence that mGluR1a immunoreactivity declines within 3 days after sciatic axotomy in rat.[148]

There is an ever-growing list of AMPA receptor properties and processes that might be physiologically relevant points of entry for regulating synaptic function. Included are changes in number, distribution, and recycling of the receptors in the postsynaptic membrane, and changes in heteromeric subunit composition that can result from alternative splicing and RNA editing. Recent reports can be consulted for a description of these features of AMPA receptors and for citations to earlier works.[149–154] Our investigation of glutamatergic mechanisms underlying Ia* EPSP enlargement began with examination of the density and composition of AMPA subunits in MNs at early time points following sciatic nerve section in adult rats.[155] Antibodies to glutamate receptor (GluR) subunits were used to detect subunits GluR1, GluR2/3, and GluR4 with immunohistochemistry. The intensity of immunostaining was quantified by densitometric analysis and used to estimate the amount of GluR expression. Untreated MNs showed intense immunoreactivity (ir) for both GluR2/3 and GluR4, but only weak GluR1-ir. The reader should note that staining was restricted to cytosolic regions of MNs, and the relationship of GluRs in this cellular compartment to the membrane-bound GluRs, which were not stained by these procedures, remains to be determined. After 3 days of axotomy, MNs exhibited significant declines in staining intensity for all subunits, with a disproportionately large decrease in GluR2/3-ir. Figure 12.7 shows the reduction in GluR2/3-ir selectively for those MNs in the right dorsolateral (DL) ventral horn that were axotomized. These findings largely confirm earlier studies of both untreated and nerve-sectioned adult rats.[156–161]

We extended examination of the change in MN GluRs by showing that application of TTX to the sciatic nerve had little effect on GluR-ir. Comparison of the

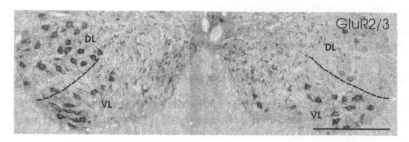

FIGURE 12.7 Axotomy reduces motoneuron immunoreactivity (ir) for the glutamate receptor subunits 2/3 (GluR2/3). Serial sections of lumbar segment 4/5 of spinal cord immunostained for GluR2/3 in a rat 7 days after sciatic nerve cut. GluR2/3-ir was strongly reduced among dorsolateral (DL) motoneurons that were axotomized by sciatic nerve section (ventral horn (right)), but not among ipsilateral ventrolateral (VL) motoneurons and contralateral DL and VL motoneurons, all of which were uncut. (From Alvarez, F.J. et al., *J. Comp. Neurol.*, 426, 229, 2000. With permission.)

effects of axotomy vs. TTX suggests that physical disconnection of MNs from muscle and/or overt physical injury (unique to nerve section), and not muscle paralysis or elimination of impulse-evoked release from MN terminals (common to nerve section and TTX treatment) are responsible for the change in GluR-ir profile. The early and apparently unbalanced loss of GluR-ir may be yet another feature of the axon reaction[58,59] expressed by axon-damaged neurons. Most relevant to the central topic of this chapter, the axotomy-induced change in GluR expression suggests a candidate mechanism for Ia* EPSP enlargement. In addition, these findings provide further indirect evidence that Ia* EPSP enlargement after nerve section and TTX treatment occur by different mechanisms (see also 12.4.2.1.3).

A decrease in GluR2-ir early after sciatic nerve section (recently supported using GluR2 specific antibody in unpublished studies of Dr. F.J. Alvarez and colleagues) generates an exciting possible explanation for Ia* EPSP enlargement. AMPA receptors that either lack GluR2 or contain unedited GluR2 are Ca^{++} permeable.[150,162,163] Jonas and Burnashev[162] estimate that homomeric unedited AMPA receptor channels yield 3 to 4% more Ca^{++} entry than heteromeric channels. The acquisition of Ca^{++} permeability and associated Ca^{++} current at Ia-MN synapses in response to axotomy has the potential to alter synaptic strength directly by increasing inward current through the AMPA receptor channel and/or indirectly via a variety of other mechanisms.[162] Indeed, the activation of Ca^{++}-permeable AMPA receptors is shown to enhance synaptic strength in dorsal horn neurons in the developing spinal cord[164] and to mediate long-term potentiation in slices of basolateral amygdala from young rats.[165] Synaptic enhancement by this mechanism requires, however, that synapses remain at least moderately active in order to relieve the channel from polyamine block.[166] All considered, these observations suggest that the acquisition of Ca^{++}-permeable AMPA receptors by axotomized MNs might enhance transmission from those Ia afferents that remain active. It is important to remember, however, that Ia* EPSP enlargement also occurs in uncut MNs, wherein we detected no change in GluR-ir (Fig. 12.7 ventrolateral (VL) MNs in right ventral horn). These findings indicate that a change in GluR composition is not a necessary condition for Ia*

EPSP enlargement, but it may be responsible for amplifying the enlargement above the level obtained by afferent axotomy alone (see Fig. 12.3).

12.5 CLOSING REMARKS

In this chapter, we examine factors that may regulate the strength of transmission *in vivo* at a mature synapse in the mammalian central nervous system. Specifically, we exploit the early, injury-evoked increase in Ia* EPSP amplitude as a means of investigating these factors. Studies from our laboratory and others yield data to suggest that Ia* EPSP enlargement is a unique form of synaptic plasticity, one in which short-term presynaptic inactivity strengthens transmission with postsynaptic neurons that remain active. In addition, there is evidence that injury-evoked changes in neurotrophin expression might participate in altering Ia* EPSP amplitude. Whatever signals induce the change in synaptic function, there is evidence to suggest that the underlying mechanism(s) involves alterations in presynaptic neurotransmitter release and/or postsynaptic neurotransmitter receptor function. Although these assertions are reasonably well supported by available evidence, we note many sources of ambiguity that limit the strength of conclusion. Indeed, these limitations may prove difficult to overcome using existing methodologies for studying the central nervous system in living animals. Despite the problems, however, several avenues for *in vivo* study of adult mammalian synapses remain, and we are motivated to pursue these studies by their unique physiological relevance to nervous system function.

ACKNOWLEDGMENTS

The authors gratefully acknowledge Drs. Kathrin Engisch, Valerie Haftel, and Marty Pinter, Ms. Paige Riley and Anne Shirley, and Mr. Jon Prather for valuable contributions to the work presented here and/or to the preparation of this document. This work has been supported by grants from the National Institutes of Health (NS38693; NS31563; NS21023).

REFERENCES

1. Miyata, Y. and Yasuda, H., Enhancement of Ia synaptic transmission following muscle nerve section: dependence upon protein synthesis, *Neurosci. Res.*, 5, 338, 1988.
2. Manabe, T., Kaneko, S., and Kuno, M., Disuse-induced enhancement of Ia synaptic transmission in spinal motoneurons of the rat, *J. Neurosci.*, 9, 2455, 1989.
3. Seburn, K.L. and Cope, T.C., Short-term afferent axotomy increases both strength and depression at Ia-motoneuron synapses in rat, *J. Neurosci.*, 18, 1142, 1998.
4. Brock, L.G., Coombs, J.S., and Eccles, J.C., The recording of potentials from motoneurones with an intracellular electrode, *J. Physiol.*, 117, 431, 1952.
5. Henneman, E. and Mendell, L.M., Functional organization of motoneuron pool and its inputs, in *Handbook of Physiology. The Nervous System. Motor Control*, Brookhart, J.M. and Mountcastle, V.B., Eds., American Physiological Society, Bethesda, MD, 1981, chap. 11.

6. Burke, R.E., Motor units: Anatomy, physiology, and functional organization, in *Handbook of Physiology. The Nervous System. Motor Control*, Brookhart, J.M. and Mountcastle, V.B., Eds., American Physiological Society, Bethesda, MD, 1981, 345.

7. Burke, R.E. and Rudomin, P., Spinal neurons and synapses, in *Handbook of Physiology. The Nervous System. Cellular Biology of Neurons*, Brookhart, J.M. and Mountcastle, V.B., Eds., American Physiological Society, Bethesda, MD, 1977, chap. 24.

8. Redman, S., Junctional mechanisms at group Ia synapses, *Prog. Neurobiol.*, 12, 33, 1979.

9. Kuno, M., *The Synapse: Function, Plasticity, and Neurotrophism*, Oxford University Press, Oxford, 1995.

10. Rudomin, P., Romo, R., and Mendell, L., *Presynaptic Inhibition and Neural Control*, Oxford University Press, New York, 1998.

11. Burke, R.E., Fleshman, J.W., and Segev I., Factors that control the efficacy of group Ia synapses in alpha-motoneurons, *J. Physiol.*, 83, 133, 1988.

12. Eccles, J.C., *The Physiology of Synapses*, Academic Press, New York, 1964.

13. Lin, J.H. et al., Functionally related motor neuron pool and muscle sensory afferent subtypes defined by coordinate ETS gene expression [see comments], *Cell*, 95, 393, 1998.

14. Brown, A.G., *Organization in the Spinal Cord*, Springer-Verlag, Berlin, 1981.

15. Mendell, L.M. and Henneman, E., Terminals of single Ia fibers: location, density, and distribution within a pool of 300 homonymous motoneurons, *J. Neurophysiol.*, 34, 171, 1971.

16. Prochazka, A., Ensemble inputs to alpha-motoneurons during movement, in *The Motor Unit — Physiology, Diseases, Regeneration*, Dengler, R., Ed., Urban & Schwarzenberg, Munich, 33.

17. Scott, J.G. and Mendell, L.M., Individual EPSPs produced by single triceps surae Ia afferent fibers in homonymous and heteronymous motoneurons, *J. Neurophysiol.*, 39, 679, 1976.

18. Fleshman, J.W., Munson, J.B., and Sypert, G.W., Homonymous projection of individual group Ia-fibers to physiologically characterized medial gastrocnemius motoneurons in the cat, *J. Neurophysiol.*, 46, 1339, 1981.

19. Harrison, P.J. and Taylor, A., Individual excitatory post-synaptic potentials due to muscle spindle I-a afferents in cat triceps, *J. Physiol.*, 312, 455, 1981.

20. Cope, T.C., Hickman, K.R., and Botterman, B.R., Acute effects of spinal transection on EPSPs produced by single homonymous Ia-fibers in soleus alpha-motoneurons in the cat, *J. Neurophysiol.*, 60, 1678, 1988. [published erratum appears in *J. Neurophysiol.*, 61(3), 1989].

21. Eccles, J.C., Eccles, R.M., and Lundberg, A., The convergence of monosynaptic excitatory afferents on to many different species of alpha motoneurones, *J. Physiol.*, 137, 22, 1957.

22. Burke, R.E., Group Ia synaptic input to fast and slow twitch motor units of cat triceps surae, *J. Physiol.*, 196, 605, 1968.

23. Peshori, K.R., Collins, W.F., III, and Mendell, L.M., EPSP amplitude modulation at the rat Ia-alpha motoneuron synapse: effects of GABA-B receptor agonists and antagonists, *J. Neurophysiol.*, 79, 181, 1998.

24. Burke, R.E., Synaptic efficacy and the control of neuronal input-output relations, *TINS*, 10, 42, 1987.

25. Lawson, S.N. and Waddell, P.J., Soma neurofilament immunoreactivity is related to cell size and fiber conduction velocity in rat primary sensory neurons, *J. Physiol.*, 435, 41, 1991.

26. Watt, D.G.D. et al., Analysis of muscle receptor connections by spike-triggered averaging. 1. Spindle primary and tendon organ afferents, *J. Neurophysiol.*, 39, 1375, 1976.

27. Munson, J.B. and Sypert, W., Properties of single central Ia afferent fibers projecting to motoneurons, *J. Physiol.*, 296, 315, 1979.

28. Munson, J.B. et al., Monosynaptic projections of individual spindle group II afferents to type-identified medial gastrocnemius motoneurons in the cat, *J. Neurophysiol.*, 48, 1164, 1982.

29. Stauffer, E.K. et al., Analysis of muscle receptor connections by spike-triggered averaging. 2. Spindle group II afferents, *J. Neurophysiol.*, 39, 1393, 1976.

30. Eccles, J.C., Eccles, R.M., and Lundberg, A., Synaptic actions on motoneurons in relation to the two components of the group I muscle afferent volley, *J. Physiol.*, 136, 527, 1957.

31. Eccles, J.C., Eccles, R.M., and Lundberg, A., Synaptic actions on motoneurones caused by impulses in golgi tendon organ afferents, *J. Physiol.*, 138, 227, 1957.

32. Fetz, E.E. et al., Autogenetic inhibition of motoneurones by impulses in group Ia muscle spindle afferents, *J. Physiol.*, 293, 173, 1979.

33. Edwards, F.R. et al., Reduction by baclofen of monosynaptic EPSPs in lumbosacral motoneurones of the anaesthetized cat, *J. Physiol.*, 416, 539, 1989.

34. Heckman, C.J. and Binder M.D., Analysis of effective synaptic currents generated by homonymous Ia afferent fibers in motoneurons of the cat, *J. Neurophysiol.*, 60, 1946, 1988.

35. Nichols, R., Receptor mechanisms underlying heterogenic reflexes among the triceps surae muscles of the cat, *J. Neurophysiol.*, 81, 467, 1999.

36. Lee, R.H. and Heckman, C.J., Adjustable amplification of synaptic input in the dendrites of spinal motoneurons *in vivo, J. Neurosci.*, 20, 6734, 2000.

37. Kullmann, D.M., Martin, R.L., and Redman, S.J., Reduction by general anaesthetics of group Ia excitatory postsynaptic potentials and currents in the cat spinal cord, *J. Physiol.*, 412, 277, 1989.

38. Fetz, E.E. and Gustafsson, B., Relation between shapes of post-synaptic potentials and changes in firing probability of cat motoneurones, *J. Physiol. (Lond.)*, 341, 387, 1983.

39. Gustafsson, B. and McCrea, D., Influence of stretch-evoked synaptic potentials on firing probability of cat spinal motoneurones, *J. Physiol.*, 347, 431, 1984.

40. Cope, T.C., Fetz, E.E., and Matsumura, M., Cross-correlation assessment of synaptic strength of single Ia fiber connections with triceps surae motoneurones in cats, *J. Physiol. (Lond.)*, 390, 161, 1987.

41. Clark, B.D. and Cope, T.C., Frequency-dependent synaptic depression modifies postsynaptic firing probability in cats, *J. Physiol. (Lond.)*, 512, 189, 1998.

42. Curtis, D.R. and Eccles J.C., Synaptic action during and after repetitive stimulation, *J. Physiol.*, 150, 374, 1960.

43. Honig, M.G., Collins, W.F., III, and Mendell, L.M., α-Motoneuron EPSPs exhibit different frequency sensitivities to single Ia-afferent fiber stimulation, *J. Neurophysiol.*, 49, 886, 1983.

44. Lev-Tov, A., Pinter, M.J., and Burke, R.E., Posttetanic potentiation of group Ia EPSPs: Possible mechanisms for differential distribution among medial gastrocnemius motoneurons, *J. Neurophysiol.*, 50, 379, 1983.

45. Luscher, H.-R., Ruenzel, P., and Henneman, E., How the size of motoneurones determines their susceptibility to discharge, *Nature*, 282, 859, 1979.

46. Luscher, H.-R., Ruenzel, P., and Henneman, E., Composite EPSPs in motoneurons of different sizes before and during PTP: implications for transmission failure and its relief in Ia projections, *J. Neurophysiol.*, 49, 269, 1983.

47. Mendell, L.M., Modifiability of spinal synapses, *Physiol. Rev.*, 64, 260, 1984.

48. Baldissera, F., Hultborn, H., and Illert, M., Integration in spinal neuronal systems, in *Handbook of Physiology*, Waverly Press, Baltimore, MD, 1981, chap. 12.

49. Hayward, L., Breitbach, D., and Rymer, W.Z., Increased inhibitory effects on close synergists during muscle fatigue in the decerebrate cat, *Brain Res.*, 440, 199, 1988.

50. Nichols, T.R., The organization of heterogenic reflexes among muscles crossing the ankle joint in the decerebrate cat, *J. Physiol. (Lond.)*, 419, 463, 1989.

51. Dacko, S.M., Sokoloff, A.J., and Cope, T.C., Recruitment of triceps surae motor units in the decerebrate cat. I. Independence of type S units in soleus and medial gastrocnemius muscles, *J. Neurophysiol.*, 75, 1997, 1996.

52. Devor, M., Abnormal excitability in injured axons, in *The Axon: Structure, Function and Pathophysiology*, Waxman, S.G., Kocsis, J.D., and Stys, P.K., Eds., Oxford University Press, New York, 1995, 530.

53. Seburn, K.L. et al., Decline in spontaneous activity of group Aalphabeta sensory afferents after sciatic nerve axotomy in rat, *Neurosci. Lett.*, 274, 41, 1999.

54. Haftel, V., *The Effects of Removal of Homonymous Afferent Input on Recruitment Order and Firing Rate of Medial Gastrocnemius Motoneurons in the Decerebrate, Paralyzed Cat*, Ph.D. thesis, Emory University, Atlanta, GA, 1999.

55. Michaelis, M., Liu, X., and Janig, W., Axotomized and intact muscle afferents but no skin afferents develop ongoing discharges of dorsal root ganglion origin after peripheral nerve lesion, *J. Neurosci.*, 20, 2742, 2000.

56. Gordon, T. et al., Long-term effects of axotomy on neural activity during cat locomotion, *J. Physiol.*, 303, 243, 1980.

57. Whelan, P.J. and Pearson, K.G., Plasticity in reflex pathways controlling stepping in the cat, *J. Neurophysiol.*, 78, 1643, 1997.

58. Titmus, M. and Faber, D., Axotomy-induced alterations in the electrophysiological characteristics of neurons, *Prog. Neurobiol.*, 35, 1, 1990.

59. Gillen, C., Korfhage, C., and Muller, H.W., Gene expression in nerve regeneration, *Neuroscientist*, 3, 112, 1997.

60. Gallego, R. et al., Disuse enhances synaptic efficacy in spinal mononeurones, *J. Physiol.*, 291, 191, 1979.

61. Sleeper, A.A. et al., Changes in expression of two tetrodotoxin-resistant sodium channels and their currents in dorsal root ganglion neurons after sciatic nerve injury but not rhizotomy, *J. Neurosci.*, 20, 7279, 2000.

62. Jeftinija, S. and Urban, L., Repetitive stimulation induced potentiation of excitatory transmission in the rat dorsal horn: an *in vitro* study, *J. Neurophysiol.*, 71, 216, 1994.

63. Carr, P.A. et al., Effect of sciatic nerve transection or TTX application on enzyme activity in rat spinal cord, *Neuroreport*, 9, 357, 1998.

64. Kanda, K. et al., The effects of blocking nerve conduction on retrograde HRP labeling of rat motoneuron, *Neurosci. Lett.*, 99, 153, 1989.

65. Sala, C. et al., Calcitonin gene-related peptide: possible role in formation and maintenance of neuromuscular junctions, *J. Neurosci.*, 15, 520, 1995.

66. Snider, W.D. and Harris, G.L., A physiological correlate of disuse-induced sprouting at the neuromuscular junction, *Nature*, 281, 69, 1979.

67. Tsujimoto, T., Umemiya, M., and Kuno, M., Terminal sprouting is not responsible for enhanced transmitter release at disused neuromuscular junctions of the rat, *J. Neurosci.*, 10, 2059, 1990.

68. Webb, C.B. and Cope, T.C., Modulation of Ia EPSP amplitude: the effects of chronic synaptic inactivity, *J. Neurosci.*, 12, 338, 1992.
69. Fields, R.D., Yu, C., and Nelson, P.G., Calcium, network activity, and the role of NMDA channels in synaptic plasticity *in vitro*, *J. Neurosci.*, 11, 134, 1991.
70. Stent, G.S., A physiological mechanism for Hebb's postulate of learning, *Proc. Natl. Acad. Sci. U.S.A.*, 70, 997, 1973.
71. Black, I.B., Trophic regulation of synaptic plasticity, *J. Neurobiol.*, 41, 108, 1999.
72. McAllister, A.K., Katz, L.C., and Lo, D.C., Neurotrophins and synaptic plasticity, *Annu. Rev. Neurosci.*, 22, 295, 1999.
73. Schuman, E.M., Neurotrophin regulation of synaptic transmission, *Curr. Opin. Neurobiol.*, 9, 105, 1999.
74. Lu, B. and Chow, A., Neurotrophins and hippocampal synaptic transmission and plasticity, *J. Neurosci. Res.*, 58, 76, 1999.
75. Kang, H. and Schuman, E.M., Long-lasting neurotrophin-induced enhancement of synaptic transmission in the adult hippocampus, *Science*, 267, 1658, 1995.
76. Henderson, C.E., Role of neurotrophic factors in neuronal development, *Curr. Opin. Neurobiol.*, 6, 64, 1996.
77. Goldring, J.M. et al., Reaction of synapses on motoneurones to section and restoration of peripheral sensory connexions in the cat, *J. Physiol.*, 309, 185, 1980.
78. Mendell, L.M. et al., Rescue of motoneuron and muscle afferent function in cats by regeneration into skin. II. Ia-motoneuron synapse, *J. Neurophysiol.*, 73, 662, 1995.
79. Munson, J.B., Johnson, R.D., and Mendell, L.M., NT-3 increases amplitude of EPSPs produced by axotomized group Ia afferents, *J. Neurophysiol.*, 77, 2209, 1997.
80. Mendell, L., Johnson, R., and Munson, J., Neurotrophin modulation of the monosynaptic reflex after peripheral nerve transection, *J. Neurosci.*, 19, 3162, 1999.
81. Barde, Y.A., Trophic factors and neuronal survival, *Neuron*, 2, 1525, 1989.
82. Korsching, S., The neurotrophic factor concept: a reexamination, *J. Neurosci.*, 13, 2739, 1993.
83. Davies, A.M., The neurotrophic hypothesis: where does it stand? *Phil. Trans. R. Soc. Lond. B*, 351, 389, 1996.
84. Conner, J.M., Lauterborn, J.C., and Gall, C.M., Anterograde transport of neurotrophin proteins in the CNS — a reassessment of the neurotrophic hypothesis, *Rev. Neurosci.*, 9, 91, 1998.
85. Funakoshi, H. et al., Differential expression of mRNAs for neurotrophins and their receptors after axotomy of the sciatic nerve, *J. Cell Biol.*, 123, 455, 1993.
86. Griesbeck, O. et al., Expression of neurotrohpins in skeletal muscle: quantitative comparison and significance for motoneuron survival and maintenance function, *J. Neurosci.*, 42, 21, 1995.
87. Ernfors, P. et al., Molecular cloning and neurotrophic activities of a protein with structural similarities to nerve growth factor: developmental and topographical expression in the brain, *Proc. Natl. Acad. Sci. U.S.A.*, 87, 5454, 1990.
88. Maisonpierre, P.C. et al., NT-3, BDNF, and NGF in the developing rat nervous system: parallel as well as reciprocal patterns of expression, *Neuron*, 5, 501, 1990.
89. Yamamoto, M. et al., Expression of mRNAs for neurotrophic factors (NGF, BDNF, NT-3, and GDNF) and their receptors (p75NGFR, trkA, trkB, and trkC) in the adult human peripheral nervous system and nonneural tissues, *Neurochem. Res.*, 21, 929, 1996.
90. Fernyhough, P., Diemel, L.T., and Tomlinson, D.R., Target tissue production and axonal transport of neurotrophin-3 are reduced in streptozotocin-diabetes rats, *Diabetologia*, 41, 300, 1998.

91. Funakoshi, H. et al., Muscle-derived neurotrophin-4 as an activity-dependent trophic signal for adult motor neurons, *Science*, 268, 1495, 1995.
92. Koliatsos, V.E. et al., Evidence that brain-derived neurotrophic factor is a trophic factor for motor neurons *in vivo*, *Neuron*, 10, 359, 1993.
93. Maisonpierre, P.C. et al., Neurotrophin-3: a neurotrophic factor related to NGF and BDNF, *Science*, 247, 1446, 1990.
94. Junier, M.P. et al., Regulation of growth factor gene expression in degenerating motoneurons of the murine mutant wobbler: a cellular patch-sampling/RT-PCR study, *Mol. Cell Neurosci.*, 12, 168, 1998.
95. Kobayashi, N.R. et al., Increased expression of BDNF and trkB mRNA in rat facial motoneurons after axotomy, *Eur. J. Neurosci.*, 8, 1018, 1996.
96. Scarisbrick, I., Isackson P., and Windebank, A., Differential expression of brain-derived neutrophic factor, neurotrophin-3, and neurotrophin-4/5 in the adult rat spinal cord: regulation by the glutamate receptor agonist kainic acid, *J. Neurosci.*, 18, 7757, 1999.
97. Buck, C.R., Seburn, K.L., and Cope, T.C., Neurotrophin expression by spinal motoneurons in adult and developing rats, *J. Comp. Neurol.*, 416, 309, 2000.
98. Copray, S. and Kernell, D., Neurotrophins and trk-receptors in adult rat spinal motoneurons: differences related to cell size but not to 'slow/fast' specialization, *Neurosci. Lett.*, 289, 217, 2000.
99. Karchewski, L.A. et al., Anatomical evidence supporting the potential for modulation by multiple neurotrophins in the majority of adult lumbar sensory neurons, *J. Comp. Neurol.*, 413, 327, 1999.
100. Li, B., Wang, Z., and Zhu, P., [Changes of BDNF mRNA by molecular hybridization during embryonic spinal cord repairing injury of adult rats], *Chung-Hua I Hsueh Tsa Chih [Chin. Med. J.]*, 77, 516, 1997.
101. Zhou, X.F. et al., Satellite-cell-derived nerve growth factor and neurotrophin-3 are involved in noradrenergic sprouting in the dorsal root ganglia following peripheral nerve injury in the rat, *Eur. J. Neurosci.*, 11, 1711, 1999.
102. Zhou, X.F. and Rush, R.A., Localization of neurotrophin-3-like immunoreactivity in the rat central nervous system, *Brain Res.*, 643, 162, 1994.
103. Nishio, T., Sunohara, N., and Furukawa, S., Neutrophin switching in spinal motoneurons of amyotrophic lateral sclerosis, *Neuroreport*, 9, 1661, 1998.
104. Dreyfus, C.F. et al., Expression of neurotrophins in the adult spinal cord *in vivo*, *J. Neurosci. Res.*, 56, 1, 1999.
105. Elkabes, S., Peng, L., and Black, I.B., Lipopolysaccharide differentially regulates microglial trk receptor and neurotrophin expression, *J. Neurosci. Res.*, 54, 117, 1998.
106. Hendry, I.A., Developmental changes in tissue and plasma concentrations of the biologically active species of nerve growth factor in the mouse, by using a two-site radioimmunoassay, *Biochem. J.*, 128, 1265, 1972.
107. Zhang, S. et al., Neurotrophin 4/5 immunoassay: identification of sources of errors for the quantification of neurotrophins, *J. Neurosci. Meth.*, 99, 119, 2000.
108. Zhang, S.H. et al., Measurement of neurotrophin 4/5 in rat tissues by a sensitive immunoassay, *J. Neurosci. Meth.*, 89, 69, 1999.
109. Balkowiec, A. and Katz, D.M., Activity-dependent release of endogenous brain-derived neurotrophic factor from primary sensory neurons detected by ELISA *in situ*, *J. Neurosci.*, 20, 7417, 2000.
110. Cohen, S., Levi-Montalcini, R., and Hamburger, V., A nerve growth-stimulating factor isolated from sarcomas 37 and 180, *Proc. Natl. Acad. Sci. U.S.A.*, 40, 1014, 1954.

111. Chao, M.V. and Hempstead, B.L., p75 and Trk: a two-receptor system, *Trends Neurosci.*, 18, 321, 1995.

112. Johnson, H., Hokfelt, T., and Ulfhake, B., Decreased expression of TrkB and TrkC mRNAs in spinal motoneurons of aged rats, *Eur. J. Neurosci.*, 8, 494, 1996.

113. Johnson, H., Hokfelt, T., and Ulfhake, B., Expression of p75(NTR), trkB and trkC in nonmanipulated and axotomized motoneurons of aged rats, *Brain Res. Mol. Brain Res.*, 69, 21, 1999.

114. Bergman, E., Fundin, B.T., and Ulfhake, B., Effects of aging and axotomy on the expression of neurotrophin receptors in primary sensory neurons, *J. Comp. Neurol.*, 410, 368, 1999.

115. Lu, B. et al., Expression of NGF and NGF receptor mRNAs in the developing brain: evidence for local delivery and action of NGF, *Exp. Neurol.*, 104, 191, 1989.

116. Schecterson, L.C. and Bothwell, M., Novel roles for neurotrophins are suggested by BDNF and NT-3 mRNA expression in developing neurons, *Neuron*, 9, 449, 1992.

117. Acheson, A. and Lindsay, R.M., Non-target-derived roles of the neurotropins, *Phil. Trans. R. Soc. Lond. B*, 351, 417, 1996.

118. Zhou, X. and Rush, R.A., Endogenous brain-derived neurotrophic factor is anterogradely transported in primary sensory neurons, *Neuroscience*, 74, 945, 1996.

119. Schutte, A. et al., The endogenous survival promotion of axotomized rat corticospinal neurons by brain-derived neurotrophic factor is mediated via paracrine, rather than autocrine mechanisms, *Neurosci. Lett.*, 290, 185, 2000.

120. Xu, B. et al., The role of brain-derived neurotrophic factor receptors in the mature hippocampus: modulation of long-term potentiation through a presynaptic mechanism involving TrkB, *J. Neurosci.*, 20, 6888, 2000.

121. Zhang, Q. et al., Effect of growth factors on substance P mRNA expression in axotomized dorsal root ganglia, *Neuroreport*, 6, 1309, 1995.

122. Zhang, Y. et al., Cell surface Trk receptors mediate NGF-induced survival while internalized receptors regulate NGF-induced differentiation, *J. Neurosci.*, 20, 5671, 2000.

123. Tsui-Pierchala, B.A., Putcha, G.V., and Johnson, E.M., Jr., Phosphatidylinositol 3-kinase is required for the trophic, but not the survival-promoting, actions of NGF on sympathetic neurons, *J. Neurosci.*, 20, 7228, 2000.

124. Ernfors, P. et al., Expression of nerve growth factor receptor mRNA is developmentally regulated and increased after axotomy in rat spinal cord motoneurons, *Neuron*, 2, 1605, 1989.

125. Bussmann, K.A. and Sofroniew, M.V., Re-expression of p75NTR by adult motor neurons after axotomy is triggered by retrograde transport of a positive signal from axons regrowing through damaged or denervated peripheral nerve tissue, *Neuroscience*, 91, 273, 1999.

126. Munson, J.B., Shelton, D.L., and McMahon, S.B., Adult mammalian sensory and motor neurons: roles of endogenous neurotrophins and rescue by exogenous neurotrophins after axotomy, *J. Neurosci.*, 17, 470, 1997.

127. Rutherford, L.C., Nelson, S.B., and Turrigiano, G.G., BDNF has opposite effects on the quantal amplitude of pyramidal neuron and interneuron excitatory synapses, *Neuron*, 21, 521, 1998.

128. Eriksson, N.P., Lindsay, R.M., and Aldskogius, H., BDNF and NT-3 rescue sensory but not motoneurones following axotomy in the neonate [see comments], *Neuroreport*, 5, 1445, 1994.

129. Groves, M.J., An S.F., Giometto B., et al., Inhibition of sensory neuron apoptosis and prevention of loss by NT-3 administration following axotomy, *Exper. Neurol.*, 155, 284, 1999.
130. Ljungberg, C. et al., The neurotrophins NGF and NT-3 reduce sensory neuronal loss in adult rat after peripheral nerve lesion, *Neurosci. Lett.*, 262, 29, 1999.
131. Oyelese, A.A. et al., Differential effects of NGF and BDNF on axotomy-induced changes in GABA(A)-receptor-mediated conductance and sodium currents in cutaneous afferent neurons, *J. Neurophysiol.*, 78, 31, 1997.
132. Thoenen, H., Neurotrophins and neuronal plasticity, *Science*, 270, 593, 1995.
133. Skup, M. et al., Locomotion induces changes in Trk B receptors in small diameter cells of the spinal cord, *Acta Neurobiol. Exper.*, 60, 371, 2000.
134. Collins, W.F., III and Honig, M.G., Mendell L.M., Heterogeneity of group Ia synapses on homonymous a-motoneurons as revealed by high-frequency stimulation of Ia afferent fibers, *J. Neurophysiol.*, 52, 980, 1984.
135. Davis, B.M., Collins, W.F., III, and Mendell, L.M., Potentiation of transmission at Ia-motoneuron connections induced by repeated short bursts of afferent activity, *J. Neurophysiol.*, 54, 1541, 1985.
136. Thies, R.E., Neuromuscular depression and the apparent depletion of transmitter in mammalian muscle, *J. Neurophysiol.*, 28, 427, 1965.
137. Dobrunz, L.E. and Stevens, C.F., Heterogeneity of release probability, facilitation, and depletion at central synapses, *Neuron*, 18, 995, 1997.
138. Hsu, S.-F., Augustine, G.J., and Jackson, M.B., Adaptation of Ca2+-triggered exocytosis in presynaptic terminals, *Neuron*, 17, 501, 1996.
139. Bellingham, M.C. and Walmsley, B., A novel presynaptic inhibitory mechanism underlies paired pulse depression at a fast central synapse, *Neuron*, 23, 159, 1999.
140. Otis, T., Zhang, S., and Trussell, L.O., Direct measurement of AMPA receptor desensitization induced by glutamatergic synaptic transmission, *J. Neurosci.*, 16, 7496, 1996.
141. Nelson, S.G. et al., Immediate increase in Ia-motoneuron synaptic transmission caudal to spinal cord transection, *J. Neurophysiol.*, 42, 655, 1979.
142. Engberg, I. et al., An analysis of synaptic transmission to motoneurones in the cat spinal cord using a new selective receptor blocker, *Acta Physiol. Scand.*, 148, 97, 1993.
143. Walmsley, B. and Bolton P.S., An *in vivo* pharmacological study of single group Ia fiber contacts with motoneurones in the cat spinal cord, *J. Physiol.*, 481, 731, 1994.
144. Pinco, M. and Lev-Tov, A., Modulation of monosynaptic excitation in the neonatal rat spinal cord, *J. Neurophysiol.*, 70, 1151, 1993.
145. Ziskind-Conhaim, L., NMDA receptors mediate poly- and monosynaptic potentials in rat embryos, *J. Neurosci.*, 10, 125, 1990.
146. Arvanov, V.L., Seebach, B.S., and Mendell, L.M., NT-3 evokes an LTP-like facilitation of AMPA/kainate receptor-mediated synaptic transmission in the neonatal rat spinal cord, *J. Neurophysiol.*, 84, 752, 2000.
147. Jahr, C.E. and Yoshioka, K., Ia afferent excitation of motoneurones in the *in vitro* new-born rat spinal cord is selectively antagonized by kynurenate, *J. Physiol.*, 370, 515, 1986.
148. Alvarez, F.J. et al., Downregulation of metabotropic glutamate receptor Ia in motoneurons after axotomy, *Neuroreport*, 8, 1711, 1997.
149. Luscher, C. et al., Role of AMPA receptor cycling in synaptic transmission and plasticity, *Neuron*, 24, 649, 1999.

150. Seeburg, P.H., Higuchi, M., and Sprengel, R., RNA editing of brain glutamate receptor channels: mechanism and physiology, *Brain Res. Brain Res. Rev.*, 26, 217, 1998.
151. Nusser, Z., AMPA and NMDA receptors: similarities and differences in their synaptic distribution, *Curr. Opin. Neurobiol.*, 10, 337, 2000.
152. Turrigiano, G.G., AMPA receptors unbound: membrane cycling and synaptic plasticity, *Neuron*, 26, 5, 2000.
153. Carroll, R.C. et al., Dynamin-dependent endocytosis of ionotropic glutamate receptors, *PNAS*, 96, 14112, 1999.
154. Kim, J.H. and Huganir, R.L., Organization and regulation of proteins at synapses *Curr. Opin. Cell Biol.*, 11, 248, 1999. [Published erratum appears in *Curr. Opin. Cell Biol.* 11(3), 407, 1999.]
155. Alvarez F.J. et al., Factors regulating AMPA-type glutamate receptor subunit changes induced by sciatic nerve injury in rats, *J. Comp. Neurol.*, 426, 229, 2000.
156. Furuyama, T. et al., Region-specific expression of subunits of ionotropic glutamate receptors (AMPA-type, KA-type and NMDA receptors) in the rat spinal cord with special reference to nociception, *Brain Res. Mol. Brain Res.*, 18, 141, 1993.
157. Tachibana, M. et al., Light and electron microscopic immunocytochemical localization of AMPA- selective glutamate receptors in the rat spinal cord, *J. Comp. Neurol.*, 344, 431, 1994.
158. Popratiloff, A. et al., Glutamate receptors in spinal motoneurons after sciatic nerve transection, *Neuroscience*, 74, 953, 1996.
159. Kennis, J.H.H. and Holstege, J.C., A differential and time-dependent decrease in AMPA-type glutamate receptor subunits in spinal motoneurons after sciatic nerve injury, *Exper. Neurol.*, 147, 18, 1997.
160. Tang, F. and Sim, M., Expression of glutamate receptor subunits 2/3 and 4 in the hypoglossal nucleus of the rat after neurectomy, *Exp. Brain Res.*, 117, 453, 1997.
161. Robinson, D. and Ellenberger, H., Distribution of N-methyl-D-aspartate and non-N-methyl-D-aspartate glutamate receptor subunits on respiratory motor and premotor neurons in the rat, *J. Comp. Neurol.*, 389, 94, 1997.
162. Jonas, P. and Burnashev, N., Molecular mechanisms controlling calcium entry through AMPA-type glutamate receptor channels, *Neuron*, 15, 987, 1995.
163. Swanson, G.T., Kamboj, S.K., and Cull-Candy S.G., Single-channel properties of recombinant AMPA receptors depend on RNA editing, splice variation, and subunit composition, *J. Neurosci.*, 17, 58, 1997.
164. Gu, J.G. et al., Synaptic strengthening through activation of Ca2+-permeable AMPA receptors, *Nature*, 381, 793, 1996.
165. Mahanty, N.K. and Pankaj, S., Calcium-permeable AMPA receptors mediate long-term potentiation in interneurons in the amygdala, *Nature*, 394, 683, 1998.
166. Rozov, A. et al., Facilitation of currents through rat Ca2+-permeable AMPA receptor channels by activity-dependent relief from polyamine block, *J. Physiol. (Lond.)*, 511, 361, 1998.

13 The Organization of Distributed Proprioceptive Feedback in the Chronic Spinal Cat

T. Richard Nichols and Timothy C. Cope

CONTENTS

13.1 INTRODUCTION

Interneurons in the mammalian spinal cord receive convergent, sensory input from many sources, including muscles of the limbs and trunk, joints, and skin, and from a wide variety of receptors in these structures.[1,2] This convergence constitutes the substrate for an extensive neural network in the spinal cord. This network links sensory information with the motor apparatus and is thought to modulate central commands,[3] regulate central pattern generators,[4] and provide postural regulation during different motor behaviors.[5–8] In order to better understand the functions of this distributed network, knowledge of at least three aspects of the system is required. The first aspect comprises the dynamic properties of the component synaptic linkages and of the musculoskeletal apparatus. These dynamic properties include the nonlinear and time-varying transformations between sensory input and motor output as well as the dependence of these transformations on activation history.[9,10] The second aspect is the state-dependence of sensory–motor transformations. The state can be defined in terms of behavioral context,[4,11] the lengths and forces of the relevant muscles,[12,13] and state variables representing nonmechanical modalities such as temperature and metabolite concentrations. The third kind of information required for an understanding of this system is the spatial organization of sensory convergence. That is, it is crucial to have the map that links specific receptors and anatomical locations to specific motor nuclei.[6,14]

Progress has been made in the explication of these three aspects with respect to cutaneous afferents and the muscle proprioceptors, muscle spindles, and Golgi tendon organs.[1,2,4,6,15–17] For example, afferent information from muscle spindle receptors serves to regulate the mechanical properties of joints in a directionally specific manner and to increase mechanical coupling between joints by virtue of the dynamic properties and projections of these receptors. The dynamic properties of primary receptors in muscle spindles and the properties of skeletal muscle are matched to result in spring-like behavior.[1,2,4,6,15–20] Regulation of the mechanical properties of muscle occurs for a wide range of forces and lengths in muscle[20,21] as well as for different behavioral contexts.[22,23] During locomotion, continuous motion causes muscles to be more intrinsically spring-like and the reflex contributions to muscular stiffness to decrease.[10,24] In terms of spatial distribution, length feedback to a given motor pool originates from the parent muscle and from muscles with closely related mechanical functions.[6,7,25,26] The result is that length feedback regulates muscular stiffness in a directionally specific way at a given joint and also enhances the mechanical coupling between joints through the actions of biarticular muscles.

A similar analysis has been applied to feedback arising from tension receptors in skeletal muscle. Feedback from Golgi tendon organs originates mainly from heteronymous sources, but is integrated postsynaptically with feedback from muscle spindle receptors. In the decerebrate state without locomotion, this force feedback is inhibitory and increases with the background tension in the muscle of origin independently of the length of that muscle.[16] The inhibitory force feedback develops more slowly than the length feedback and so contributes significantly to intermuscular coordination after the initial rapid response due to muscle spindle receptors. Force feedback arises from muscles that span different joints and different axes of rotation and, therefore, tends to regulate the coupling of these degrees of freedom.[7,27–30] Finally, under conditions of locomotion, excitatory pathways from muscle spindle receptors and Golgi tendon organs are opened and enhance the load-bearing capacity of the limbs.[4,8] These examples illustrate that knowledge of the aspects of dynamic properties, state dependence, and spatial distribution of proprioceptive feedback has led to the hypothesis that these pathways regulate the stiffness of limbs and interjoint coordination. This system may underlie the regulation of intersegmental dynamics[31] and more complex postural responses involving the four limbs and trunk.[32,33]

13.2 THE CLASP-KNIFE RESPONSE

In spinal injury, a constellation of additional reflex pathways becomes activated or inappropriately amplified.[34-36] One of the most thoroughly studied of these reactions is the clasp-knife response,[37] in which an abrupt reduction in force results from either the stretch of an extensor muscle or forcible flexion of an intact limb. Recent work has shown that this response is mediated by group III and IV muscle afferents and resembles a flexion-withdrawal reflex evoked by muscle stretch.[38-40] Clasp-knife responses also include autogenic inhibition,[36,39] and stretch of extensor muscles leads to widespread inhibition of other extensors.[39] Clasp-knife inhibition is also thought to require rather large stretches and forces for expression and adapts with repeated application of the stimulus.[39] This reflex may have a protective function against musculoskeletal injury in normal subjects, but it can be evoked in neurologically damaged subjects in the absence of muscle damage.[39]

Although the receptor mechanisms underlying the clasp-knife response are better understood now, a number of issues remain unresolved. First, it is not clear how clasp-knife inhibition is distributed among different categories of muscles, such as stabilizing muscles and biarticular muscles. Second, the apparent requirement for high forces and large stretch amplitudes requires reinvestigation to check whether the relevant receptors are activated during a wide range of physiological conditions. Since clasp-knife inhibition is expressed with little delay after section of the spinal cord, the receptors respond even without any damage to the muscle. A more detailed assessment of their response properties may provide insights into the normal functions of these pathways. Third, it is not clear how clasp-knife inhibition is integrated with force-dependent inhibition from Golgi tendon organs. Clasp-knife inhibition includes an autogenic component[36,39] while force-dependent inhibition does not,[16] but it is not clear how these pathways are combined for muscles receiving both. Information on this issue is important to understand how clasp-knife inhibition interacts with other postural mechanisms.

Our investigations on animals with chronic spinal injuries were motivated by the need for (1) a global perspective on the distribution of reflexes among muscle species, (2) a more detailed description of the dynamics and state dependence of pathways released in spinal injury, and (3) information concerning the changes that occur with time in the days and weeks following spinal injury. This information is needed to guide investigations of abnormal reflex mechanisms at the cellular level and to further understand the processing of information from group III and IV receptors in the spinal cord. Finally, these data provide a baseline description of reflex organization of the damaged spinal cord that can be used to test the success of attempts at repair and rehabilitation. Animals with long-standing spinal injuries are characterized by a poverty of reflex pathways[41] unless some stance training has been provided.[42] An evaluation of spinal pathways including clasp-knife inhibition, therefore, provides a measure of the effectiveness of rehabilitation.

13.3 METHODS

The studies reported here were conducted using five animals subjected to complete spinal transection at the T13 level under deep surgical anesthesia. Following recovery from the surgery and administration of appropriate antibiotics and analgesics, the animals were housed in pairs in large cages containing 12 in of shredded paper. These measures promoted movement of the animals and prevented the formation of decubitus ulcers. The animals showed little sign of distress under these conditions. Bladders were expressed manually twice daily, and the animals were allowed to move outside the cage every day. Survival times ranged from 6 to 28 days.[6,14,17,22,28] At the end of the survival period, terminal experiments were performed in which the animals were decerebrated under deep surgical anesthesia. All brain tissue rostral to the intercollicular transection was removed from the cranium before anesthesia was withdrawn. The tendons of selected muscles crossing the ankle joint and the quadriceps muscles were isolated and attached in a pair-wise fashion to two stretching devices for the evaluation of autogenic and heterogenic reflexes.[12,16,27]

Muscles were activated in sets using electrical stimulation of ipsilateral or contralateral posterior tibial nerves. During decaying crossed extension or flexion reflexes, a muscle pair was subjected to stretches consisting of a 4-mm lengthening completed in 100 ms, a 300-ms hold, and a return to the original length (see Fig. 13.1). The stretches were delivered according to one of three protocols. Either one muscle was stretched repeatedly (protocol 1), one muscle was stretched in alternation with the stretch of both muscles (protocol 2), or each muscle was stretched individually followed by stretch of both muscles (protocol 3). These procedures allowed the evaluation of both autogenic and heterogenic reflexes with the same data sets. The detailed temporal features of the responses were extracted from the computerized records. The influence of state was examined by controlling initial muscle length and allowing background force to vary, and by comparing results from animals with spinal injury to results obtained from control decerebrate animals. The spatial distribution of pathways was investigated by measuring autogenic and heterogenic reflexes in of a number of muscles in a given preparation.

13.4 RESULTS

13.4.1 DYNAMIC FEATURES OF CLASP-KNIFE RESPONSES

A hallmark of clasp-knife inhibition after spinal injury was profound autogenic inhibition that occurs with a latency exceeding 80 ms (Fig. 13.1A). This autogenic inhibition could be observed in the soleus muscle (SOL) during ongoing contraction up to at least 4 weeks after the transection (Fig. 13.1A). In this short-term chronic state, relatively modest forces (approximately 7 N) and stretch amplitudes (4 mm) could elicit clasp-knife inhibition. Furthermore, reciprocal inhibition received from the tibialis anterior muscle (TA) was unaffected by the lesion[43] and could combine with autogenic inhibition (Figs. 13.1A, 13.2A). In contrast, TA did not exhibit autogenic inhibition for any of the survival periods (Fig. 13.1B). This observation

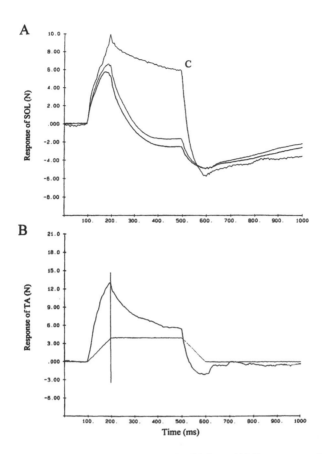

FIGURE 13.1 Autogenic inhibition following spinal injury. (A) Force traces from the soleus muscles (SOL) of a control decerebrate animal (C) and from another decerebrate animal 4 weeks following spinal transection at the T13 level obtained during crossed-extension reflex (electrical stimulation of contralateral posterior tibial nerve at 40 Hz). The force traces represent responses to ramp and hold stretches with the same temporal parameters and amplitude (4 mm) as the length record shown in (B). The background forces were subtracted from all traces. The steeper initial trajectory of the control trace (C) probably resulted from the slightly higher background tension for this response (7.4 N) than the matched responses for the spinalized animal (6.3 and 6.2 N). The heavier trace was obtained during simultaneous stretch of the tibialis anterior muscle (TA) and illustrates the presence of control levels of reciprocal inhibition. (B) Response of TA during a flexion withdrawal reflex that shows the adaptation of the stretch reflex typical of the control decerebrate preparation. The corresponding length record is also shown.

is consistent with previous findings that flexor muscles in general are unaffected by the lesion.[39]

When soleus or quadriceps (QUAD) muscles were subjected to repeated stretches during a contraction, autogenic inhibition did not progressively diminish but instead remained unchanged for the duration of the contraction (Fig. 13.2A,B). It has been suggested that the adaptation of clasp-knife inhibition with repeated

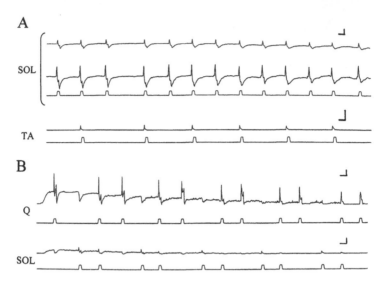

FIGURE 13.2 Undiminished clasp-knife inhibition during ongoing contraction. (A) Responses of SOL and TA during a prolonged rebound contraction with protocol 2. The force traces for SOL show autogenic inhibition for a series of 13 consecutive stretches. The increased inhibition for the even-numbered records represents reciprocal inhibition from TA. The 5 traces are (1) SOL force; (2) amplified SOL force with background subtracted; (3) SOL length; (4) TA force; (5) TA length. Survival, 28 d. Calibration bars apply to the unamplified traces and represent 5 N and 1 s. (B) Responses of SOL and QUAD during crossed-extension reflex using protocol 3. Autogenic inhibition for both muscles and bidirectional heterogenic inhibition are evident. Note that autogenic inhibition on QUAD (shown in records 1, 4, 7, ...) and heterogenic inhibition on QUAD (records 2, 5, 8, ...) combine when both muscles are stretched together (records 3, 6, 9, ...). Heterogenic inhibition most likely consists of both clasp-knife inhibition and force feedback from Golgi tendon organs. The traces are from top to bottom: QUAD force; QUAD length; SOL force; SOL length. Survival: 17d. Calibration bars represent 5 N and 1 s.

stretch requires the complete relaxation of the muscle between perturbations.[38,39] The present result confirms this suggestion and indicates that the internal mechanical environment of the muscle is critically important to the response properties of the receptors. During ongoing postural regulation or movement, the receptors remain capable of responding indefinitely to modest mechanical inputs. In addition, autogenic inhibition was expressed even as background force decayed to low levels (Fig. 13.2B). This observation indicates that the receptors responsible for clasp-knife inhibition were responsive to mechanical changes well within the normal physiological range.

The widespread distribution of clasp-knife inhibition was also observed, as illustrated by the interactions between SOL and QUAD (Fig. 13.2B). These muscles are normally linked by inhibitory force feedback from Golgi tendon organs,[30] but the inhibitory interactions are greatly exaggerated following spinal injury (Fig. 13.2B). The heterogenic inhibitory responses were large enough to reduce the force in the destination muscle to nearly zero. The increased inhibition most likely resulted from the addition of autogenic and heterogenic components of clasp-knife

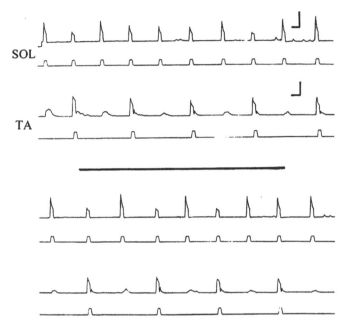

FIGURE 13.3 Clasp-knife excitation and adaptation of receptors. Stretch responses of SOL and TA according to protocol 2 during quiescent background conditions. During stretch of SOL alone (odd records), the isometric responses of TA are excitatory. During successive repetition of the stretch sequence, the isometric responses of TA (odd records) diminish. During combined stretch (even records), the responses of TA are prolonged by clasp-knife excitation. Comparison of odd and even records for SOL reveals reciprocal inhibition from TA that resembles results from control decerebrate animals. Survival, 28 d. The traces are from top to bottom: SOL force; SOL length; TA force; TA length. The lower panel shows the continuation of the results in the upper panel. Calibration bars represent 10 N for trace 1, 5 N for trace 3, and 1 s.

inhibition and force-dependent inhibition from Golgi tendon organs. It was not possible to distinguish this possibility from an increase in the more rapid force-dependent inhibition from Golgi tendon organs since the force records did not generally show two distinct phases of inhibition. However, the autogenic and heterogenic components of inhibition onto QUAD were clearly additive (Fig. 13.2B). Since force-dependent inhibition from Golgi tendon organs is most likely postsynaptic,[16] it is parsimonious to conclude that all three forms of inhibition add together.

In addition to these inhibitory actions that appear following spinal injury, stretch of the same muscles leads to excitation of flexors.[39] This organizational feature was confirmed in the present study when stretches were applied to SOL or the gastrocnemius muscles. Given the normally reciprocal patterns of activation of SOL and TA, clasp-knife excitation was most readily observed with quiescent backgrounds in the two muscles (Fig. 13.3). Magnitudes of reciprocal inhibition from TA to SOL were similar to those observed in control decerebrate preparations,[43] while the normally small reciprocal inhibition from SOL to TA[43] was replaced or outweighed by clasp-knife excitation (Fig. 13.3, odd records). Under the conditions of quiescent

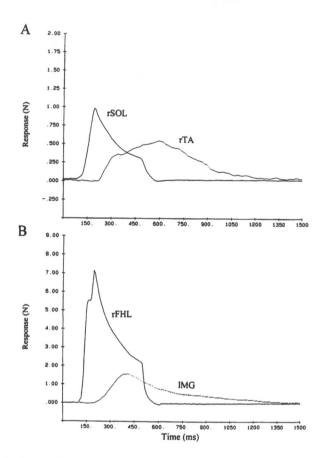

FIGURE 13.4 Clasp-knife excitation. (A) Responses of SOL and TA of the right hindlimb to stretch of SOL, selected from the data shown in Fig. 13.3. The excitatory response of TA occurred with a latency of approximately 100 ms. The vertical scale applies to the response of TA only. The response of SOL was compressed 10 times and included in order to compare the timing of the two responses. (B) Responses of the flexor hallucis longus muscle (FHL) and the contralateral medial gastrocnemius muscle (MG) to stretch of FHL. The excitatory response of the left MG occurred with a latency of approximately 100 ms.

background, the adaptation of the group III and IV receptors of origin was also apparent during successive stretches of S. When both muscles were stretched together, the response of TA was prolonged apparently due to the reciprocal excitation from SOL (Fig. 13.3, even records). The latency of clasp-knife excitation was approximately 100 ms and comparable to that observed for autogenic inhibition (Fig. 13.4A).

It was also observed that stretch of antigravity muscles evoked excitatory responses in the contralateral limb (Fig. 13.4B). Stretch of either QUAD or FHL led to an excitatory response in the contralateral medial gastrocnemius muscle with a latency of approximately 100 ms. This latency is similar to that of the excitatory response of TA to stretch of either SOL or G. The latency of approximately 100 ms for clasp-knife inhibition and excitation suggests that group IV receptors play a prominent role in mediating these responses. Contralateral responses are usually not observed in control decerebrate animals.

13.4.2 Dependence of Clasp-Knife Responses on Input Parameters and State

13.4.2.1 Amplitude

We reinvestigated the range of amplitudes, lengths, and forces over which clasp-knife responses are observed in actively contracting muscles to determine if the adequate stimuli for the associated receptors fell within the normal physiological range. Previous studies in acutely spinalized animals indicated that large stretch amplitudes and forces were required to evoke clasp-knife responses.[39] Since a functional interpretation of clasp-knife responses and of the normal actions of the associated pathways depend critically upon the range of conditions over which the receptors are activated, it was important to extend the investigation to conditions of ongoing contraction and widely varying forces. A survival time of even a few days between the spinal transection and terminal experiment allowed substantially higher forces than was possible with acute spinalization.

In an experiment performed on an animal spinalized 14 days before the terminal experiment, stretches of as little as 1 mm were sufficient to evoke clasp-knife responses in SOL (Fig. 13.5). Responses of muscles in spinal and control animals were undistinguishable for stretches of 0.5 and 1 mm, but profound inhibition of long latency appeared for responses to stretches greater than 2 mm (Fig. 13.5A). Plots of force responses vs. stretch amplitude revealed the failure of stiffness regulation[20] in the presence of clasp-knife inhibition (Fig. 13.5B). This breakdown of stiffness regulation was particularly apparent for responses measured 150 and 300 ms following initiation of the ramp, as expected from the long delay associated with clasp-knife inhibition.

The preceding result demonstrated that clasp-knife inhibition could be evoked by stretches as little as 1 mm for SOL, or about 2.5% of muscle fiber length.[44] Since the active lengthening of the soleus muscle during walking and trotting amounts to approximately 4 mm,[45] or 10% of muscle fiber length, the receptors in question are activated well within the physiological range of muscle length changes.

13.4.2.2 Force and Length

The next question was to determine the range of forces and lengths over which clasp-knife inhibition was expressed. In order to investigate the effective range of forces and lengths, the reflex interactions between SOL and the gastrocnemius muscles (G) were studied. Four findings resulted from this investigation. First, the clasp-knife reflex was shown to depend upon both length and force. Second, the effective lengths and forces were well within ranges that occur during natural movements. Third, the autogenic component of clasp-knife inhibition for G, but not for S, declined with survival period. Fourth, stretch of G still provoked greater than normal inhibition in SOL even though G did not show autogenic inhibition.

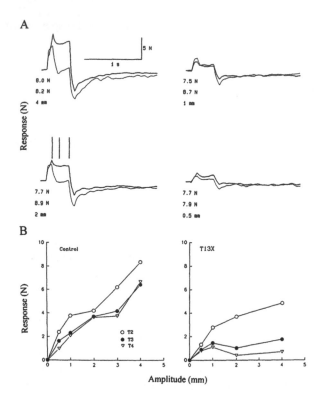

FIGURE 13.5 Dependence of clasp-knife inhibition on stretch amplitude. Responses from SOL in spinal (T13X) and control decerebrate animals to stretches of various amplitudes on background tensions close to 8 N. (A) Responses for matched amplitudes and background forces. Heavy lines, control data. Light lines, data from animals spinalized 14 days prior to terminal experiment. Note clasp-knife inhibition for responses to amplitudes greater than 2 mm. (B) Linearity plots of response amplitude vs. stretch amplitude. Responses were measured at the end of the ramp phase of stretch (T2), during the ramp plateau (T3), and at the end of the plateau (T4). These times are indicated by the three vertical lines above the 2-mm response. The plots were quasi-linear for the control muscle, indicating stiffness regulation by the stretch reflex.[20] The plots departed strongly from linear behavior for amplitudes greater than 1 mm for the spinalized animal, particularly for T3 and T4.

Autogenic clasp-knife inhibition was well developed in G for the survival time of 6 days (Fig. 13.6). The responses of G to stretch were characterized by an initial excitatory component followed by a large adaptation and small static response. Correspondingly, SOL received inhibition large enough to bring its own force to zero (Fig. 13.6A). Analysis of individual responses showed bidirectional inhibition between SOL and G (Fig. 13.6). Stretch of SOL caused initial excitatory responses in both SOL and G, followed by clasp-knife inhibition (Figs. 13.6B and C). Similar results followed the stretch of G (Figs. 13.6D and E). Although SOL receives force-dependent inhibition from G in the control decerebrate animal, this inhibition was more modest and was rarely large enough to bring the force in SOL to zero.[16] Furthermore,

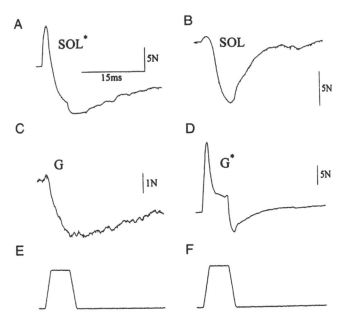

FIGURE 13.6 Clasp-knife inhibition in a biarticular muscle, gastrocnemius (G), and SOL during a crossed-extension reflex. The left panels indicate responses of SOL (A) and G (C) to stretch of SOL. (Right) Responses of SOL (B) and G (D) to stretch of G. Asterisks indicate the stretched muscles. (E and F) Length records from SOL (E) and G (F). Survival time: 6 d. In all cases, responses consisted of initial monosynaptic excitation followed by inhibition, or large adaptation (D). Same animal as shown in (A).

G receives only excitation from SOL in the control decerebrate preparation.[16] Therefore, the inhibitory responses observed in chronic spinal injury cannot be explained simply by an enhancement of the force feedback attributed to Golgi tendon organs, although the two sources of inhibition appeared to blend nearly seamlessly.

For survival times beyond 6 days, autogenic clasp-knife inhibition declined in G. In the experiment for survival time of 28 days, responses of G showed no sign of the clasp-knife response (Fig. 13.7). As the initial length of G was increased (Fig. 13.7 A–C), the responses of G increased in magnitude and showed no sign of clasp-knife inhibition. In contrast, heterogenic clasp-knife inhibition onto SOL remained strong (Fig. 13.7). As force declined during crossed-extension reflexes, the inhibition remained at constant amplitude, increased slightly, or increased in duration (Fig. 13.7A). These force-dependent properties contrast with those observed for the inhibitory force feedback arising from Golgi tendon organs,[16] for which responses decline as force decreases. The inhibitory force responses in SOL also increased with initial length of G. It was not possible to determine from this experiment whether the inhibitory responses in SOL depended upon the initial length of G or the force responses of G, since both increased together. The increased inhibition could have been due to increases in either length or the magnitudes of the force responses of G.

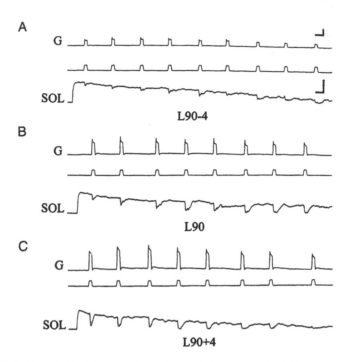

FIGURE 13.7 Clasp-knife inhibition from G to SOL increases with initial length. The initial length of G was set at 3 lengths, L90-4 mm (A), L90 (maximum physiological extension) (B), and L90 + 4 (C). Autogenic clasp-knife inhibition did not appear in G even though the force responses of G increased more than 2-fold. Strong inhibition in SOL was observed, however, and this inhibition increased as initial length was increased. Although the inhibition onto SOL could not be temporally distinguished from force-dependent inhibition, the increase in magnitude and duration with descending force is not a feature of the force-dependent feedback from Golgi tendon organs. Since the autogenic responses of G also increased with length, it was not possible to determine whether the increase in inhibition depended upon the length or force responses of G. Survival time: 28 d.

In additional experiments in which SOL was stretched and G remained isometric, clasp-knife inhibition was expressed autogenically in SOL and heteregenically in G (Fig. 13.8). Earlier during a crossed-extension reflex when SOL was developing approximately 15 N of background tension, excitatory responses occurred in both muscles as in the case for the control decerebrate preparation. As force declined, however, the baseline force in both became irregular and clasp-knife inhibition appeared in both muscles. These inhibitory responses were observed as force decayed toward rest. Since G receives only excitatory inputs from SOL in the control decerebrate preparation, and since the inhibitory responses in G appeared simultaneously with the appearance of clasp-knife inhibition in SOL, it is concluded that both autogenic and heterogenic responses arise from similar interneuronal mechanisms. This experiment also showed that clasp-knife inhibition is expressed at low and intermediate forces but not necessarily high forces. It is possible that the absence of the clasp-knife response at high background forces was due to competition or

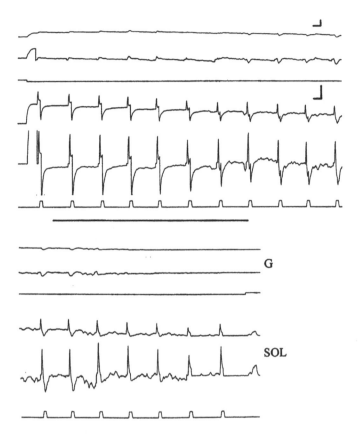

FIGURE 13.8 Force dependence of clasp-knife inhibition. SOL was stretched during a decaying crossed-extension reflex and responses were recorded from SOL and the isometric G (protocol 1). Clasp-knife inhibition evoked by the stretch of SOL appeared in both muscles at intermediate forces and remained as force declined toward rest. (Bottom) Continuation of upper panels. Trace 1, force of G; 2, force of G amplified and with baseline reset before each response; 3, force of SOL; 4, force of SOL amplified and reset; 5, length of SOL. Calibration bars correspond to 5 N for G 10 N for SOL and 1 s. Survival time: 28 d.

mutual inhibition between pathways mediating clasp-knife and flexion withdrawal reflexes. When the flexion withdrawal reflex adapted sufficiently, the pathways mediating clasp-knife inhibition were expressed. It will be important to check in future studies whether the background force per se or the pattern of activity associated with the flexion withdrawal reflex is responsible for the suppression of the clasp-knife response at higher forces.

The experiment shown in Fig. 13.8 was repeated using two other initial lengths of SOL (Fig. 13.9). At the shortest initial length of SOL (Fig. 13.9A), the stretch responses of SOL declined at the lowest forces but otherwise resembled those obtained in control decerebrate animals. Similarly, the isometric responses of G remained excitatory for most of the force range. For the intermediate initial length (Fig. 13.9B; original data shown in Fig. 13.8), clasp-knife inhibition appeared at

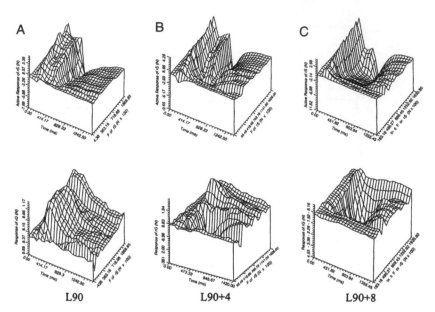

L90   L90+4   L90+8

FIGURE 13.9 Dependence of clasp-knife inhibition on force and length. Composite diagrams showing the dependence of force responses of SOL and G on time and background force. SOL was stretched during decaying crossed-extension reflexes starting from three initial lengths, L90 mm (A), L90 + 4 (length of SOL at 90° ankle angle) (B), and L90 + 8 mm (C). The upper diagrams represent data from SOL and the lower diagrams represent data from G. To construct each diagram, the amplified and reset traces for a given muscle were plotted against background tension. The data points were fitted to a surface using the method of kriging. Note that the responses of G became inhibitory when clasp-knife inhibition appeared in SOL. Survival time: 28 D.

intermediate forces in both muscles. At the longest initial length of SOL (Fig. 13.9C), the inhibition appeared at higher forces in both muscles. For similar background force ranges in SOL, the inhibition was stronger at the longest initial length of SOL. The data for each initial length show that clasp-knife inhibition is force dependent, and comparison of the data for the three initial lengths shows that the inhibition is also length dependent. The latter conclusion is possible because the force responses of SOL do not progressively increase with initial length. Since similar force ranges were obtained at each length and the magnitudes of the initial force responses in SOL were similar or smaller as length was increased, the larger inhibitory responses in both muscles were probably influenced by the initial length.

The major result of the experiments described in this section is that during ongoing muscle activity in injured animals, clasp-knife inhibition was expressed at low and intermediate forces and with relatively small amplitudes of stretch. Surprisingly, clasp-knife responses were not expressed at higher forces in the soleus muscle. This set of findings suggests that the receptors mediating clasp-knife responses are responsive to mechanical changes in muscles that occur during normal movements, and that the spinal lesion releases the associated pathways abnormally. The significance of this conclusion is that if these pathways are used to signal abnormal levels of stress or strain within the muscle, the detector for such abnormal levels must lie within the spinal cord rather than in the receptors themselves. It has not been established that these receptors can detect changes in force or length as small as those detected by Golgi tendon organs[46] or muscle spindle receptors,[47] but it seems apparent that they can respond well within normal physiological ranges.

An additional finding from the experiments described in this section is that autogenic clasp-knife inhibition declines in the gastrocnemius muscles 2 to 3 weeks following spinal injury, while the levels of this inhibition remain constant in the soleus muscle. This observation can be considered in light of other differences in reflex organization between these two muscle groups. Although G and SOL are synergists in the sense that they exchange feedback from Ia afferents,[26,48] there exists a uni-directional inhibitory pathway from G to SOL mediated by Golgi tendon organs.[12] This inhibition may enhance coupling between the ankle and knee at high forces by virtue of the biarticular linkages of G.[6,7] Clasp-knife inhibition differs from force feedback in that it extends in both directions between the two muscle groups. However, the reduction in autogenic inhibition in G suggests that this muscle receives less total inhibition than SOL. Therefore, even though antigravity muscles throughout the limb may be inhibited, the relative sparing of the bi-articular muscles leads to some coordination among the joints as the collapse is progressing. Further studies are needed to determine if similar partitioning of inhibition occurs between the bi-articular rectus femoris and uni-articular vastus muscles.

13.4.3 INTERMUSCULAR DISTRIBUTION OF CLASP-KNIFE RESPONSES

The above results suggest that clasp-knife inhibition is distributed within and between antigravity muscles and is directed most powerfully toward single joint muscles. In a complementary fashion, long-latency excitatory responses are directed at flexor and contralateral antigravity muscles. Additional experiments were performed in the same animals to determine whether clasp-knife inhibition was expressed in stabilizing muscles of the ankle. These muscles serve to control movements of the ankle in the transverse plane.[49] In addition, an opposing pair of them (tibialis posterior and peroneus brevis) are linked by reciprocal inhibition, apparently to enhance the lateral stabilization of this joint.[28] No evidence of clasp-knife inhibition was found for either of these two muscles. In addition, clasp-knife inhibition was absent in two other muscles that exert substantial forces in the transverse plane, namely, peroneus longus and flexor digitorum longus. The latter muscle flexes the toes with FHL and shares feedback from group Ia afferents with this muscle. The lack of clasp-knife inhibition in flexor digitorum longus and the presence in FHL correlates with the antigravity actions of the latter. Taken together, these results demonstrate that clasp-knife inhibition is specific to antigravity muscles, and clasp-knife responses (inhibitory or excitatory) are specific to muscles that act about the flexion/extension axis.

The intramuscular and intermuscular distribution of clasp-knife inhibition differs markedly from the pattern of force dependent feedback from Golgi tendon organs (Fig. 10). Inhibitory force feedback is not expressed autogenically or between muscles that cross the same joints and exert forces in similar directions. Instead, force

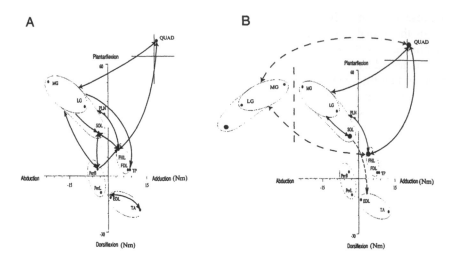

FIGURE 13.10 Summary diagram showing the intermuscular distributions of inhibitory force feedback from tendon organs (A) and clasp-knife responses (B) for muscles crossing the ankle as well as QUAD and contralateral MG. The data points are torques exerted by the named muscles about two axes of rotation. The axis denoted "plantarflexion/dorsiflexion" represents torques exerted in the sagittal plane, and "abduction/adduction" represents torques exerted in the transverse plane.[49] The axes are shown with different scales for clarity. Muscles grouped by ellipses are linked by monosynaptic Ia connections.[7] Lines with arrows (A) indicate the distribution of inhibitory feedback attributed to Golgi tendon organs.[7,27,28] Lines with arrows in (B) indicate clasp-knife responses. Solid lines indicate inhibition and dashed lines excitation. The filled circles indicated autogenic clasp-knife inhibition. This diagram indicates the distribution of clasp-knife reflexes for the longer survival times after the loss of autogenic clasp-knife inhibition in G. Note that force feedback links muscles crossing different joints or exerting actions about different axes of rotation. Clasp-knife reflexes link antigravity muscles and pretibial flexors, but not ankle stabilizers. Clasp-knife reflexes also link antigravity muscles across limbs unlike short-latency force feedback. MG (medial gastrocnemius); LG (lateral gastrocnemius); PLN (plantaris); FHL (flexor hallucis longus); FDL (flexor digitorum longus); TP (tibialis posterior); PerB (peroneus brevis); PerL (peroneus longus); EDL (extensor digitorum longus).

feedback links muscles across joints and axes of rotation (Fig. 10A).[6,7] In contrast, clasp-knife inhibition is expressed autogenically in antigravity muscles and particularly single joint muscles. Clasp-knife pathways also link antigravity muscles to other antigravity muscles by inhibition and antigravity muscles to flexors by excitation (Fig. 10B). Excitation also extends to antigravity muscles in the contralateral limb (Fig. 10B). In summary, clasp-knife inhibition differs from inhibitory force feedback not only in latency and state dependence, but in intermuscular distribution as well.

The overall effect of the distribution of clasp-knife inhibition would be to promote a flexion response or collapse of the limb along the major flexion-extension axis, while preserving lateral stability and some coupling between joints. The muscles that stabilize the ankle are not strongly activated by flexion withdrawal reflexes[28] so both clasp-knife and flexion withdrawal reflexes appear to act in a directionally specific manner. One difference in the muscular distribution of the two reflexes is that although G receives weaker inhibition during flexion-withdrawal reflexes than SOL, this muscle appears to be spared from the clasp-knife response for the longer survival times. Despite the general similarities between the two responses in terms of muscular distribution, the findings that clasp-knife responses can be evoked with small stretches at moderate values of force and length show that the adequate stimuli are very different from those provoking flexion-withdrawal responses. These considerations leave open the questions of the role of the relevant receptors in the normal regulation of motor output and of the conditions under which exaggerated clasp-knife responses are expressed.

13.5 IMPLICATIONS

13.5.1 THE CLASP-KNIFE RESPONSE AS A PROTECTIVE MECHANISM

A conclusion from this and previous studies is that the clasp-knife response can be evoked in the absence of muscle damage.[36,39,40] However, previous studies did lead to the conclusion that large forces and lengths are required to elicit this response.[39] This conclusion at least suggests that the high threshold of the relevant receptors make these sensors, rather than Golgi tendon organs,[40,46] good candidates for detecting conditions that could lead to muscle damage. The present results suggest instead that the receptors mediating the clasp-knife response, like Golgi tendon organs, have a lower threshold for activation than had been previously thought. This observation leads to a modified view of the clasp-knife response as a protective mechanism. If the pathways mediating the clasp-knife response were opened by peripheral inputs in the presence of generalized damage to a limb, then the response would be evoked, not by damaging levels of stress within the muscle, but by more modest mechanical changes. In this way the response would help to prevent further damage.

The finding that the clasp-knife response is evoked by small stretches and modest forces and lengths also suggests that the underlying pathways may have a regulatory role under normal conditions and may not be reserved solely as a global protective mechanism. In a number of control decerebrate preparations, which generally do not exhibit clasp-knife responses, long-latency, inhibitory responses in the vastus lateralis, but not vastus medialis, muscle have been detected following stretch of the vastus intermedius muscle.[29,30] A proposed action of this pathway would be to help balance the force responses of the more massive vastus lateralis muscle with the force responses of the less massive vastus medialis muscle to improve patellar tracking and prevent asymmetrical wear on the patella.[30] This observation suggests that that pathways included in the clasp-knife response may be expressed individually in the normal animal rather than within a global and exaggerated response.

13.5.2 THE CLASP-KNIFE RESPONSE IN SPINAL INJURY

The expression of the clasp-knife response is important to consider in the rehabilitation of spinal injury. If this response is triggered by modest stresses within muscle following spinal injury, then the response would interfere with the ability of the subject to regulate posture either in the face of mechanical perturbations during standing or during locomotion. Following prolonged stance training, spinalized cats were able to able to stand for 35 to 40 min/d supporting their own weight, but control of lateral stability, particularly in the face of stepping and platform translations, was severely compromised.[50] Reflex analysis of one of these animals showed full expression of clasp-knife responses as well as reflexes arising from muscle spindle receptors and Golgi tendon organs.[42] These results showed that stance training can maintain the integrity of spinal circuitry,[42] but the results also suggest that management of clasp-knife responses may be important to restore normal balance and postural control.

In additional studies of animals with complete spinal transections, responses to platform translations occurred mainly in muscles that were active during quiet standing.[51,52] Ground reaction force vectors in the horizontal plane were directed more laterally and medially than in normal animals,[51] which may indicate the actions of stabilizing muscles that are not strongly affected by clasp-knife inhibition. It is possible that the reduced participation of the antigravity muscles in postural stabilization arose in part because of inhibitory influences of interneurons that mediate the clasp-knife response.

Animals subjected to spinal transection can be trained to step[53-55] as well as stand;[50,52,56,57] however, evidence suggests that training is specific. Training in stepping did not enhance the ability to stand.[58] When stance training was facilitated by mechanical tail stimulation, stance required mechanical tail stimulation.[56] It would be important to know what effect a specific training protocol would have on the expression of the clasp-knife response. If, for example, mechanical stimulation of the tail led to a decreased expression of the clasp-knife response, then the failure to restore control of standing without tail stimulation would follow.

13.5.3 THE FRA CONCEPT

Flexor reflex afferents arise from many types of receptors that may produce flexion withdrawal reflexes, including high threshold muscle, cutaneous, and joint afferents.[3,59] The term "FRA" is retained mainly for historical reasons, since these afferents have other actions as well.[60] Specialized actions of pathways arising from skin or muscle[17,61-64] indicate that a monolithic flexion withdrawal reflex is not the primary function of these pathways.

Superficially, the clasp-knife response seems to fall into the category of a flexion withdrawal reflex, so the underlying pathways might be considered components of the FRA system. However, the lack of participation of biarticular muscles after a short chronic period indicates that the clasp-knife response comprises a more selective activation of muscles than the flexion withdrawal reflex. In addition, the apparent competition between flexion withdrawal and clasp-knife responses at high background forces (see above) indicates that these pathways are independent. The clasp-knife response constitutes another specialized pathway, suggesting further that the FRA system is not a single entity but actually a complex network characterized by a variety of sensory modalities and destinations.

The model of a monolithic flexion withdrawal response is perhaps even less applicable to the role of the pathways underlying the clasp-knife response in the normal animal. The low threshold for activation is a requirement for a role during normal movements. In addition, the independent expression of specific components of the response, such as the long-latency inhibition from the vastus intermedius to the vastus lateralis muscle (see above), indicates that the clasp-knife response itself consists of a set of more specialized pathways.

An important characteristic of the FRA system is the wide convergence of feedback from high threshold receptors onto the relevant interneurons.[3] The pathways underlying the clasp-knife response are also characterized by considerable convergence, as are the pathways underlying inhibitory force feedback (see above). However, the specific muscular distributions as well as the adequate stimuli of these three systems are markedly different. It seems that more understanding of the normal functions of these systems is to be gained by investigating these differences and their interactions in the spinal cord than treating them as a single entity.[65]

ACKNOWLEDGMENT

This work was supported by NS20855.

REFERENCES

1. Baldissera, F., Hultborn, H., and Illert, M., Integration in spinal neuronal systems, in *Handbook of Physiology, The Nervous System, Vol. II, Motor Control*, Brooks, V.B., Ed., American Physiological Society, Bethesda, 1981.
2. Jankowska, E., Interneuronal relay in spinal pathways from proprioceptors, *Progr. Neurobiol.*, 38, 335, 1992.
3. McCrea, D.A., Can sense be made of spinal interneuron circuits?, *Behav. Brain Sci.*, 15, 633, 1992.
4. Pearson, K.G., Proprioceptive regulation of locomotion, *Curr. Opin. Neurobiol.*, 5, 786, 1995.
5. Macpherson, J.M., Strategies that simplify the control of quadrupedal stance II. Electromyographic activity, *J. Neurophysiol.*, 60, 218, 1988.
6. Nichols, T.R., Cope, T.C., and Abelew, T.A., Rapid spinal mechanisms of motor coordination, *Exerc. Sport Sci. Rev.*, 27, 255, 1999.
7. Nichols, T.R., A biomechanical perspective on spinal mechanisms of coordinated muscular action: an architecture principle, *Acta Anat.*, 151, 1, 1994.
8. Prochazka, A., Proprioceptive feedback and movement regulation, in *Handbook of Physiology, Exercise: Regulation and Integration of Multiple Systems*, Rowell, L.B. and Shepherd, J.T., Eds., Oxford, New York, 1996.
9. Heckman, C.J. and Lee, R.H., Synaptic integration in bistable motoneurons, in *Progr. Brain Res.*, Binder, M.D., Ed., Elsevier, Amsterdam, 1999, 49.
10. Nichols, T.R., Lin, D.C., and Huyghues-Despointes, C.M.J.I., The role of musculoskeletal mechanics in motor coordination, in *Peripheral and Spinal Mechanisms in the Neural Control of Movement*, Binder, M.D., Ed., Elsevier, Amsterdam, 1999.
11. Pearson, K.G., Neural adaptation in the generation of rhythmic behavior, *Ann. Rev. Physiol.*, 62, 723, 2000.
12. Nichols, T.R., The organization of heterogenic reflexes among muscles crossing the ankle joint in the decerebrate cat, *J. Physiol.*, 410, 463, 1989.

13. Houk, J.C. and Rymer, W.Z., Neural control of muscle length and tension, in *Handbook of Physiology, The Nervous System, Vol. II. Motor Control,* Brooks, V.B. Ed., American Physiological Society, Bethesda, MD, 1981, 257.

14. He, J., Levine, W.S., and Loeb, G.E., Feedback gains for correcting small perturbations to standing posture, *I.E.E. Trans. Auto. Contr.,* 36, 322, 1991.

15. Gandevia, S.C., Kinesthesia: roles for afferent signals and motor commands, in *Handbook of Physiology, Exercise: Regulation and Integration of Multiple Systems,* Rowell, L.B. and Shepherd, J.T., Eds., Oxford, New York, 1996, 128.

16. Nichols, T.R., Receptor mechanisms underlying heterogenic reflexes among the triceps surae muscles of the cat, *J. Neurophysiol.,* 81, 467, 1999.

17. Siegel, S.G., Nichols, T.R., and Cope, T.C., Reflex activation patterns in relation to multidirectional ankle torque in decerebrate cats, *Motor Contr.,* 3, 135, 1999.

18. Cope, T.C., Bonasera, S.J., and Nichols, T.R., Reinnervated muscles fail to produce stretch reflexes, *J. Neurophysiol.,* 71, 817, 1994.

19. Houk, J.C., Crago, P.E., and Rymer, W.Z., Function of the spindle dynamic response in stiffness regulation — a predictive mechanism provided by non-linear feedback, in *Muscle Receptors and Movement,* Taylor, A. and Prochazka, A., Eds., Macmillan, London, 1981, 299.

20. Nichols, T.R. and Houk, J.C., The improvement in linearity and regulation of stiffness that results from action of the stretch reflex, *J. Neurophysiol.,* 39, 119, 1976.

21. Hoffer, J.A. and Andreassen, S., Regulation of soleus muscle stiffness in premammillary cat intrinsic and reflex components, *J. Neurophysiol.,* 45, 267, 1981.

22. Sinkjaer, T., Muscle, reflex and central components in the control of the ankle joint in healthy and spastic man, *Acta Neurol. Scand.,* 96, 1, 1997.

23. Huyghues-Despointes, C.M.J.I., Effects of movement history on the intrinsic properties and the neural regulation of feline skeletal muscle, Ph.D. dissertation, Emory University, Atlanta, 1998.

24. Kirsch, R.F., Boskov, D., and Rymer, W.Z., Muscle stiffness during transient and continuous movements of cat muscle: perturbation characteristics and physiological relevance, *IEEE Trans. Biomed. Eng.,* 41, 758, 1994.

25. Eccles, R.M. and Lundberg, A., Intergrative pattern of Ia synaptic actions on motoneurons of hip and knee muscles, *J. Physiol.,* 144, 271, 1958.

26. Eccles, J.C., Eccles, R.M., and Lundberg, A., The convergence of monosynaptic excitatory afferents onto many different species of alpha motoneurons, *J. Physiol.,* 137, 22, 1957.

27. Bonasera, S.J. and Nichols, T.R., Mechanical actions of heterogenic reflexes linking long toe flexors and extensors of the knee and ankle in the cat, *J. Neurophysiol.,* 71, 1096, 1994.

28. Bonasera, S.J. and Nichols, T.R., Mechanical actions of heterogenic reflexes among ankle stabilizers and their interactions with plantar flexors of the cat hindlimb, *J. Neurophysiol.,* 75, 2050, 1996.

29. Wilmink, R.J.H., Huyghues-Despointes, C.M.J.I., Abelew, T.A., and Nichols, T.R., Non-uniform distribution of neural feedback among the quadriceps and triceps surae muscles of the cat, *Soc. Neurosci. Abstr.,* 22, 2042, 1996.

30. Wilmink, R.J.H., Organization and modulation of excitatory and inhibitory spinal reflexes in cats and humans, Ph.D. dissertation, *Center for Sensorimotor Interaction,* Aalborg University, Aalborg, 1998.

31. Nichols, T.R., Burkholder, T.J., and Wilmink, R.J.H., The multidimensional and temporal regulation of limb mechanics by spinal circuits, in *Progress in Motor Control-II: Structure-Function Relationships in Voluntary Movements,* Latash, M.L., Ed., Human Kinetics, Champaign, in press.

32. Macpherson, J.M., Changes in postural strategy with inter-paw distance, *J. Neurophysiol.*, 71, 931, 1994.
33. Macpherson, J.M., Strategies that simplify the control of quadrupedal stance I forces at the ground, *J. Neurophysiol.*, 6, 204, 1988.
34. Young, R.R., Spasticity: a review, *Neurology*, 44(9), S12, 1994.
35. Mailis, A. and Ashby, P., Alterations in group Ia projections to motoneurons following spinal lesions in humans, *J. Neurophysiol.*, 64, 637, 1990.
36. Burke, D., Knowles, L., Andrews, C., and Ashby, P., Spasticity, decerebrate rigidity, and the clasp knife phenomenon: an experimental study in cat, *Brain*, 95, 31, 1972.
37. Creed, R.S., Denny-Brown, D., Eccles, J.C., Liddell, E.G.T., and Sherrington, C.S., *Reflex Activity of the Spinal Cord*, University Press, Oxford, 1972.
38. Cleland, C.L., Hayward, L., and Rymer, R.W., Neural mechanisms underlying the clasp-knife reflex in the cat. II. Stretch-sensitive muscular-free nerve endings, *J. Neurophysiol.*, 64, 1319, 1990.
39. Cleland, C.L. and Rymer, W.Z., Neural mechanisms underlying the clasp knife reflex in the cat. I. Characteristics of the reflex, *J. Neurophysiol.*, 64, 1303, 1990.
40. Rymer, W.Z., Houk, J.C., and Crago, P.E., Mechanisms of the clasp-knife reflex studied in an animal model, *Exp. Brain Res.*, 37, 93, 1979.
41. Cope, T.C. and Nichols, T.R., Reflex organization among ankle extensors and pretibial flexors in the chronic spinal cat, *Soc. Neurosci. Abstr.*, 14, 795, 1988.
42. Bonasera, S.J., Pratt, C.A., Price, C.M.J.I., Cope, T.C., and Nichols, T.R., Stance training preserves intermuscular reflexes and muscle properties in chronic spinal cats, *Soc. Neurosci. Abstr.*, 20, 572, 1994.
43. Nichols, T.R. and Koffler-Smulevitz, D., Mechanical analysis of heterogenic inhibition between soleus muscle and the pretibial flexors in the cat, *J. Neurophysiol.*, 66, 1139, 1991.
44. Sacks, R.D. and Roy, R.R., Architecture of the hind limb muscles of cats: functional significance, *J. Morph.*, 173, 185, 1982.
45. Goslow, G.E., Reinking, R.M., and Stuart, D.G., The cat step cycle: hind limb joint angles and muscle lengths during unrestrained locomotion, *J. Morph.*, 141, 1, 1973.
46. Houk, J. and Henneman, E., Responses of Golgi tendon organs to active contractions of the soleus muscle of the cat, *J. Neurophysiol.*, 30, 466, 1967.
47. Hasan, Z. and Houk, J.C., Transition in sensitivity of spindle receptors that occurs when muscle is stretched more than a fraction of a millimeter, *J. Neurophysiol.*, 38, 673, 1975.
48. Scott, J.G. and Mendell, L.M., Individual EPSPs produced by single triceps surae Ia afferent fibers in homonymous and heteronymous motoneurons, *J. Neurophysiol.*, 39, 679, 1976.
49. Lawrence, J.H.I., Nichols, T.R., and English, A.W., Cat hindlimb muscles exert substantial torques outside the sagittal plane, *J. Neurophysiol.*, 69, 282, 1993.
50. Pratt, C.A., Fung, J., and Macpherson, J.M., Stance control in the chronic spinal cat, *J. Neurophysiol.*, 71, 1981, 1994.
51. Macpherson, J.M. and Fung, J., Weight support and balance during perturbed stance in the chronic spinal cat, *J. Neurophysiol.*, 82, 3066, 1999.
52. Fung, J. and Macpherson, J.M., Attributes of quiet stance in the chronic spinal cat, *J. Neurophysiol.*, 82, 3056, 1999.
53. Lovely, R.G., Gregor, R.J., Roy, R.R., and Edgerton, V.R., Effects of training on the recovery of full-weight-bearing stepping in the adult spinal cat, *Exp. Neurol.*, 92, 421, 1986.

54. de Leon, R.D., Hodgson, J.A., Roy, R.R., and Edgerton, V.R., Locomotor capacity attributable to step training vs. spontaneous recovery after spinalization in adult cats, *J. Neurophysiol.*, 79, 1329, 1998.
55. Rossignol, S., Neural control of stereotypic limb movements, in *Handbook of Physiology. Exercise: Regulation and Integration of Multiple Systems,* Rowell, L.B. and Shepherd, J.T., Eds., Oxford, New York, 1996.
56. Edgerton, V.R. et al., Use-dependent plasticity in spinal stepping and standing, *Adv. Neurol.*, 72, 233, 1997.
57. de Leon, R.D., Hodgson, J.A., Roy, R.R., and Edgerton, V.R., Full weight-bearing hindlimb standing following stand training in the adult spinal cat, *J. Neurophysiol.*, 80, 83, 1998.
58. Edgerton, V.R., Roy, R.R., de Leon, R., Tillakaratne, N., and Hodgson, J.A., Does motor learning occur in the spinal cord?, *Neuroscientist*, 3, 287, 1997.
59. Eccles, R.M. and Lundberg, A., Supraspinal control of interneurones mediating spinal reflexes, *J. Physiol.*, 147, 565, 1959.
60. Windhorst, U.R. et al., Group report: What are the output units of motor behavior and how are they controlled?, in *Motor Control: Concepts and Issues,* Humphrey, D.R. and Freund, H.-J., Eds., John Wiley & Sons, New York, 1991.
61. Engberg, I., Reflexes to foot muscles in the cat, *Acta Physiol. Scand.*, 62, 235, 1, 1964.
62. Schouenborg, J. and Kalliomaki, J., Functional organization of the nociceptive withdrawal reflexes. I. Activation of hindlimb muscles in the rat, *Exp. Brain Res.* 83, 67, 1990.
63. Nichols, T.R., Lawrence, J.H.I., and Bonasera, S.J., Control of torque direction by spinal pathways at the cat ankle joint, *Exp. Brain Res.*, 97, 366, 1993.
64. Hagbarth, K.-E., Excitatory and inhibitory skin areas for flexor and extensor motoneurons, *Acta Physiol. Scand. Suppl.*, 94, 1, 1952.
65. Matthews, P.B.C., *Mammalian Muscle Receptors and Their Central Actions*, Williams and Wilkins, Baltimore, 1972.

Index

A

Acetylcholine, 71, 240

Achilles tendon, 95, 217

Action potentials
backpropagation in dendrites, 31
measurement for motor unit isolation, 108–109
motoneuron transfer function and, 143–144
post-axotomy distal dendritic arborizations, 264–265
single motoneuron selection, 109
site of initiation, 22

Afterhyperpolarization (AHP), 123, 124

4-Aminopyridine, 239–240

AMPA receptors, 293–294, See Glutamate receptors

Amyotrophic lateral sclerosis (ALS), 232

Anesthetics, 90–91, 276, 277

Ankle extensors
afferent feedback during walking, 215–226
clasp-knife inhibition and, 319–321
correlational studies of pattern generation during fictive locomotion, 151–153, 156–162
embryo reflex studies, 176
spinal muscular atrophy studies, 236

Anxiety, 50

Astrocytes, 256

Astroglial cells, 285

Auto-correlation function, 137, 207

Average common excitatory (ACE) potential, 138, 139–140

AxoClamp, 96–98

Axonal abnormalities, in hereditary canine spinal muscular atrophy, 243–244

Axotomy-induced effects on motoneuron structure, 251–266
action potentials, 264–265
dendritic growth and dendraxons, 253–256
dendritic tree expansion, 257–259
dendritic tree shrinkage, 252–253
effects of proximity of axotomy to soma, 265
functional synapse, 264
loss of synaptic integration, 253
mitochondria clusters, 254, 262
myelination, 256, 260–261

neuronal polarity concept, 252, 256, 257, 263
summary of, 263–264
supernumerary axons, 256–257, 264
unusual distal dendrites, 253–256, 259–263
electron microscopy, 259–261
light microscopy, 259–261

Axotomy-induced effects on synaptic strength, 271–272, 275–295
afferent vs. motoneuron, 278
EPSP enlargement phenomenon, 275–279
neurotrophin effects, 272, 284–290
axotomy-induced changes, 287–288
effects of manipulating neurotrophins, 288–289
expression and cellular localization, 285–287
synaptic activity relationship, 289–290
trophic dependence of synaptic function, 284–285
synaptic inactivation effects, 280–284
axotomy, 280–282
neurotrophin relationship, 289–290
TTX treatment, 282–283, 293–294

B

Background motoneuron discharge rate, 124–125

Background synaptic noise, See Synaptic noise

Backpropagating action potentials, in dendrites, 31

Bandpass filtering, 109

Barbiturates, 276, 277

Basis functions, 150–151

Biceps femoris, 151–153, 156–159

Bicuculline, 156

Bistability, 91, 93, 100

Blastomere injection, 14

Botulinum toxin, 252

Brain-derived neurotrophic factor (BDNF), 284, 285, 287–289

C

Cable theory, 30, 89, 253

Cajal, R. Y., 251

Calcium imaging, 9–12, 13

Milton Keynes UK
Ingram Content Group UK Ltd.
UKHW031127141024
449569UK00006B/389